Occupational Therapy with Children

Occupational Therapy with Children

Helen Clancy MA DipOccThy

Michele J. Clark BOccThy(Hons) BA

MELBOURNE EDINBURGH LONDON AND NEW YORK 1990

CHURCHILL LIVINGSTONE
Medical Division of Longman Group UK Limited

Distributed in Australia by Longman Cheshire Pty Limited,
Longman House, Kings Gardens, 95 Coventry Street, South
Melbourne 3205, and by associated companies, branches and
representatives throughout the world.

© Longman Group UK Limited 1990

First published 1990

ISBN 0-443-03437-0

British Library Cataloguing in Publication Data
Clancy, Helen
   Occupational therapy with children.
   1. Children. Occupational therapy
   I. Title   II. Clark, Michele J.
   615.8515

Library of Congress Cataloging in Publication Data
Clancy, Helen.
   Occupational therapy with children/Helen Clancy, Michele J..Clark.
      p.   cm.
   ISBN 0–443–03437–0
   1. Occupational therapy for children.   I. Clark, Michele J.
   II. Title.
   [DNLM: 1. Child Behavior Disorders — rehabilitation.   2. Child
Development Disorders — rehabilitation.   3. Learning Disorders —
rehabilitation.   4. Occupational Therapy — in fancy & childhood.
WS 350.2 C5870]
RJ53.025C53   1990
615.8′515′083 — dc20
DNLM/DLC
for Library of Congress   90–1805

Produced by Longman Singapore Publishers (Pte) Ltd.
Printed in Singapore

Preface

The object of this book is to present theories and principles underlying the practice of occupational therapy with children. The book is designed for use by undergraduate students and therapists who are new to this specialist area. However, other health professionals and parents may also find that there is much to interest them.

Our central tenet is that the family — however it is culturally defined — is the appropriate unit of therapeutic intervention with children. We have attempted to convey our belief that productive therapy is most likely to result when specialists respect the child and family members as partners in the process — hence our choice of the title *Occupational Therapy with Children*.

We have assumed that you, the reader, will already have some preparation in the basic sciences such as anatomy and neuroanatomy. However, we have not assumed any preparation in the specialist field of occupational therapy with children.

Textbooks can be so boring. We were determined not to write a boring book. We hope that when you pick up this book you will not only be challenged by it and learn from it, but that you will also enjoy it. To this end we have tried to write simply, in ordinary understandable English, yet mindful of the need to introduce you to the professional terminology.

This is not a recipe book and we have not attempted to address every specialist area in the field of practice with children. Some of our reviewers asked us to include detailed 'how to' treatment ideas for children in particular diagnostic categories. We chose not to do so because we believe very strongly that it is dangerous for any specialist to approach a clinical situation with a 'Standard Operating Procedures' mentality. Rather we have presented ways of thinking about problems and arriving at practical solutions to clinical needs.

Brisbane   H. C.
1990   M. J .C.

Acknowledgements

We would like to thank Frances Forbes and Sylvia Roger for their contribution to the preparation of Chapters 14 and 17; our clinical and academic colleagues for their continuing encouragement and sound advice throughout the preparation of the manuscript; Sally McMahon for her delightful cartoons; and The Women's College within The University of Queensland, for providing a conducive working environment.

We are indebted to Heather Cunningham, whose professional typing skills, dedication and attention to detail made us believe that this book would really happen.

There are not words that can adequately express our gratitude and appreciation to Glenorchy McBride for his unflagging enthusiasm, encouragement and practical support for us and our seemingly endless project.

Every effort has been made to trace the copyright holders of material reproduced in this book. If oversights or omissions have occurred the authors and publishers would be pleased to hear from copyright holders.

Contents

PART I

PRINCIPLES OF THERAPY

For therapy to be more than the mechanical application of standard operating procedures, there must be understanding of general principles which determine the form of procedures. General principles are influenced by the philosophical frame of reference of the person designing the therapeutic approaches. Equipped with a clearly defined frame of reference, and an understanding of appropriate general principles, a therapist can exercise flexibility, variation and imagination in the design and implementation of therapeutic approaches. Chapters 1 to 3 provide a statement of the philosophy for this book, and trace the historical evolution of paediatric occupational therapy with children. Chapter 3 provides a brief but comprehensive overview of the areas of basic knowledge which is essential for safe and effective practice.

The therapy process always occurs in an environment or context. There is the physical environment, for example the Occupational Therapy Department, or the hospital ward, or the school room, or other space. There is the social context — the behavioural interaction between the therapist and the child, alone or with other children or specialists. Then there is the activity which a therapist uses to focus the child and family's effort, in order to facilitate the achievement of therapeutic objectives. Chapters 4 and 5 examine the contexts of therapy.

Introduction

1. Goals of therapy

READERS' OBJECTIVES

After reading this chapter, you should be able to:
1. Describe the philosophical tenets of occupational therapy which have influenced the approach taken in this book.
2. Compare and contrast different views of the concept of 'competence'.
3. Describe and discuss the factors which may influence therapy outcome.

PHILOSOPHY

The position taken throughout this book is that therapy of any kind should influence the development and maturation of the whole child, in his or her real world setting, which is chiefly the family. Occupational therapy represents one component in a co-operative effort involving a range of specialists, the child and the family. The corporate goal is a life-style for the child and family which is personally satisfying, and attracts respect from others. Occupational therapy is an action-oriented process, which typically involves learning through doing (Cynkin 1979, Mosey 1981), direct experience, real performance, and practice by child and family (Nuse-Clarke 1979). Rogers (1982) has restated the important philosophic tenets of our profession thus:

1. That there is healing value in occupation.
2. That client competence, physical and social, is to be pursued in the therapeutic process.
3. That there is a natural man–environment interaction, which should be capitalized in the therapeutic process (i.e., man inherently seeks to interact with the environment).

Because this book aims to introduce you, the reader to the 'whys' and 'hows' of current occupational therapy with children, many different views of therapy will be presented. However, Rogers' three statements of philosophy will provide the point of reference for all discussion.

The domain of concern for occupational therapy with children is the same as it is with adult patients or clients (see Fig. 1.1). However, the characteristics of the therapeutic relationship and process differ widely. For the child is no longer regarded as a miniature adult, as was the case up to the 20th century. Often therapeutic techniques, media and objectives that are suitable for the adult client are inappropriate for the child or require adaptation. This is so even when the disease process is recognizably the same, for example, rheumatoid arthritis.

Therapy may be perceived as habilitation or re-habilitation. 'Habilitation', the process of developing new skills and behaviours, is *always* part of the therapeutic programme with the developing child. One example would be a child, born with a developmental disability, learning to tie shoe laces.

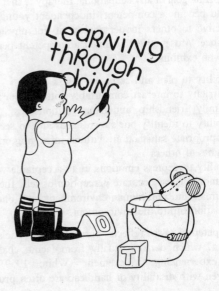

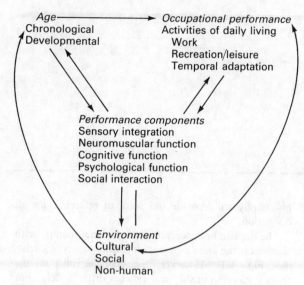

Fig. 1.1 Domain of concern for occupational therapy. Reproduced by permission from Mosey A C 1981 Configuration of a profession. Raven Press, New York (p. 75)

'Rehabilitation', the *re*-development or relearning of a lost skill or behaviour, on the other hand is less often the case. One example of rehabilitation would be a child relearning to walk after sustaining a head injury in a car accident.

Competence

The prime goal of all occupational therapy is that a child should become a competent, independent young adult, attractive to others in personality, if not physical appearance. Mosey (1981) defined a competent person as one who exhibits:

— ability to plan and carry out a task
— capacity to interact comfortably with others, in family, friendship, and group relationships
— ability to identify one's own needs and to seek appropriate satisfaction, without infringing on the rights of others
— ability to express emotions in an acceptable way
— a more or less accurate perception of self, the human and non-human environment, and one's relationship to the environment.

'Competence' also reflects perception of one's self-esteem, which derives usually from facing challenges and experiencing achievement (White 1959). Yet children with disability or handicap are often protected from the usual challenges of tasks and social encounters. Thus, it will be proposed that therapy programmes should incorporate challenge to the child, and lead to observable achievement.

Realism

Competence must be defined humanely and realistically for each child, with a view to enriched quality of life of the child and family. For example, in absolute developmental terms it is realistic to define competence in mobility as, 'walking or moving around one's environment without any assistance'. However, even when a child has the potential ability to achieve such an absolute developmental goal, it is not necessarily in the child's best interests to aim for it. Take the case of the cerebral palsied young person who can walk alone, though slowly and painfully. To get to lunch, the child leaves the school room half an hour earlier than others in order to walk the short distance independently. She/he loses time from school learning, and arrives at lunch tired from the effort and pain. The costs of independent walking are high for this child, and it is difficult to argue that quality of life is enhanced by its achievement. It may be more realistic to define competence in mobility for this cerebral palsied child as being able to get to meals in ten minutes by operating an electrically driven wheelchair.

When making important decisions about defining objectives in terms of competent behaviour, the demands of the therapy process must be clearly distinguished from the end points. Effort and some temporary pain may be unavoidable in the process required to reach the end points. However, excessive effort and pain as an unavoidable part of the therapy end point is unacceptable. The costs must always be balanced against the achievements to be sought.

Holistic therapy

In the broad sense an occupational therapist takes a holistic view of the developing child, and seeks to promote competence in physical self-care skills, in play and leisure skills, and in home, school and work skills. At each stage of the child's maturation the skills can be defined precisely in terms of 'developmental tasks' (Havighurst 1952). A developmental task is 'a task which arises at, or about a certain period in the life of the individual', for example, learning to take solid food in the second year of life. Havighurst says that successful mastery of age appropriate tasks is necessary for continuing maturation of an individual. Havighurst's developmental tasks are listed in Appendix III.

FACTORS WHICH INFLUENCE THERAPY OUTCOME

There are two factors that have particular importance in therapy with children: (a) the power of the child's experience to shape future development; (b) the level of social skill achieved. Each factor is worth examination.

Experience

Experience will always influence a child's future, and sometimes in a detrimental way. Where uncontrolled experience has produced undesirable distortions in a child's behaviour, specialists face a dual task. It becomes necessary to undo or modify such distortions in the child's behaviour and social interactions. Concurrently, intervention must provide controlled experience to inhibit further distortions from developing and becoming the 'norm' for the child and family. This is particularly the case where a child has been affected by some problem, or situation from earliest infancy, for example, when a child is developmentally disabled by spina bifida or intellectual handicap. Experience and time combine to influence the pattern of a child's developing skills.

Time

'Time' can be the child's enemy, for maturation proceeds relentlessly, whether or not for the child's good. Equally, time may be considered an ally allowing external forces, such as therapy, to be brought to bear on a child's emerging skills; to shape them to his/her advantage, now and in the future. It follows logically that strenuous efforts should be made to identify potential, or actual problems, as soon as concern is expressed by those in contact with a child. Equally logically, it follows that to be most effective, intervention should also begin as early as possible in an identified child's life (AOTA Position Statement 1986). Indeed, the concept of 'early intervention' is now a widely accepted one, and has coloured the approach taken throughout this book.

Social skill

The second important determinant of the long-term effectiveness of therapy is the level of the child's social skill development. Successful acquisition of a range of social skills is the basis for comfortable, unobtrusive integration into society, and should thus be a basic goal of therapy. Also social skills are the basis for developing bonded, long-lasting relationships with others, as in friendships.

In spite of disability, some children do become socially accomplished without special help. Yet, both environmental factors and the child's own self perceptions may operate to hinder social development. For example, there are studies which suggest that whenever a child perceives him/herself as 'different' from peers, she/he develops patterns of social behaviour which are effectively isolating (Bryne et al 1968). Again, other studies suggest that children who look different are avoided both by peers and adults (Puchinger et al 1975).

Therapy and other specialty processes may hinder social maturation by maintaining the child in a separate, artificially cocooned world — quite unintentionally. Often it happens that so much *giving* is done to and for the disabled or sick child, that she/he tends to develop 'receiver', but not 'giver' skills. The full extent of the social handicaps of being a receiver, but not a giver, only becomes apparent as childhood gives way to adulthood. It is not easy to modify adult social behaviour so that it does not seem contrived. It is much simpler, though rather tedious, to mould the developing child's social skill repertoire.

To ensure that therapy works *for* and *not* against the child, we suggest that the therapeutic design must always specify a social context in which all therapy occurs. The context should embrace the child's usual world — his family and their social environment — as agents of therapy. This idea is more fully developed in Chapter 4. In this view of therapy, social skills are regarded as interdependent with performance skills, each requiring procedures which are applied in parallel. In this way therapy cannot become overly concerned with promoting the child's performance skills alone, in an environment which is separated from the real world.

SUMMARY

The ideas presented in this introduction to occupational therapy with children are important for you to think about, though you may not necessarily agree with them. Here follows a summary of the more important ideas.

1. Therapy of any kind should promote the maturation of the whole child in real world settings, chiefly the family.
2. Occupational therapy represents one component in a co-operative effort involving a range of specialists, the child and the family. The corporate goals for the child and family are two-fold; both should enjoy a life-style which is personally satisfying, and which attracts respect for the child.
3. There should always be a designed social context for therapy. Special techniques and procedures should be applied in the designed social context.

4. The occupational therapy medium is activity, usually play, which is familiar and attractive to children, incorporates challenge, and which leads to observable achievement.
5. The use of direct experience, real performance and practice by the child and the family is

emphasized, for it is these factors which distinguish occupational, from other therapies.

These five statements about therapy apply whatever the period of therapy, or the nature of the child's physical or behavioural disability or problems receiving attention.

REFERENCES

American Occupational Therapy Association 1986 Roles and function of occupational therapy in early childhood intervention. American Journal of Occupational Therapy 40: 835–837

Bryne D, London D, Reeves K 1968 The effects of physical attractiveness, sex and attitudes similarity on interpersonal attraction. Journal of Personality, 36: 259–271

Cynkin S 1979 Occupational therapy: towards health through activities. Little Brown, Boston

Havighurst R J 1952 Developmental tasks and education. Longmans Green, London

Mosey A C 1981 Occupational therapy — configuration of

a profession. Raven Press, New York

Nuse-Clarke P 1979 Human development through occupation, parts 1 and 2. American Journal of Occupational Therapy 33 (8), 33 (9)

Puchinger B, Zimprich H, Reiss-Patzak E 1975 Empirical analysis of the behaviour of nursing staff in a children's hospital. Paediatric and Padologie 10 (1): 55–65

Rogers J 1982 The spirit of independence: the evolution of a philosophy. Paper presented to 62nd Conference American Occupational Therapy Association Philadelphia PA

White W 1959 Motivation reconsidered: the concept of competence. Psychological Review 66: 313–324

2. Evolution of paediatric occupational therapy

READERS' OBJECTIVES

After reading this chapter, you should be able to:
1. Present a critical evaluation of the evolution of occupational therapy with children.
2. Discuss the role of research in occupational therapy practice with children.
3. Compare and contrast modern occupational therapy with children in a residential institution, and in a community context e.g. the school system.

In two short decades there have been dramatic changes in societal thinking about health and disease, health care delivery, and consequently, the various therapies. New areas of occupational therapy practice with children have opened up, and new techniques abound. Practice is both exciting and experimental, and we have reached a point of needing carefully constructed evaluation studies to identify and validate effective techniques and regimes. The clinician and the research specialist should truly become 'partners in research', for the ultimate benefit of the client — the child and his family.

FACTORS INFLUENCING PRESENT DAY PRACTICE

Altered views of childhood

The rapid changes in occupational therapy practice with children also reflect major changes in the study of children, and the practice of medical 'paediatrics'. Until quite recently children were regarded as expendable commodities to be traded, or otherwise used to ensure that adult members of their family unit survived. Indeed, in many modern societies such a view still prevails. Our current interest in children, and concern for their welfare and rights, is unique to highly industrialized and materially wealthy societies. Connell's (1982) important and fascinating account of the child in history is highly recommended to the reader. Modern knowledge about children, though still limited, has dramatically influenced the type of medical care given to them.

Changes in medical paediatrics

Morbidity and mortality have been so reduced that the model of medical intervention in acute crisis or medical care for chronic and/or terminal conditions has given way to a new model. Health and disease are now regarded as inter-related, and the current model is that of intervention to promote health *before* an acute medical crisis arises. Moreover, current society's view of 'health' embraces behavioural, psychosocial and developmental dysfunction beyond the usual scope of the medical practitioner (Hamburg 1985). Acceptance of this model is expressed in the significant change of facility name throughout the world from 'paediatric unit' implying pathology and its care, to 'child health' unit or department.

Apart from altered societal perception of children as possessions, specifically 'assets', other major reasons for change have been identified. These include improved standards of living, with better nutrition, less overcrowding, immunization, and a better educated society (Robinson 1980). The application of statistics and epidemiological procedures to clinical medicine have resulted in clearer understanding of various disease processes. Disease and abnormality control mechanisms have become more effective with our advance in technology, and understanding of the biological and social processes at work. For example, neonatal jaundice, once a common cause of cerebral palsy, deafness, and intellectual retardation, has been largely controlled (Robinson 1980).

Developmental paediatrics

A new type of paediatric practice has arisen — 'developmental paediatrics'. This discipline is concerned with understanding maturational processes, from fetal viability to full growth, as well as the structure and function of normal and abnormal children. Sheridan (1962) cites three goals of the discipline:

1. To promote optimal physical and mental health for all children
2. To ensure early diagnosis and effective treatment of handicapping conditions of body, mind and personality
3. To discover the cause and means of preventing such handicapping conditions.

HISTORICAL PERSPECTIVES

Changes in occupational therapy practice with children parallel and reflect changes in medical and societal thinking and knowledge. Previously, the main context in which occupational therapists practised with children was the hospital for acutely ill children. The majority of clients were children with chronic conditions such as osteomyelitis, polio, tuberculosis, infantile eczema, or kidney disease, who often spent months and even years in a hospital. Here are some examples of objectives of therapy thirty years ago:

a. To provide experience and an environment that will encourage normal development
b. To aid in diagnosis and treatment by learning to know and understand the child, through observation of his play
c. To arrange a plan of activity which will retain or restore the sence of security missed by the child when removed from the home surroundings.

Therapists may write more sophisticated objectives today, but the intentions expressed in those early objectives also remain valid. Time has produced a remarkable change in the pattern of diseases and problems confronting a paediatric occupational therapist, and in approaches to caring for sick children. For example, the average length of a child's hospital stay for a simple operation has been reduced from one or two weeks to 48 hours. Moreover, 25 years ago, hospitals generally followed a policy of restricted visiting. Sheppard (1982) recalls that only parents — not even brothers and sisters — could visit the sick child, and then only at weekends. Nowadays, in most children's hospitals throughout the world, administrators not only allow but actively encourage unrestricted visiting, at least by the child's family.

Children who could not survive previously, e.g., those with spina bifida, or the cancers of childhood, now do so, but with attendant long-term sequelae. Non-educable mentally retarded children who were either tucked away in an institution or at home, now receive vigorous educational and therapeutic attention. Non-accidental child injury — or child abuse, as it is colloquially called — was hardly discussed, whereas now it is a major cause of societal and medical concern. Behaviour disorders which were then regarded as 'exotica' are now rather commonplace.

With these dramatic changes, there has been a corresponding shift and expansion of the services of occupational therapists. Medical advances, and societal change in perception of childhood and children's rights and needs have helped to influence the shift from a primary medical care model where specialists react to events, to a proactive health oriented model where specialists promote well-being.

Another important trend has been a shift in focus from the child as the unit of treatment to the family as the unit of the treatment. The acute medical setting is still an important context, but the occupational therapist is now also to be found in a number of settings. For example, such settings include the school system; community health centres; specialist private organizations; large state institutions; obstetric hospitals; and high density living apartment blocks. A brief overview of the currently accepted roles of therapists in these new occupational therapy contexts sets the scene for the more specialized and detailed discussion throughout the book.

MODERN ROLES AND CONTEXTS

Llorens (1973) observed that broadening in both roles and contexts of occupational therapy with children, has led to a change in the point at which therapists first interact with potential clients. Llorens identified the old and new entry points of therapy with a shift from a medical to a health care model (see Table 2.1).

Table 2.1 Entry points for therapy: From a medical to a health care model (after Llorens 1973)

Previous entry point	Proposed entry point	Proposed follow-through
Illness	Early Detection	Health Maintenance
Treatment	Screening	Programming
Rehabilitation	Prevention	Consultation
	Programming	
Supervision	Consultation	

The scope for occupational therapy with children is broad, and therapists have become specialized in dealing with different client groups: for example, children with school learning difficulties. Inevitably, at any given time there will be 'fashions' in the selection of therapy systems and media. However, care must always be exercised to ensure that such fashionable approaches are not the only ones used in therapy with children. Therapy services may include any combination of the following media, methods, and techniques identified by Reed (1983):

— analysis and training of daily living skills for the development, restoration or maintenance of self-care, work, and play occupations
— design, fabrication, and application of orthotic and prosthetic devices to assist or substitute for functional performance
— analysis, selection, and use of adaptive or assistive equipment or devices for functional performance
— selected application of sensorimotor, cognitive or psychosocial activities to develop, or redevelop specific performance components
— use of therapeutically analysed crafts, games, or toys to promote purposeful actions which can be organized into performance components
— analysis of talks, development of play, and prevocational and avocational skills to facilitate the organization of performance components into occupational areas
— adaptation of the physical environment to improve the health, well-being and functional performance of all people.

Reed noted that these services are part of the problem solving process of occupational therapy which includes:

1. acceptance of a person for screening evaluation: *the referral step*
2. evaluation of that person's occupational performance: *the formative evaluation step*
3. analysis of results to identify performance problems and planning of a programme to improve, maintain, or promote occupational performance: *the therapy design step*
4. implementation of that programme: *the treatment or management step*
5. assessment of the results of the programme: modification of the programme if needed: *the summative evaluation step*
6. analysis for dismissal of the person: *the discharge step*.

The remainder of this discussion focuses on the various contexts as the setting for different functions of paediatric occupational therapists.

Children's hospital settings

Attending to the effects of the hospital and the separation experience among young children is an important function of the occupational therapist. Such work is also performed by a new group of people who wear various names, for example, 'play leader'. The reduction in length of hospital stay evolved, not only because of advanced medical techniques, but also from general acceptance of the theories and research studies of Bowlby (1952; 1969), Robertson (1952; 1962) about the mother and child bonds and the impact of interruption of this bond on the child's development. Other workers (for example, Klaus & Kennell 1976) also made important contributions to our understanding of the subtle and influential role of the early establishment of a bond, especially in unusual situations such as premature birth. These studies demonstrated that there could be long-ranging harmful effects to the young child, as an outcome of separation from the family unit during a stressful period of hospitalization. Citizen groups have developed throughout the world, e.g. the Association for the Welfare of Children in Hospital (AWCH), whose function is to protect children's welfare in hospitals, and to influence administrators to effect change. For example, as a result of pressure from AWCH, provision is now being made for mothers of sick children to 'room-in' with their young child. Unfortunately the practice of 'rooming-in' is still rare in western societies, and confined largely to middle-class families.

There has been an expansion of the occupational therapist's functions with these young clients. The therapist still provides compensatory support for the separated child, and may also provide 'preparation for hospital' programmes for families. In such programmes the therapist may counsel parents about possible predictable responses by the young child to the separation experience (see Chapter 14). Occupational therapists are wise to develop close and complementary working relationships with such groups as AWCH and the new 'play leaders'; there are never enough workers, and each group has some unique expertise to offer.

Hospitals for acutely sick children are still the major foci for the treatment of unusual and/or difficult medical, surgical and orthopaedic conditions of childhood. Thus occupational therapists still work with such children, but the range of conditions has changed. Most hospitals now have special units, for example, for the study and care of children with childhood cancers, or severe behaviour disorders. Also, there has been a change in the balance between the proportion of children seen in hospital as inpatients, and those seen as outpatients. Nowadays, in many locations, half or more of the client care load would be outpatient children and their families. Further, there is an area of overlap between hospitals and Community Health Centres where children with similar problems are seen, e.g. those with sensorimotor and learning disabilities. Occupational therapy settings must share certain client-types because of the low ratio of therapists available to meet community demands.

Therapists still attend children with burns, rheumatoid arthritis and diabetes. For example, today's occupational therapist working with a diabetic child might contribute to the evaluation process, by organizing a daily activity programme in the hospital closely resembling the child's usual daily activity programme at home. The information gained from observing the child and measuring behavioural responses would allow medication to be monitored accurately. One goal is to reduce the number of hospital visits needed by the child to achieve stabilization of the medication. Thus, realistic stabilization must reflect the situation to which the child will return from hospital.

In therapy the diabetic child will be taught how to plan interest and recreational activities compatible with physical abilities and a continuing medical regime. Such programmes still require long-term contact with the child and family, and provide an interesting example of developmentally oriented therapy.

Community settings

The strict separation between hospital and community settings has broken down. Care is no longer seen as ending at the front gate. Therapists from general hospitals assess clients in community settings, while community centre therapists attend case conferences in hospitals. Community Health Centres and community health promotion programmes are phenomena of the 1970s. Governments established Community Health Centres to monitor and promote health, and lessen the incidence of acute hospital care. Children are a major client group in Community Health Centres, in particular two groups: (a) those identified as *learning disabled*; and (b) those identified as *developmentally disabled*.

The designation of *learning disabilities* has replaced other unsatisfactory terms such as 'hyperactivity'. The newer term simply identifies a child who is failing in the formal school learning situation — for reasons which are complex, varied, and not always clear.

The term *developmental disability* replaces certain

medical diagnostic labels such as 'cerebral palsy', and relates to events which occur early in life and have long-lasting effects on a child's developmental process. The new classification reflects a change in thinking from concern with signs and symptoms, to concern about the effects of the medically defined condition. There is a full discussion of developmental disabilities provided in Chapter 13.

New intervention teams have developed in Community Health Centres. Medical and educational specialists work to detect, minimize or prevent handicapping conditions which might restrict a child from realizing and using potential abilities. Occupational therapists have been called on to develop skills of appraising developmental progress, and of working with families, rather than the child, as the unit of therapy.

Prophylactic programs in the community

Our professional role in helping children has expanded to embrace intervention programmes with those who, at birth, can be identified as being 'at risk' of interruption to their normal developmental process.

For example, there has been much basic research in the past ten years about how mothers and babies form their special relationship, 'the bond', which is regarded as critical for normal maturation. It is now possible to predict when a child may be unable to engage fully in that special relationship — thereby leading to less than optimal development. Premature infants and their mothers have greater difficulty in establishing the initial smooth bonded interaction than do normal full-term in-

---

Example 2.1 An intervention program
One very interesting example is a program in Boston USA using the model of a 'drop-in' neighbourhood coffee house in a poor, largely black persons suburb (Finn 1973). The aim of the specialist team on the project was to reach people in their own environment in a non-medical manner, free of bureaucracy. The health objectives were to screen and monitor children's health and development; and to provide general education about house and budget management, and child rearing. In addition, specific therapy was available as a service. The mode of reaching the people was to run regular free coffee mornings in a local well-known church building, with attendant play groups for children. Anyone might join by simply walking in. The program was designed as a long-term one, requiring commitment from the staff. The ultimate or terminal goal was that the general health and life quality of the people in that community should improve. Occupational therapists were important members of the specialist team.

fants and their mothers (Kennell & Klaus 1971). For example, when an infant is born prematurely — or with the Down syndrome (mongolism). In these particular cases therapeutic intervention begins with the family from the time of the child's birth. We call some of the techniques used 'teaching mothers to be more motherly'.

The school system

Appointment of occupational therapists and other specialists to the normal school system also reflects the increased attention and emphasis that society places on the nurturing of children. The intention was that specialists should monitor all of the children's maturation, in order to identify and correct developmental deviations before they could have serious effects on formal school learning. However, in practice therapists are still primarily engaged in identifying and treating those children who are already in the school system. This situation should change as therapists become established in screening children before they go to school. The ideal of developmentally screening all children in the kindergarten and preschool years, and providing intervention at this point, has yet to be realized.

Residential institutions

In the early 1960s Barker and colleagues (1963) demonstrated the impact that the physical and social environment has on an individual's behaviour. Since then a strong movement has developed in which specialists in a range of disciplines (for example, psychology, architecture, anthropology) have developed methodologies that allow study of the man–physical environment interaction. This movement has particular importance for paediatric occupational therapists who often work in large institutions, where environmental influences can be as powerful as any designed therapy regime. It is clear that there will be a continuing need for some residential institutions. Because there are rarely enough professional people to cope with resident numbers and needs, the more traditional approach of individual client intervention becomes a futile, despairing exercise. Programmes which use and manipulate the physical environment so that it becomes a positive therapeutic agent offer an exciting avenue for new occupational therapy strategies (Clancy 1976). Some useful programmes are discussed in Chapter 15.

Research in occupational therapy

Occupational therapists have been very active in clinical research about the possible reasons underlying learning difficulties. For example, the role of sensory integration and dysfunction in the production of learning difficulties has received considerable attention both inside and beyond the profession. Sensory integration therapy is still experimental, and for that reason exciting. The objectives are to take data about a given child's sensory perceptual and motor functions, as discovered on standardized tests, and systematically design treatment measures to deal with the problems discovered by the tests. The accompanying therapy is important as an example of the profession seeking to be more systematic and rational in treatment designs. Data is being amassed to allow objective evaluation of the theory and arguments. The theory of sensory integration, and its attendant therapy practices remains controversial. Regardless of the final research outcome, occupational therapists have established themselves as valuable members of the educational team in the school system (Knickerbocker 1980).

THE FUTURE

Changes in the role and functions of occupational therapists working with children are represented in Table 2.2.

Historically it is clear that technological advances in medicine have wiped whole groups from the occupational therapy client population, e.g., children with chronic suppurative bone disease. But at the same time new client groups have been added, e.g., the non-accidentally injured child, the normal child at school and the child with Acquired Immune Deficiency Syndrome (AIDS). Other client groups have gained in visibility and importance e.g. developmentally disabled children and their parents. Parent and consumer advocacy groups are becoming more politically sophisticated and articulate. It is not only such groups who are helping to mould the future shape of the profession, but policy makers are also inviting specialists such as occupational therapists to participate in the design of new policy.

From a thoughtful analysis of societal and technological trends it may be possible to predict what kind of future paediatric occupational therapy services the community at large will seek, require, and value. Some predictive attempts will allow therapists to prepare for possible future demands — to be professionally 'in the right place at the right time'. Therapists should pay careful attention to trends reflected in the child development and paediatric clinical research literature. For example, as skill developed in keeping more sick, frail

Table 2.2 A comparison of the historical and modern functions of the occupational therapist

| Historical role | | Modern role | |
Function	Context	Function	Context
		Evaluate developmental abilities of both well and sick children	
Treat functional loss through infection or accident	Acute illness hospital	*Treat* acutely and chronically ill child – with family as a unit of therapy	Acute illness hospital Community health centre
Train functional skills	Institutions for chronically ill, physically disabled, and mentally retarded children	*Develop programmes* through consultation e.g. with community self-help groups	Specialist organizations e.g. Society for Long Stay Residences Private Practice
		Research questions of theoretical and clinical importance	Universities Research institutes Clinic

infants alive and we grew to understand the infant–mother attachment process, specialists recognized the necessity for special therapy with infants and their families (Andrews et al 1982). At least in Western nations children are no longer traded, exploited, or ignored in quite the same way as used to be the case. Nonetheless, Connell (1982) makes some sobering observations about growing up in today's world. 'It is estimated that 46% of children born in the '70s have been, or will be, affected by divorce or separation of their parents. School leavers, disillusioned about the prospects of finding work, turn to the streets. Big business corporations, well aware of the impact advertising has on young minds and how susceptible parents are to pestering by children to buy commodities, use mass media mercilessly, guiding children toward consumer-oriented and competitive attitudes. The same media teach that "crime does pay".' Again, it appears that there may be a relationship between unemployment and a variety of social trends, e.g., extramarital births, non-accidental injury to children. There is every reason to believe that general community unemployment will remain high, and may even increase over the next decade. Could we occupational therapists develop experimental community programmes to help forestall the devastating effects of unemployment on family life, and thus inevitably on children? In this age of the microchip what will be our contribution to technological development which will ease daily effort and enhance the quality of life for physically disabled children?

Direct service delivery to clients has been our traditional priority. However, increasingly we are being asked to show professional accountability. It will be necessary to demonstrate that therapy strategies and programmes are based on verifiable theory, and empirical evaluation. Both therapeutic effectiveness and economic viability of service will need to be apparent. Clinicians of the future will need to possess basic skills in research, so that at the very least, they may consult with research specialists about programme evaluation (see Kannegieter 1980).

Thus, throughout this text an attempt has been made to link theory to practice, to show what is the state of our theoretical knowledge in relation to empirical studies supporting practice, and to clarify what practice is still experimental.

REFERENCES

Andrews S R Blumenthal J B, Johnson D L et al 1982 The skills of mothering: a study of parent child development centers. Monograph of The Society for Research in Child Development No 198, Vol 47, No 6

Barker R G (ed) 1963 The stream of behaviour. Appleton-Century-Crofts, New York

Bowlby J 1952 Child care and the growth of love. Penguin, Harmondsworth

Bowlby J 1969 Attachment and loss Vol 1. The Hogarth Press & the Institute of Psychoanalysis, London

Clancy H G 1976 Integrating the environment in therapy. Man–Environment Systems 6: 305–312

Connell H M 1982 Suffer the little children: society and the child, an historical perspective. Records of the Adelaide Children's Hospital 3: 3–15

Finn G 1973 The children's developmental workshop. In: Llorens L (ed) Consultation in the Community: occupational therapy in child health. Kendall/Hunt, Dubuque, Iowa

Hamburg B A 1985 Comments on the relationship of child development to modern child health care. SRCD 50th Anniversary Special Edition Newsletter, Society for Research in Child Development

Kannegieter R 1980 Environmental interactions in psychiatric occupational therapy: some inferences. American Journal of Occupational Therapy 34(11): 715

Kennell J H, Klaus M H 1971 Care of the mother of the high risk infant. Clinical Obstetrics and Gynecology 14(3): 926–954

Klaus M H, Kennell J H 1976 Maternal infant bonding. C V Mosby, St Louis

Knickerbocker B M 1980 A holistic approach to the treatment of learning disorders. Charles B Slack, Thorofare, New Jersy

Llorens L 1973 Occupational therapy in community child health. In Llorens L (ed) Consultation in the community. Kendall/Hunt, Dubuque, Iowa

Reed K L 1983 Concepts of occupational therapy. Williams & Wilkins, Baltimore

Robertson J 1952 A two year old goes to hospital (16 mm sound film with guidebook). Child Development Unit, Tavistock Clinic, London

Robertson J 1962 Hospitals and children: a parents-eye view. Gollanz, London

Robinson M J 1980 The year in paediatrics. Medical Journal of Australia 14 June 580–584

Sheppard P M 1982 Interview in Hospital Journal of Australia. November pp 16–17

Sheridan M D 1962 Infants at risk of handicapping conditions. Monograph of the Bulletin of the ministry of Health 21: 238

3. Foundations of therapy

READERS' OBJECTIVES

After reading this chapter, you should be able to:
1. **Discuss the objectives of normal growth and development.**
2. **Describe the principles governing normal and abnormal growth and development.**
3. **Know the forces that shape and influence the socialization of the child.**
4. **Discuss the potential impact of illness, disability and/or handicap on the developing child and family system.**
5. **Discuss the role of the central nervous system maturation and integrity on childhood development and behaviour.**
6. **Differentiate between 'cortical level learning' and sub-cortical level learning.**

In the following discussions an attempt has been made to identify and discuss developmental issues which have particular relevance to the practice of occupational therapy with children. Four issues have been identified, each reflecting a knowledge base essential to effective therapy. The four issues are:

1. The objective of normal growth and development.
2. The accepted principles governing normal and abnormal growth and development.
3. Environment, family, and maturation.
4. The role of brain plasticity in acquiring environmental mastery and adaptive skill.

The recent explosion of research data about human development (Smuts & Hogan 1986) confronts the busy clinician with the practical problem of keeping abreast of new knowledge. One workable solution is to monitor one or two comprehensive, respected journals. For example, the journal *Child Development* provides an excellent coverage of important research issues. *Developmental Medicine and Child Neurology* is an excellent clinical interdisciplinary journal, providing discussion of basic research applied to clinical questions. As well, a therapist should maintain one general textbook in child development as an essential resource, and update it about every five years. Some recommended general texts and journal resources are noted at the end of this chapter.

THE OBJECTIVE OF NORMAL GROWTH AND DEVELOPMENT

There is enormous effort involved in nurturing young children through to adulthood. The objective is that the child will become a valued, contributing member of our social community. The passport to membership is the acquisition of a complex network of skills: social, communicative, motor and cognitive. The process through which the cultural passport is gained is called *socialization* and is ongoing throughout the life cycle.

Socialization

The forces that shape and influence socialization are depicted in Table 3.1.

How is socialization initiated? For every newborn child, the bridgehead into the social culture is the special bond developed with the family, especially with the mother (Sluckin et al 1983). To what extent is it necessary that there should be an enduring relationship with one particular mother or caretaker remains controversial, but there can be no doubt that the child's emotional, cognitive development and social situation are all closely interwoven (Bowlby 1969, 1971; Bretherton & Waters 1985; Dubois 1968; Hinde 1974). Park (1981) has stressed the importance of stable social relationships surrounding the child — which also have the flexibility to allow change within him or her. The bond represents safety and security for the child, and as such it is the child's early learning environment. The

Table 3.1 The process and components of socialization

The raw material	Will be socialized along these dimensions	While selectively acquiring	In dynamic interaction with people and forces	Limited by these individual attributes	To form these life stages systems of behaviour	That will form the adult
The newborn organism with physical needs and inherited characteristics	Emotional Social Cognitive Perceptual Intellectual Behavioural Expressive	Skill Knowledge Attitudes Values Motives Habits Beliefs Needs Interests Ideals	*Agents* Parents Siblings Peers Relatives Teachers *Forces* Social class Religion Race School Community Mass media Voluntary groups	Age Sex Development rate stage Constitution Intelligence	Oral stage Anal stage Sexuality Aggression Achievement Affiliation Self-esteem	Trait Character Personality Role preference Goals

Reproduced by permission from McNeil E B 1969 Human Socialization. Brooks/Cole, Pacific Grove, California

child is led — gently — to explore and master an ever widening set of experiences (Anderson 1972).

The behaviour of infants is most intelligible within the context of the family, of which she/he is an integral part. The idea that 'the family' is one unit is an important one for therapy. When behavioural abnormality is seen in a young infant or child, the whole family interactive pattern around the infant–mother axis is affected.

The process of socialization is not normally a one-sided affair (Barrera et al 1986; McNeil 1969), and neither is the child a 'clean slate'. Blauvelt (1928) and Blauvelt & McKenna (1961) observed and filmed a human neonate crawling unassisted up the mother's body and orienting to her breast, within minutes of being born. Other similar occurrences have been reported and such information, though scanty, emphasizes the potentially two-way nature of the bonding process, from the moment of birth.

The infant's contribution

From birth both infant and mother reciprocally seek physical closeness (Brazelton et al 1974), and their developing attachment is implied by their behaviours which promote proximity and contact. Human infants have an early behaviour repertoire comprising a variety of cries, and facial and body movements, and later on approaching following and clinging to a significant person (Ainsworth 1972; Ainsworth et al 1971; Richards 1974; Tinbergen 1951). Bowlby (1969) called the re-

pertoire 'primary instinctual response systems'. The interactive properties of the early behaviour emerge as the infant matures. For example, by the age of five to eleven weeks the reflexive smiling response becomes linked with a specific visual cue, the human face. From six to sixteen months the infant responds preferentially to individual faces (Ambrose 1961; Brackbill 1958; Rheingold 1961; Salzen 1968 Spitz 1945). The maternal or caregiver behavioural repertoire includes, eye contact, kissing fondling, talking and feeding (Blurton-Jones 1972; Papousek & Papousek 1977; Todd & Palmer).

Sex differences

Sex difference studies are confusing in their details, but support the notion of general differences in social behaviour between males and females. For example, there is some evidence from sex difference studies to suggest that smiling is important to producing cuddling. In fact, Freedman (1971) and Garai & Scheinfield (1968) found quite distinct sex differences in all areas of early affiliative behaviour. For example, newborn girls 'smile', eyes closed, more than boys, and this is also true of later social smiling (McLean 1970). Freedman (1971) observed further that by six months, normal girls show a preference for gazing at social objects, while boys quite definitely do not. Other workers, for example, Stott (1962) had drawn attention to the higher vulnerability of boys to a wide range of physical conditions and problems in the neonatal period. Then Schaffer (1971) reported that a higher proportion of normal boys than girls actively avoided or passively tolerated cuddling.

Several workers have commented that infants of either sex who failed to achieve eye-to-eye gaze, whatever the reason, were less likely to achieve a normal attachment to their mother (Moss & Robson 1968; Rheingold 1961). While it is rash to draw a direct cause and effect inference, such studies emphasize the important role of eye contact in establishing and maintaining social interaction. Because of the reciprocal nature of the mother–child interaction, it seems likely for example, that a smiling or cuddly baby receives more physical contact than does a solemn or non-cuddly infant. Again, the quiet child might receive less maternal attention than the noisy one (Gewirtz 1961).

Stranger response

Over time, new behaviours appear in the child's repertoire, signalling the successful culmination of many individually insignificant but interrelated experiences, in new phases of socialization. The appearance of the 'stranger response', first described by Spitz (1945) is one such major event announcing that the primary caretaker, usually the mother, has special significance distinct from all others (Ainsworth et al 1971; Schaffer & Emerson 1964; Scott 1967). Again, Freedman (1971) noted a sex difference, namely that girls were more sensitive than boys to strangers entering the home in the first year of life. The phenomenon of intense attachment on the infant's part serves at least one important function, namely to keep the child close by mother over the period of rapidly developing locomotor abilities, which could otherwise lead him or her into dangerous exploration. It is increasingly clear that our understanding of the stranger response phenomenon and its functions is in its infancy.

Interaction of socialization and development

Much emphasis has been given to the child in his/her social world in the present discussion because the social world, chiefly the family, is probably the major determinant of the course that maturation will take (Lewis & Rosenblum 1979; Parmelee 1982; Taylor 1981). However, it is necessary to understand how interaction between the developing child and his/her social world promotes central nervous and other bodily system maturation. Several elegant studies of the effects produced by an infant crying provide a useful discussion point (Korner 1984; Korner & Grobstein 1966; Korner & Thoman 1972). It was observed that normally, the first effort made to comfort a crying infant is to pick the infant up and hold him or her upright over an adult's shoulder (usually mother). As well as serving social and emotional needs for comfort and company, the change to upright posture stimulates CNS structures, specifically the vestibular apparatus, which provides sensory feedback to the child about balance, posture and visual orientation. Repeated practice (following crying) reinforces maturing visual attention, and postural skills — a situation which appears to encourage the child to become even more adventurous. So, new motor skills appear and are practised and reinforced similarly. In all, there are cross-modal sensory, affective, and potentially cognitive experiences involving the tactile, proprioceptive, visual, motor and auditory systems. Bower (1977) has also provided important insights and evidence about the role of practice and repetitive processes in development, especially related to maturing perceptual and cognitive capacities and behaviour. The hypothesized effects of reciprocal interaction between infant and the environment on maturation of the central nervous system, and thus continuing development will be discussed later in this chapter.

Korner (1984) makes an important observation for therapists with the statement that 'it is through visual exploration that motorically helpless infants are most apt to get acquainted with their environment, including the mother'. Wilbarger (1984) advocates a 'gestalt' approach when an infant or young child presents with problems related to touching and movement. She advises therapists to pay attention to the *pattern* of a child's sensory processing problems. Furthermore, she advocates intervention through the provision of what is called a 'sensory diet' — experiences sustained through the sensory modalities in varying combinations of stimuli. In summary, a therapist who understands the influences at work in the socialization process can maximize their effects in intervention with child and family.

PRINCIPLES GOVERNING NORMAL AND ABNORMAL GROWTH AND DEVELOPMENT

Principles are important because once grasped, they enable the therapist to make sense of a child's observed/reported behaviour, and to design appropriate assessment and therapy. Naturally, principles may change in the light of new theories, models and empirical research information. For a comprehensive overview of theories of child development the work of Crain (1980) is highly recommended. For example, it has been a generally accepted principle that growth proceeds in a cephalo-caudal (i.e., head to feet) direction. More recent studies question this accepted belief (Brinkman & Kuypers 1973; Loria 1980; Parmelee 1982), though there is as yet no conclusive evidence against. The outcome of these studies will be of practical importance to therapists. For example, some therapy practices rest on the theory that postural skills must be achieved before fine manipulative skills are promoted. However, Prechtl & Beintema (1964) advocated the concept of system, as preferable to the notion of horizontal versus vertical hierarchies in CNS development. Twitchell (1970) quotes them thus, 'If we think of it as a network, then the network of the young infant is far less complex because there are fewer connections.'

Terminology

Growth refers usually to the increase and change in size and composition of the body *structure*. Growth can be measured objectively, for example by reference to head circumference, and height.

Development refers usually to the gradual elaboration and increased complexity of *function*. Development can also be 'measured' objectively by observing behaviour representing function in developmental assessment tests.

Maturation refers usually to the total process in which genetic and environmental influences combine so that the underlying structures and functions of the nervous system become differentially more complex and integrated — leading to the adult form. Though there is no one accepted definition of maturation, the following essential characteristics are recognizable (Espenchade & Eckert 1980):

- sudden appearance of new patterns of growth and development
- The appearance of particular abilities without benefit of previous practice
- The consistency of these patterns in different individuals of the same species
- The orderly sequence in the manifestation of different patterns
- The gradual course of physical and biological growth towards the attainment of mature status

Heredity determines the limits of each individual child's capacity to achieve optimal structural and functional maturity.

Environment determines the extent to which each child can fulfil his potential capacity (Sheridan 1977).

Normal: usual, typical, regular, healthy, free of abnormality. 'Normal' is a descriptive term which be applied to any child who shows typical characteristics for his age.

Average: the calculated point around which other values are dispersed. The term 'average' is derived from statistics and implies that measurements have been taken of some particular feature.

Normal growth and development

1. Normal development depends primarily on maturation of the brain and central nervous system.
2. Growth and development are the result of interaction between the individual's genetic endowment (heredity), and the physical and social environment (nature and nurture).
3. Growth and development occur in predictable sequences for all children, though the rate will vary from child to child. For example, the average age at which children walk is 12.5 months, but the normal range is 10–15 months.
4. Structure must always change before the child achieves functional competence. For example, an infant can sit upright only once certain primitive reflexes have become integrated, others have appeared, and neck and trunk muscles have developed strength.
5. It is necessary for earlier phases of growth to be negotiated satisfactorily, if later phases are to proceed normally.
6. There appear to be times during growth which are optimal for the acquisition of new behaviours. These times are called *sensitive periods*, or sometimes 'critical periods'.

   The term derives from the study of a phenomenon first called 'imprinting' by Lorenz (1970). He observed that young birds needed certain experiences at particular times after hatching, in order for the bird to learn an essential behaviour. The concept of 'sensitive periods' has been studied carefully by others (e.g., Hess 1973; Hinde 1961; Sluckin et al 1983) and confirmed for a range of animals. The situation appears to be more flexible for humans. Infants deprived of some experience, such as moving about freely, may still develop normal motor behaviour, though later, and with less ease than is normally the case (Provence & Lipton 1967, Rutter 1972).

Abnormal growth and development

1. Abnormal growth or development may occur locally or generally.
2. Abnormality is manifested by precocity, delay, exaggeration, dimunition, absence, duplication, or distortion.
3. Abnormal growth in one system tends to affect growth in related systems.
4. Failure of appropriate stimulation of a developing system tends to produce a reduction of functional capacity in that system.

5. Excessive stimulation of a developing system may lead to hypertrophy or increase of function up to a point, after which atrophy or reduction of function may ensue.
6. Decline from a point of peak function proceeds by the processes of:
   (a) diminution;
   (b) re-differentiation;
   (c) disintegration.
7. Lack of appropriate stimulation at, or exposure to inappropriate or excessive stimulation at a sensitive period in the development of a system, may lead to irreversible functional impairment in that system or related systems.
8. Growth failure, precocity, delay or distortion are due to an abnormality in the genes, or in the environment, or both.

Norms of growth and development

Growth and development may be considered at any or several of the following micro- or macro-systematic levels: biochemical, cellular, mass, intrapsychic, interpersonal, social. Each system has its own growth rate pattern, which is not linear, and is independent of the other systems.

One can only judge behaviour and thus development, to be 'abnormal' or 'deviant' by reference to some established and agreed standards of what constitutes 'normality'. Gesell et al (1934, 1940) laid the foundations for the study of behavioural development, leading to the presentation of 'norms of development'. Such norms are not absolute; they may change over time in response to environmental factors such as nutrition, or child rearing practices.

The general sequence and timing of behavioural norms and development are outlined in Appendices I–III. In clinical practice a therapist will probably refer to such charts quite often, as it is difficult to memorize such information accurately.

Sequence and timing of behavioural development is generally presented in the following areas:

— Gross motor skills
— Eye–hand co-ordination and fine motor skills
— Communication and language skills
— Personal-social skills
— Performance and adaptation skills

The prenatal period of development is summarised in Appendix I. It appears that in-utero behaviour development follows a trend of progression from diffuse to specific, gross to fine responses, traditionally thought

Definitions

There are conventions about the names designated to ages and stages in a child's development. The following definitions express general usage (Turner & Helms 1979, Barnes et al 1982).

Prenatal period

Gestation: period of intrauterine development from conception to birth.
Embryo: denotes the organism during initial period of cell differentiation following ovum implantation, from about second to eight week.
Fetus: the developing organism from about the eighth week of gestation until birth.

Neonatal and postnatal period

Infancy: generally considered to be the first two years of life.
Neonate: generally considered to be the newborn infant from birth to the end of the second week.
Premature infant: a viable infant with a gestational period of less than 38 complete weeks.

Term infant: a viable infant with a gestational period of 38–42 weeks.

Childhood

Toddler: the period between two and three years of age.
Early childhood: second through sixth year.
Middle childhood: seventh through ninth year, or 6 to 12 years depending on whether the terms 'late childhood' or 'preadolescence' are used.
Late childhood (if used): 10 to a maximum of 15 years (female); 10 to a maximum of 16 years (male).

Adolescence

Generally the teenage years (13–19) or commencing with the onset of puberty to emancipation from parents or to commitment to work.

Adulthood

Young: 20 to 40 years
Middle aged: 40 to 65 years
Elderly: 65 years and over, the retirement years — though recently there has been further refinement of this classification.

to be in a cephalo-caudal, proximal-distal direction. The primitive reflexes which constitute a significant component in the newborn infant's behavioural repertoire are clearly apparent and well established before birth (28 weeks gestation).

Appendices II and III present a summary of significant developmental milestones from birth onwards. Behavioural development in the first five years is emphasized, as it is during this period that new skills are acquired progressively by the child. Behavioural development from about four years onward generally reflects elaboration and refinement of the basic skill repertoire attained in the early years.

ENVIRONMENT, FAMILY AND MATURATION

Any physical or psychological trauma related to disease, injury, environmental influence or intrapersonal vulnerability can interrupt the growth process (Llorens 1970). Three groups of factors will be reviewed, namely:

1. Adverse experiences in the family context.
2. Adverse factors associated with physical disability and handicap.
3. Adverse affects of separating young children from a stable family context.

Adverse experiences in the family context

Families are not necessarily loving caring clans, nor are they any longer traditional units of mother, father and children. Indeed, there is really no such thing any more as a 'typical' family; for example the Australian Bureau of Statistics reported in 1986 that the traditional nuclear family is now only 27% of households. There is an increasing number of single parent families — mothers or fathers raising their children alone — divorcees, unmarried mothers and widowers. 18.6% of Australian children under 18 years live in one-parent (usually mother) households. An even more sobering statistic is the prediction that 45% of children born in 1977 will live in one-parent families before reaching 18 years. Grandparents raise their grandchildren, couples foster children, while others choose not to, or cannot have children. Children from non-English speaking migrant families present a particular dilemma and challenge. In such diverse family types the old known rules, guides, and supports for rearing children no longer seem to be adequate (UNESCO Report 1983). There is increased opportunity for a child to encounter adverse developmental experiences. The various adverse factors which may operate in the family are summarized by Nurcombe (1972) as follows:

Parental attitudes/expectations

Faulty parental attitudes in otherwise stable well in-

tegrated family units can present possible adverse developmental experiences for a child (Peterson & Koulack 1969). Most common are rejection, overdomination, overambition, overprotectiveness and faulty discipline. Overdomination and protectiveness are interesting examples of well-meaning motivation turned sour. Usually it is a mother who exhibits the behaviour, and her wish is to prevent any harm, physical and emotional from possible contact with her child. The result for such a child is restriction on normal maturational desire to become independent. The mother may become excessively indulgent of the child's stated wishes, and may exaggerate childish physical complaints. The child's response is usually to become insatiable in demands until finally mother's tolerance dissolves and the two become locked in conflict. An overambitious parent on the other hand, can foster an excessively submissive child, or an overtly rebellious one, or a passively negative, dawdling deceitful child. All such behaviours are counterproductive to healthy independent maturation (Cialdin et al 1981).

Parental personality disorder

Such disorder may take various forms, namely, intellectual inadequacy, emotional immaturity and disorder, and overt psychiatric illness.

Children of intellectually handicapped parents face the potential danger of an inadequate and/or inappropriate physical environment, social, cultural and cognitive experiences. The problems are serious ones, whether the child is similarly handicapped, or of normal intelligence thereby quickly outstripping the parents(s).

Nurcombe (1972) defines the socially immature person as one who has not completed earlier developmental tasks (see Appendix III, Havighurst 1952), and has for example, married in response to social pressures. The children of such unions face dangers similar to those associated with family dissolution.

Emotionally disordered parents may also communicate their own particular difficulties to their children. For example, a mother who is phobic about mess and dirt may forbid her child to explore any 'messy' activities, and may also transmit her own feelings of anxiety to the child. Again, a parent who identifies a 'bad' aspect of him/herself in a particular child may attempt to stamp it out of their child by inappropriately harsh measures. Radke-Yarrow et al (1985) found that the young children of clinically depressed mothers were more likely to show insecure behaviour attachments.

Gross personality disorders, alcoholism, drug addiction, and psychosis in a parent renders a child particularly vulnerable to extreme experiences. Some examples include deprivation, separation, non-accidental physical and psychological injury, and the possibility of genetic influences for some disorders, e.g., manic-depressive psychosis. Musick et al (1984) report effective intervention with families where the mother is mentally ill, in a project called 'Thresholds Mothers Project' in Chicago USA. Initially the children showed delay in intellectual performance, social competence, and normative development when compared with matched children of well mothers. After intervention over 9 to 30 months the authors reported significant developmental gains across a variety of measures for half the treatment group. The authors continued the study in an effort to identify factors associated with gains made by the children showing improvement. It was found that the primary factor was what they called 'the enabling quality of the child's relationship with the mother'. In general such mothers, even with their mental illness, showed the following characteristics:

— used the programme and showed some personal improvement in psychosocial functioning
— were less self-involved, made friends, showed thoughtfulness about and interest in others
— displayed more positive affect and interested attention toward their children, even when depressed, and at some times were able to enjoy their children and become actively involved with them in an activity requiring joint attention and engagement
— may have viewed their children as burdens, but not as agents of their mental illness and other troubles, to be victimized.

The mothers were able — at least for some brief periods — to perceive their children as separate people with their own needs. The authors report that the mothers were able to recognize that many of their children's problems were direct results of understimulation, repeated separations, and exposure to a somewhat unpredictable environment. Also they concluded that enabling mothers had succeeded to some degree in forming an attachment with their child that somehow overrode the devastating effects of their mental illness. When given help these mothers were able to put their own needs and concerns to one side and encourage their child in growth fostering experiences.

Family dissolution

A family may dissolve as a result of parental disharmony, or the death of one or both parents. When there is dissolution because of parental disharmony the damaging experience for the child results from chronic bickering and conflict, particularly before one parent leaves the home. A parent may displace affection from their spouse to a particular child, thus using that child for gratification of needs — and placing him or her under an inappropriate degree of responsibility. Sometimes children become the mediator, and prematurely develop a need to control their own feelings. In other cases a parent may vent hostility on a child (scapegoating) especially when she/he seems to resemble the spouse or partner. The child is in danger of dividing loyalties, with attendant responses of guilt, confusion and doubts.

When the death of a parent or parents is the reason for family dissolution the child is usually unprepared for sudden and final separation and experiences bewildering grief. There is a further discussion about death and dying in Chapter 17.

Economically, the one parent family experiences financial changes in living standards — usually deprivation. More extremely, the children may face further disruption through institutionalization or fostering. For lone mothers the prime difficulty is usually to provide an adequate income, which also allows for appropriate child care of very young children. For lone fathers the prime difficulty is to provide an emotional and socially supportive home environment. All lone parents face the overwhelming problem of chronic physical fatigue from juggling several demanding daily roles. Therapists working with children from disrupted homes can show compassion for parental needs by integrating any requirements for home activities into every day tasks, rather than assigning special tasks that required extra parental time, and cost.

Adverse factors associated with physical disability and handicap

Robert Louis Stevenson, writer of magical stories that have delighted generations of children and adults alike, was chronically ill with tuberculosis — he was disabled for most of his life. Yet he said 'Life is not a matter of holding good cards, but of playing a poor hand well.' The objective for all specialists: including the occupational therapist, is that they should facilitate and support the disabled child and family, so that child and family may indeed play a 'poor hand well'. That it can be done is well documented: Beethoven was stone deaf when he wrote much of his glorious music; Van Gogh produced some of his most beautiful and challenging paintings while in the midst of florid psychotic illness episodes — in the world's eyes he was 'raving mad'.

Holt (1977) reminds us that the terms, disability, deformity, handicap, and defect are often thought to be interchangeable, when they are not.

Definitions

Defect: any abnormality of structure.

Deformity: any deviation from the normal shape and form.

Disability: any failure of function and skill.

Handicap: any condition which impedes an individual's development, opportunities, expectations, and activities.

Defects and deformities may give rise to disability, but need not necessarily do so. During the course of a chronic disorder the degrees of deformity and disability may change in opposite directions, with one improving while the other becomes worse. Holt (1963) cites the example of a cerebral palsied child who increases his speed and distance of walking; thus considerably reducing the effects of the disability. However, the increased muscular effort may result in an increase in deformity. Therapists must make clear distinctions between the concepts implied by the defining terms, and sensitively weigh factors when determining therapy. Also Holt cautions against the automatic application of the term 'multiple or multiply' to each of the defining terms.

The development of disabled, including chronically ill, children rarely proceeds along usual predictable lines. Abnormal environmental conditions impinge, for example, repeated admissions to hospital with attendant disruption and separation in family relationships; painful proceedings which cause the child to be fearful and thereby preoccupied, rather than curious and exploratory. Thus there is double jeopardy in disability: the initial effect on development of the organic non-reversible impairment, and the potentially dysfunctional interactive patterns with other people, most notably parents (Shere & Kastenbaum 1966). By way of example, these authors compared the responses of two mothers of cerebral palsied children. Mother 1 limited her reactions to meeting her two-year-old's basic physical care needs. The child was observed to be passive, 'unhappy', and uninterested in objects. Mother 2 aimed her interactions at engaging her child in social games,

and extending physical care to promote motor skills. Her child appeared 'happy, active, alert and interested in objects. Green (1981) describes parents of disabled children as being in a state of chronic sorrow. Disabled children may experience great inconsistency in their interactions with people in general and this must make the world appear a bewildering and confusing place. For example, the child may experience sympathy, even overindulgence from some, and ridicule and scapegoating from others. Sometimes the same people will give confusing responses, at different times. Such unpredictability has been demonstrated to influence a child to develop as cautious; reserved about trusting others in forming friendships and close relationships; apprehensive about taking risks. Such behaviours limit the child in the amount of scope for exploration of the physical and social world. Because the response of parents to having a disabled child is such a powerful determinant on the child's developmental experience it is worthy of examination.

Normal parental response to disability

The pattern of parental response when they are confronted by disability in their own child, in many ways parallels the pattern of response of young children who are abruptly separated from their loving family for some reason, for example hospitalization. Both groups respond initially with dismay, disbelief, anger and with vigorous behavioural attempts to deny the situation and get out of it. For parents of a disabled child, 'getting out of it' may be expressed as denial of the abnormality — the disability: or it may be expressed through refusing the child, and opting for others to take care of him/her. Those who do not elect the latter course will pass into a stage of what Green (1981) calls 're-integration'. In so doing, specialists will be the ones against whom the parents' anger will be directed. The phenomenon is a common one of parents 'shopping around' for second or third or fourth opinions which will support their denial of the disability. This is especially so if the child looks physically normal, as do some intellectually handicapped and many autistic children. Professional behaviour insists that all specialists recognize that parents are behaving normally and must be afforded patience and compassion. Specialists must gently, but firmly insist on recognizing the presence of the disability (Mattsson 1975).

If this stage is handled with sensitivity, then parents will 're-integrate' their responses and pass into the third stage of mobilizing their own practical and emotional resources to formulate a plan of how they will deal with their child's special needs. Reaching so positive an outcome does not deny the ongoing 'chronic grief', rather, it reduces the future importance of that factor.

The issue of when to tell parents that their child is disabled, if it is not glaringly apparent, and how much to tell, is an issue that concerns all specialists in a team. The primary responsibility lies with the paediatrician, but there must be close cohesion and communication between team members, to ensure that parents do not receive conflicting information and views. Green (1981) believes that, in the long run, it is more productive to inform parents of the full implications slowly, allowing them time to digest information at their own rate. The situation for non-English speaking families becomes even more complex and every endeavour should be made to provide excellent interpretation services. Even then, the subtle nuances of a counselling interaction will be very difficult to maintain.

Potentially the family unit remains the most healthy development-promoting context. Surprisingly, in view of the increasing numbers of disabled children in our societies, we know very little of the ways in which parents of disabled and normally developing children interact in their close family relationships. Barrera & Vella (1987) have reviewed the literature and provide a most useful overview of the state of research, and this review is recommended. Parents of disabled children are very stressed people, and their needs and the pressures on them must be as much the focus of therapy planning, as are the child's needs. There is no place for attitudes from specialists which allow perceptions to develop of parents as, 'non-compliant', 'resistive', 'not caring about their child', or at worst as, 'bad parents'. All parents of disabled children commence their parenthood as people who never imagined themselves coping with anything more than measles and chickenpox, the school and holiday fees, and a wedding and grandchildren in the future. Instead, measles and chickenpox become mysterious medical conditions of alarming, often life-threatening, proportions; school becomes a major time consuming, cumbersome endeavour; holidays become a 'maybe' event, while weddings and grandchildren are superseded by anxious cares for their child about socially unacceptable sexual behaviour, and unwanted pregnancy. It is indeed not only the child who is dealt 'a poor hand'.

Let us examine more closely some of the other factors which have a direct impact on the disabled child's developmental experience.

Physical attractiveness

There have been a number of imaginative and useful studies of the impact of physical attractiveness of ill and disabled children on the behaviour of caretakers (Bryne et al 1968, Puchinger et al 1975). Generally people turn away, either from embarrassment or feelings of repugnance, from those who look different. Others respond with inappropriate sympathy and solicitude. Such responses create complex problems for the physically disabled or disfigured child who has normal intellectual capacity and strivings for social intercourse with others. Nurcombe (1972) discusses the following socially handicapping effects of physical disability e.g. spine bifida, or disfigurement e.g. burns scarring.

Restriction of personality-ego development

For example, blindness, deafness, and orthopaedic abnormality may cause impoverishment or distortion of perceptual development. Again, chronic bed rest or hospitalization seriously limit the child's range of experience with persons and things. Reaction to restriction may present itself through extreme behaviours such as self-abuse. On the other hand the child may regress to immature behaviour patterns such as bed wetting.

Distortion of the child's interpersonal relationships

Parents may react with overprotectiveness, leading to infantilization of the child; permissive indulgence, leading to a child with poor impulse control; excessive demands, leading to a compulsive anxious child, or a rebellious and negativistic one; rejection and isolation, due to shame.

Distortion of the child's self-image

One's sense of self, including the 'body image', and facial expression are important influences in peer and sexual relationships. Inability to compete with the peer group, or isolation from it, may lead to defensiveness, self-isolation, self-loathing, depression and paranoid attitudes.

Narrowing of vocational choices

Dyke (1984) found that intellectual capacity was an irrelevant factor influencing occupational placement of young adults with cerebral palsy. The most influential factor used by vocational counsellors was hand function. Dyke cites the example of a severely athetoid young woman with a university honours degree who was placed vocationally in a sheltered workshop because she was judged by authorities as 'too handicapped' for open employment opportunities. These observations reinforce the view that personality distortions in handicapped young people represent, in part, responses to the attitudes of others. Such distortions do not necessarily correlate with the degree of disability per se.

Nurcombe (1972) emphasizes that more important than the specific disease or handicap are the child's adaptive capacities and those of the family as a whole. Occupational therapists have an important contribution to make by assisting the family to develop growth-promoting, coping, and adaptive strategies.

Adverse effects of separation

There is a large body of evidence drawn from both human and primate studies which confirms that there are significant developmental distortions which may result from family separation experiences. However, recent work has identified that it is not separation per se, but rather specific conditions attached to the experience which are responsible (Hinde 1974). The original work which lead to recognition of behavioural responses as syndromes was done with two groups of children. The first group comprised infants who in the aftermath of World War II were, of necessity, reared in orphanages (Bakwin 1949; Bowlby 1963; Spitz 1945). The second group were ordinary young children hospitalized for various reasons, and for periods of more than one week (Prugh 1953, Robertson 1958).

In the orphanages Spitz (1945) observed two devastating behavioural syndromes, which he associated with too few staff, clockwork caring routines, and inevitable inattention to infants' attempts to gain need fulfilment. Spitz named and described the syndromes in the following way:

Hospitalism. A syndrome apparent in infants under 6 months, characterised by listlessness, emaciation, hypotonia, immobility, quietness, failure to thrive, insomnia, 'unhappy' appearance, proneness to fever and cross infection, and the absence of spontaneous smiling.

Anaclitic depression. A syndrome apparent in infants over 6 months i.e. separation occurring after a focused relationship to the mother has developed and characterized by: child becomes weepy, ignores adults or screams at their approach, gains weight slowly, has a retarded developmental quotient and fails to thrive. If this state lasts for over three months the child may pass into an irreversible state of frozen rigidity, with expressionless face and auto-erotic rocking or body stimulation.

Such extreme syndromes though rarely seen today, represent points on a continuum. One may observe expressionless faces, inappropriate and 'shallow' social behaviour, and self-stimulating repetitive stereotyped behaviour, for example, among intellectually handicapped children living in residential institutions. There is a discussion of the environmental impact of institutional living in Chapter 14.

Impact of separation

Once a child is removed from a family — for reasons including social ones, she/he can be vulnerable to repeated fostering experiences. If fostering fails, a vicious cycle develops, with failures confirming a child's self-perceptions of incompetency and worthlessness.

Bowlby (1953) and Robertson (1958) identified a different behavioural syndrome among children from stable families, but who were separated by hospitalization — either that of child or mother. Bowlby described a process of response in the child characterized by initial protest which, if the separation continued is replaced by behaviour indicative of despair and finally detachment — often misinterpreted as acceptance by the child. Some of the early studies which followed these authors' work overstated the detrimental effects, and Rutter (1972) provides a balanced analysis of current knowledge. Such responses by normal but acutely ill children are discussed fully in Chapter 14.

BRAIN PLASTICITY AND ADAPTIVE COMPETENCE

Behavioural development of a child is the outcome of very different processes operating at different levels of biological organization. As an infant matures, the CNS network matures and a greater range of responses as well as a greater variation of responses becomes possible (Prechtl & Beintema 1964). One example is that earlier reflexes can no longer be elicited in their most predictable forms. The overall functional efficiency of the CNS is increased with improvement in its component parts. With the progressive establishment of neural networks, enriched and modified by experience, the capacity of the central processing machinery is enlarged (Connolly & Bruner 1972). The unifying theme is the interaction of the biological unit with its own effective environment (Hofer 1981). There have been various theories about relationships between CNS maturation and behaviour. The theories largely focus on localization of function to identifiable areas of the brain. The equipotential theory holds that while sensory input may be localized, perception involves the whole brain, and the effects of brain lesions depend not upon their location but upon their extent. A dominant view is that at the level of basic functional components there is a relative distribution of

Table 3.2 Major structures of the nervous system

	Structures	Function
	Central nervous system	
	Brain	
	1. Cerebrum	Sense perception; voluntary movements; learning, remembering, thinking; emotion; consciousness; personality integration
Forebrain		
	2. Thalamus	Sensory relay station on way to cerebral cortex
	3. Hypothalamus	Control of visceral and somatic function, such as temperature, metabolism, and endocrine balance
	4. Corpus callosum	Fibres connecting two cerebral hemispheres
Midbrain	5. Midbrain	Conduction and switching centre; pupillary light reflex
	6. Reticular formation	Arousal system that activates wide regions of cerebral cortex.
	7. Cerebellum	Muscle tone; body balance; co-ordination of voluntary movement, as of fingers and thumb
Hindbrain	8. Medulla	Via cranial nerves exerts important control over breathing, swallowing, digestion, heartbeat
	9. Pons	Fibres connecting two hemisphere of cerebellum
	Spinal cord	Conduction paths for motor and sensory impulses; local reflexes
	Peripheral nervous system	
	Autonomic nervous system	Autonomous or self-regulating mechanism
	1. Parasympathetic division	Operates and controls vital life functions at normal level
	2. Sympathetic division	Takes over vital life functions in stress and emergency situations; increases functions of those necessary to meet threat and decreases functions of those not necessary for survival
	Craniosacral nerves	Controls sensory nerves, motor and somatic nerves, and vagus nerve

From Kalugar G, Kalugar M F 1974 Human development: the span of life. C V Mosby, St Louis © 1985 Merill Publishing Company, Columbus Ohio. Reprinted with permission of Merill Publishing Company.

function within a region of the cerebral cortex; the more complex the function, the less localized the system and the more extensive the degree of integration. Brodmann's (1925) cytoarchitectonic mapping technique allows brain areas to be delineated by the cell types they contain. The technique represented a major advance in the study of brain organization and function across species. A review of the relationships between structure and function is presented in Table 3.2.

The classical model of brain/central nervous system functioning remains that expressed by McGraw (1974) and Hebb (1949) and it may be summarized as follows:

• There are two major divisions of the CNS controlling neuromuscular functions namely, the cerebral cortex and sub-cortical nuclei. The latter develop before the former.

• At birth, the cerebral cortex of the human infant is not functioning and behaviour patterns are mediated by sub-cortical nuclei.

• Some functions remain under sub-cortical control throughout life.

• Some behaviours of the newborn are residuals of phylogenetic functions and have no usefulness to man.

• As the cerebral cortex develops, it controls neuromuscular functions and inhibits the sub-cortical nuclei

• Developmental changes in overt behaviour are associated with advancement in cortical maturation which is reflected in suppression of some behaviours and integration of others.

• Development proceeds in a cephalo-caudal direction.

• Morphological growth does not progress uniformly.

Hebb (1949) observed that initial learning in infancy took longer than learning in maturity. The reason suggested was that initial learning occurred in a period when control over association areas was developing while learning in maturity simply reflected activation of developed neuronal pathways and associations.

Luria (1973) proposed another model of CNS organization in which the brain is organized into three functional blocks. The first block consists of the upper and lower brainstem and reticular formation and regulates the energy and tone of the cerebral cortex, thus providing a stable background for the organization of cerebral function. The second block, with highly specific functions (e.g., vision, audition, cutaneous and kinesthetic sensation) is located in the rear of the cortex where information is analysed, coded, and stored. Each area is organized in a hierarchy according to function. The primary zone sorts and records sensory information, the secondary zone organizes the information and codes it, and finally the tertiary zone integrates data from different sources to provide a foundation for behaviour. The third block which is composed of the frontal lobes, is responsible for the formation of behavioural intentions. The third block has no direct sensory or motor function but participates in every complex behavioural process. The data available on myelination supports Luria's model.

Thus it appears that integrative processes are necessary to systematic and orderly maturation of the central nervous system.

Myelination

The process of integrated reciprocal interaction between child and environment is associated with myelin deposit on neuronal pathways. Fleshig (1920) provided the first detailed study of myelination in the human nervous system. Fleshig formulated a set of 'laws of myelogeny' which remain the classical definition and description of the myelination process. The laws may be stated thus:

- Myelination of nerve fibres in the developing brain occurs in a definite sequence namely, sensory fibres prior to motor fibres, prior to association fibres.
- Fibres belonging to particular functional systems mature at the same time.
- Myelination temporarily repeats the previous formation of the axon.
- Myelination occurs at different rates which parallel cell differentiation and migration.
- Myelination is related to embryological development of the CNS.

Fleshig also noted that structures and organs related to primary functions necessary for survival, myelinate early (e.g. sucking, swallowing and breathing) and that birth accelerates the myelination process, even in prematurely born infants.

Langworthy (1933) attempted to link myelination and functional development. Sections of brain tissue of a six-, seven-, and eight-month fetus, and a full-term, one- and two-month-old infant were studied. Because examination was confined to a single series the studies did not allow for general conclusions to be made. However, Langworthy observed that traits in the tissue examined did appear to be myelinated at the same time that they became functional. It was this observation that lead Langworthy to propose sensory stimulation as the mechanism controlling maturation including myelination. He conjectured that the massive sensory input at birth might explain accelerated myelination at birth.

Yakovlev & Lecours (1967) produced a picture of the myelination process which suggests that:

1. Contrary to belief, myelination does not terminate at the first postnatal year, but extends through the third decade for pathways controlling complex behaviours.
2. Myelination is an orderly process in which functionally related systems are synchronized in rate and sequence of myelination.
3. Myelination is an important parameter of regional maturation of the central nervous system. Regional maturation, in turn, reflects the hierarchy in functional organization of the brain.

More recently Goldman-Rakic (1980) confirmed Yakovlev and Lecours' first conclusion and drew attention to the role of cortical plasticity for learning following insult or injury. There does not appear, as yet, to be any empirical evidence supporting Langworthy's (1933) proposal of sensory stimulation as the mechanism controlling myelination.

Though myelination is clearly one index of CNS maturation, Prensky et al (1978) has demonstrated that some major biochemical changes also roughly correlate with morphological development. For example, DNA correlates with an increase in number of cells, while increases in RNA and protein are indicative of cellular hypertrophy (Prensky et al 1978). Myelination results in several chemical changes as the water content of the white matter decreases and lipid content increases. Changes in the level of enzyme activity and amino acid and electrolytic concentrations during development are assumed to have some functional importance, but as yet it is not possible to correlate specific biochemical changes with functional maturity of the CNS. Another important aspect of the biochemical maturation of the brain is 'the development of systems to form, store, release and de-activate possible neurotransmitters responsible for the normal electrical activity of the brain' (Prensky et al 1978).

The two most commonly used methods to measure

electrical maturation of the central nervous system are 'evoked cortical potentials' in response to specific sensory stimuli, and electroencephalography (EEG).

Brain plasticity

The doctrine of plasticity holds that the brain is capable of modification, and that in immature individuals it is less clearly delineated into form/function related areas. Such 'plasticity' is thought to decrease with increasing age, and presumably to be influenced by environmental experiences. Thus, children have been thought to be more resilient in responding to their injury and insult than mature individuals (Bach-Y-Rita et al 1970, Held 1965, Hinde 1974). The mechanism thought to be involved is that of compensation. Other areas of existing brain take over some of the damaged area's function. However, some (e.g. Delacato 1959) have insisted that this is not the case, and that brain tissue like all others is capable of regrowth. Doman & Delacato (1968), among others, have proposed therapeutic systems built on the proposition of regrowth, stimulated by designed experience. Recently Goldman-Rakic (1980, 1982) and colleagues at Harvard University have provided the most important evidence so far on the debate about brain plasticity and regeneration following injury. Their work is of immense importance to therapists implementing programs with children (and adults) who have been subject to brain insult. The Harvard group's findings are briefly summarized.

The question asked was, 'How are the different parts of the brain connected?' The method of study used was the placement of amino-acid tracers, which change into protein that can be traced, into some parts of the cortex. Tracers were placed in opposite cortexes and the pathways by which the two sets of tracers came together in a common area were traced. The conclusions were that imput to the brain is distributed into interdigited columns; further, there is redundancy in the central nervous system, so that I after injury some of the affected function remains; it is almost never totally wiped out.

The Harvard group's work confirms that the presence of intact sub-cortical structures, particularly the caudate nucleus, is of critical importance to CNS maturation of the newborn and young infant. This finding is of practical importance to all therapists working with infants and young children with any CNS impairment. The contribution of the cortexes comes in only gradually, and where there is prenatal and early postnatal injury there is rerouting of functions to other pathways. Goldman-Rakic (1980) has demonstrated satisfactorily

that at least one component of the CNS, the cortex, is capable of 'growing' other connections to assume functions of a damaged area, and that connections can reorganize into other territories of the brain. The normal columnar pattern is preserved, and the new organization is functionally useful. From the data, Goldman-Rakic concludes that therapy in childhood — prenatal to puberty — which influences synaptic connections, is effective therapy. However, for therapists the significant question is 'What therapy strategies and interventions will influence the development of synaptic growth?' Some, such as the therapeutic school of neurobiological theorists (e.g., Ayres 1972, 1981) have made courageous attempts to define systematic therapies, but the results are as yet disappointing.

Plasticity and learning

Learning may result from a process in which the learner knows what it is that she/he is learning, what the end goals are, and how these will be achieved. This is 'cortical level or cognitive learning' and it implies that the learner contributes analytic and other cognitive skills to the process. Alternatively, the learner may reach the same end goals without having ever known that they existed. This is 'sub-cortical learning' and it is very often a feature of the occupational therapy intervention process (see Guilfoyle et al 1981). Some examples will clarify the two definitions, which represent arbitrary and convenient separate ideas to assist discussion. In reality both forms of learning coexist and proceed together, culminating in well integrated responses which are effected without conscious thought by the individual.

Let's take the simple general example of children learning formally about money management. In the cognitive learning process, the skills might be taught in a classroom maths lesson, and the goal would be quite explicit. In the sub-cortical process, the children in the classroom might be organized into game groups to play money games, e.g., 'Monopoly' or 'Poleconomy', without the goals of money management being made explicit. Provided the media are chosen appropriately, the end result from either process should be the same: the children should acquire the specified skills of money management. (See chapter 9: the example of Jenny relearning to walk by making her 'clown' crutches do tricks is a simple example of sub-cortical learning applied in therapy. The emphasis is not on walking, but on the symbolic play use of the crutches disguised gaily as clowns.)

The Peto system of 'Conductive Education' (Cotton & Kinsman 1983) provides an excellent example of cognitive learning, i.e., learning at the cortical level of organization applied to therapeutic procedures. Children perform motor actions and simultaneously verbalize exactly what is being done. 'I put my hand on the chair . . . I bend to pick up the sock . . .' and so on. Biofeedback procedures where the client focuses on the behaviour required in order to attain the desired goal, are also examples of cortically mediated cognitive learning. The learner's informed co-operation is essential to the achievement of goals. Therapies based on behavioural principles similarly emphasize cognitive awareness of behaviour through verbal instruction, e.g., 'Well done Jane, you've tried very hard and done up your coat buttons without help.'

SUMMARY

The foundations of all occupational therapy with children are that childhood developmental behaviour depends on three major considerations:

- The maturity of the central nervous system;
- The integrity of the central nervous system;
- Availability to the child of a range of environmental experiences, including that of mothering with its components of caring, security, and intellectual stimulation (Court 1981).

Immaturity in brain development, damage to the brain, developmental defects in the brain and/or sensory pathways, and an unfavourable family environment may all contribute toward delayed development and the risk of later childhood disability.

Occupational therapy is distinguished from other forms of therapy and training in that a very large proportion of our practice is mediated through the subcortical learning process.

REFERENCES

Ainsworth M D S 1972 Attachment and dependency — a comparison. In: Gewirtz J L (ed) Attachment and dependency. V H Winston & Sons, Massachusetts

Ainsworth M D S, Bell S M, Stayton D J 1971 Individual differences in strange-situation behaviour of 1 year olds. In: Schaffer H R (ed) The origins of human social relations. Academic Press, London

Ambrose J A 1961 The development of the smiling response in early infancy. In: Foss B M (ed) Determinants of infant behaviour. Methuen, London

Anderson J W 1972 Attachment behaviour out of doors. In: Blurton-Jones N (ed) Ethological studies of child behaviour. Cambridge University Press, Cambridge

Australian Bureau at Statistics 1986 Census of population and housing — a seven page summary. Australian Government Publishing service, Canberra

Ayres A J 1972 Improving academic scores through sensory integration. Journal of Learning Disabilities 5: 336–343

Ayres A J 1981 Sensory integration and the child. Western Psychological Services, Los Angeles

Bach-Y-Rita R, Collins C, Scaddeu H 1970 Display techniques in a tactile vision — substitution system. Medical Biology Illustrated 20: 6–12

Bakwin H 1949 Emotional deprivation in infants. Journal of Pediatrics 35: 512–521

Barnes M R, Crutchfield C A, Heriza C B 1982 Neurophysiological basis of patient treatment. Stokeville Publishing, Atlanta

Barrera M E, Cunningham C E, Rosenbaum P L 1986 Low birth weight and home intervention strategies: preterm infants. Journal of Developmental and Behavioural Pediatrics 7: 361–366

Barrera M E, Vella M 1987 Disabled and non-disabled infants interactions with their mothers. American Journal of Occupational Therapy 41 (3): 168–172

Blauvelt H 1928 Personal communication, Prof N Tinbergen, University of Oxford

Blauvelt H, McKenna J 1961 Mother neonate interactions: capacity of the human newborn for orientation. Methuen, London

Blurton-Jones N G 1972 An ethological study of children's behaviour. Cambridge University Press, Cambridge

Bower T G R 1977 The perceptual world of the child. Fontana/Open Books, London

Bowlby J 1953 Some pathological processes set in motion by early mother–child separation. Journal of Mental Science 99: 265–72

Bowlby J 1969 Attachment and loss, Vol 1, Attachment. Hogarth, London

Bowlby J 1971 Attachment and loss, Vol 2, Separation grief and loss. Hogarth, London

Brackbill Y 1958 Extinction of the smiling response in infants as a function of reinforcement schedules. Child Development 29: 115–124

Brazelton T B, Kloslowski B, Main M 1974 The origins of reciprocity. In: Lewis M & Rosenblaum L H (eds) The effects of the infant on its caregiver. Wiley, New York

Bretherton I, Waters E (eds) 1985 Growing points of attachment theory and research. Monographs of the Society for Research in Child Development 50: 1–2

Brinkman J, Kuypers H C 1973 Cerebral control of contralateral and ipsilateral arm, hand and finger movements in the split brain rhesus monkey. Brain 34: 459–459

Brodmann K 1925 Vergleichende Lokalisationaslehne der Grosshurnpinde 2, Auflage, J A Barth, Leipzig

Bryne D, London D, Reaves K 1968 The effects of physical attractiveness, sex and attitude similarity on interpersonal attraction. Journal of Personality 36: 259–271

Cialdin T, Getty R E, Cacioppo J T 1981 Attitude and attitude change. Annual Review of Psychology 31: 357–404

Connolly K, Bruner J 1972 The growth of competence. Academic Press, New York

Cotton E, Kinsman R 1983 Conductive education for adult hemiplegia. Churchill Livingstone, Edinburgh

Court J M 1981 Child development. Patient Management November: 21–29

Crain W C 1980 Theories of development — concepts and applications. Prentice-Hall, Englewood Heights, New Jersey.

Delacato C H 1959 Treatment and prevention of reading problems. Charles C Thomas, Springfield Illinois

Doman C, Delacato C 1968 Doman–Delacato treatment of neurologically handicapped children. Journal of Pediatrics 72: 750–752

Dubois R 1968 Environmental determinants of human life. In: Glass D C (ed) Environmental influences: Proceedings of a conference. Rockefeller University Press, New York pp 138–154

Dyke J 1984 Autonomy and disability: a study of helper influence on the life patterns of satisfaction of cerebral palsied adults, Unpublished Master Occupational Therapy thesis, University of Queensland, Brisbane

Espenchade A S Eckert H M 1980 Motor Development 2nd edn. Chas Merrill, Columbus, Ohio

Fleschig P 1920 Anatomie das Menschliechen Gehirns und Ruckenmarks auf Myelogenetischer Grundlager, I. Bd. Leipzig, Thieme

Freedman D G 1971 Human behaviour in evolutionary perspective. Basic Books, New York

Garai J E, Scheinfeld A 1968 Sex differences in mental and behavioural traits. Genetic Psychology Monographs 77: 169–299

Gesell A, Thompson H, Amatruda C S 1934. Infant behavior: its genesis and growth. McGraw-Hill, New York

Gesell A, Halvorson H, Thompson H 1940. The first five years of life. Harper & Row, New York

Gewirtz J L 1961 A learning analysis of the effects of normal stimulation and deprivation on the acquisition of social motivation and attachment. In: Foss B M (ed) Determinants of Infant Behaviour. Methuen, London

Goldman-Rakic P 1980 Morphological consequences of brain injury. Progress in Brain Research 53: 1

Goldman-Rakic P 1982 Plasticity of the central nervous system. Environmental intervention for infants at risk. Harvard Medical School and The Children's Hospital Medical Centre, Boston, Massachusetts

Green C 1981 Handicapped children: let's be more positive and practical. Medical Journal of Australia 1: 402–404

Guilfoyle E, Grady A P, Moore J C 1981 Children adapt. Charles B Slack, Thorofare, New Jersey

Havighurst R J 1952 Developmental tasks and education. David McKay, New York

Hebb D O 1949 The organisation of behaviour. Wiley, New York

Held R 1965 Plasticity in sensory-motor systems. Scientific American 213: 84–94

Hess E H 1973, Imprinting: early experience and the developmental psychology of attachment. Van Nostrand Rheinhold, New York

Hinde R A 1961 Some aspects of the imprinting problem. Symposium of Zoology Society, London 8: 129–138

Hinde R A 1974 Biological bases of human social behaviour. McGraw-Hil, London

Hofer M A 1981 The Roots of Human Behaviour. Fullman, San Francisco

Holt K 1977 Developmental pediatrics. Butterworths, London

Holt K S 1963 Deformity and disability in cerebral palsy. Developmental Medicine Child Neurology 5: 629

Kalugar G, Kalugar M F 1974 Human development — the span of life. C. V. Mosby, St Louis

Korner A F 1984 Interconnections between sensory and affective development in early infancy zero to three. Bulletin of the National Center for Clinical Infant Programs 5(1): 1–6

Korner A F, Grobstein R 1966 Visual alertness as related to soothing in neonates. Implications for maternal stimulation and early deprivation. Child Development 37(4): 867–876

Korner A F, Thoman E B 1972 The relative efficacy of contact and vestibular stimulation in soothing neonates. Child Development 43(2): 443–453

Langworthy O R 1933 Development of behaviour patterns and myelination of the central nervous system in the human fetus and infant. Contributions to Embryology. Carnegie Institute of Washington 24: 1–57

Lewis M, Rosenblum L A (eds) 1979 The child and its family. Plenum, New York

Llorens L A 1970 Facilitating growth and development, the promise of occupational therapy. American Journal of Occupational Therapy 24(2): 93–101

Lorenz K 1970 Studies in Animal and Human Behaviour, Vol I Methuen, London, pp 259–315

Loria C 1980 Relationship of proximal and distal function in motor development. Physical Therapy 60: 167–172

Luria A R 1973 The working brain. Penguin, London

McGraw D 1974 The neuro-muscular maturation of the human infant. Hafner Press, New York

McLean J D 1970 Sex correlated differences in human behaviour. Unpublished research paper for the Committee on Human Development, University of Chicago

McNeil E B 1969 Human socialization. Brooks/Cole, Pacific Grove

Mattsson A 1975 Psychophysiological study of bleeding and adaption in young haemophiliacs. In: Anthony E J (ed) Exploration in child psychiatry. Plenum Press, New York

Moss H A, Robson K S 1968 Maternal influence in early social visual behaviour. Child Development 39: 401–408

Musick J S, Stott E M, Spencer K K, Goldman J, Cohler B J 1984 The capacity for 'enabling' in mentally ill mothers. Bulletin of the National Centre for Clinical Infant Programs 4(4): 1–7

Nurcombe B 1972 An outline of child psychiatry. New South Wales University Press, Kensington

Papousek H, Papousek M 1977 Mothering and the cognitive head start: psychobiological considerations. In: Schaffer H R (ed) Studies in mother infant interaction. Academic Press, New York

Park R D 1981 Fathering. Fontana, Glasgow

Parmelee A H 1982 What are the functions of follow-up programs for high risk infants. Environmental intervention for infants at risk. Harvard Medical School and The Children's Hospital Medical Centre, Boston, Massachusetts

Peterson P D, Koulack D 1969 Attitude changes as a function of attitudes of acceptance and rejection. Journal of Personality and Social Psychology 11: 309–311

Prechtl H F R, Beintema D J 1964 The neurological examination of the full-term newborn infant. Clinics in Developmental Medicine 12 Heinemann, London

Prensky A L, Eliasson S G, Hardin W B 1978 Neurological

Pathophysiology, 2nd edn. Oxford University Press, New York

Provence S, Lipton R C 1967 Infants in institutions. International Universities Press, New York

Prugh D C 1953 Study of the emotional reactions of children and families to hospitalisation and illness. American Journal of Orthopsychiatry 13: 70–106

Puchinger B, Zimprich H, Reiss–Patzak E 1975 Empirical analysis of the behaviour of nursing staff in a children's hospital. Paediatric and Pedagogic 10(1): 55–56

Radke-Yarrow M, Cummings E M, Kuczynski L, Chapman M 1985 Patterns of attachment in two- and three-years-olds in normal families and families with parental depression. Child Development 56: 884–893

Rheingold H 1961 The effects of environmental stimulation on social and exploratory behaviour in human infants. In: Foss B M (ed) Determinants of infant behaviour. Methuen, London

Richards M P M 1974 (ed) The integration of a child into a social world. Cambridge University Press, Cambridge

Robertson J 1958 Young children in hospital. Tavistock Publications, London

Robson K, Pedersen F, Moss H 1969 Developmental observations of diadic gazing in relation to the fear of strangers and social approach behaviour. Child Development 40: 619–627

Rutter M 1972 Parent-child separation: psychological effects on the children. Journal of Child Psychology and Psychiatry 12: 233–260

Salzen E 1968 Imprinting in birds and primates. Behaviour 28: 232–254

Schaffer H R, Emerson P E 1964 The development of social attachments in infancy. Monographs of the Society for Research in Child Development 29(3): 1–94

Schaffer H R 1971 The origins of human relations. Academic Press, London

Scott J P 1967 Early experience and the organization of behaviour. Brooks/Cole, California

Shere E, Kastenbaum R 1966 Interactions in cerebral palsy: environmental and psychosocial obstacles to cognitive

development. Genetic Psychological Monographs 73–74: 257–335

Sheridan M D 1977 Spontaneous play in early childhood from birth to six years. NFER, Berkshire, England

Sluckin W, Herbert M, Sluckin A 1983 Maternal bonding. Blackwell, Oxford

Smuts A M, Hogan J W (eds). 1986 History and research in child development. Monograph of the Society for Research in Child Development. 50, Nos. 4, 5

Spitz R A 1945 Hospitalism — a follow-up report. Psychoanalytic study of the child 2: 113–117

Stott D H 1962 Abnormal mothering as a cause of mental subnormality 1. A critique of some classic studies of maternal deprivation in the light of possible congenital factors. Journal of Child Psychology and Psychiatry 3: 79–91

Taylor G 1981 The developing child. Discussion papers, International Year of the Child, National Committee of Non-Government Organisations, Canberra

Tinbergen N 1951 The study of instinct. Clarendon Press, Oxford

Todd C A, Palmer B 1968 Social reinforcement of infant babbling. Child Development 39: 592–596

Turner J S, Helms D B 1979 Life span development. W B Saunders, Philadelphia

Twitchell T E 1970 Reflex mechanism and the development of prehension. In: Connolly K J (ed) Mechanisms of motor skill development. Adademic Press, New York, 25–59

UNESCO International Symposium Report 1983 The changing family in a changing world. Newsletter of The International Society for the study Of Behavioural Development 1983, 2: 4

Wilbarger P 1984 Planning an adequate 'sensory diet' — application of sensory processing theory during the first year of life. Bulletin of the National Center for Clinical Infant Programs 5(1): 7–12

Yakovlev P, Lecours A R 1967 The myelogenetic cycles of regional maturation of the brain. In: Minkowski A (ed) Regional development of the brain. Blackwell, Oxford

RECOMMENDED READING

Child Development. Published for the Society for Research in Child Development (SRCD) 5801 Ellis Avenue, Chicago, Ill 60637 USA

Developmental Medicine and Child Neurology. Published for Spastics International Medical Publications 5A Netherhall Gardens London NW3 5RN UK

Physical & Occupational Therapy in Paediatrics. Published by The Haworth Press Inc. 75 Griswold St, Binghampton NY 13904 USA

Turner J S, Helms D B 1979 Life span development W B Saunders, Philadelphia

Kalugar G, Kalugar M F 1984. Profiles in human development. C V Mosby, St Louis

Mussen P H, Conger J J, Kagan J 1984 Child development

and personality, 6th edn. Harper & Row, New York.

Sylva K, Hunt I 1982 Child development a first course. Grant McIntyre, London

Hicks P 1981 Introduction to child development. Longman Harlow, England

The first years of life 1979 and pre-school years 1981 A handbook for parents from the Open University. In association with the Health Education Council, Ward Lock, London

Rendle-Short J 1971 The child. Wright, Bristol

Silver H K, Kempe C H Bruyn H B 1983 Handbook of paediatrics, 14th edn. Lange Medical Publications, Los Altos, California

The contexts of therapy

4. Socializing contexts: behaviour and the physical environment

READERS' OBJECTIVES

After reading this chapter, you should be able to:
1. Define 'context' 'surroundings' and 'environment', and the differences between these concepts.
2. Describe how social properties can be designed into the task context of therapy.
3. Define the features of an 'attracting environment'.
4. Discuss one model of therapy design — the 'honey-pot' model.
5. Describe the general design features of an occupational therapy facility in a general children's hospital.

Firstly, this chapter discusses briefly the way environments and surroundings become social contexts, influencing the behaviour of people, and in turn being influenced by their behaviour. The 'honey-pot model' of therapy focuses the discussion on ways to design social contexts so that practical task and personal social skills can be taught to a child in an integrated, therapeutically appropriate manner.

Secondly, there is a presentation of practical information about basic design, equipment, and materials needed in an occupational facility serving a wide range of child clients.

Contexts, surroundings and environment

Context is not the same as 'surroundings' or 'environment', and the most effective therapy outcomes are likely to be achieved if all three are designed and controlled by the therapist. The differences are expressed in the boxed definitions.

In therapy the social context can be the relationships that are developed between the child, specialists, family and peers. Also the social context can be designed into

---

Definitions

Context: a subtle concept — the meaning, associations and expectations that we attribute to places and situations. Context thus embraces space, the activities, and the social interactions and relationships that occur in it. 'Context' is different from 'surroundings' and 'environment'.

Surroundings may be thought of as the space, and everything in it around an individual, or group of people. However, we know that people either ignore or do not even notice much of their surroundings. We pay attention selectively to that which is associated with our reason for being in the space.

Environment: constitutes those parts of the surroundings to which an individual pays attention. Parts of the surroundings merit attention because of relationships that the individual has with them; relationships with other people, with sources of positive and negative reinforcement, with functional activities which take place in the surroundings.

---

activities and places to achieve therapeutic objectives. For example, by providing only one of each colour crayon to a group of young children, the social property of sharing is incorporated into play activity.

Social properties in places

Let us start with the proposition that nothing ever happens except in a social context, which is built behaviourally by people (McBride & Clancy 1975). But how? When people meet, either in pairs or groups, they interact, and a series of interactions over time will lead to the formation of a relationship or set of relationships.

Very much like a verbal conversation, behavioural interactions are full of exploratory and incomplete sentences. However, the outcome of both behavioural interactions and verbal conversations is that the participants part with greater understanding of, and adjustments made to each other. They learn about each other, and what each considers acceptable and appropriate in the particular situation. The learning and adjustments are important steps toward a relationship.

The type of reinforcement that people receive in their interactions will also influence the type of relationship which results. The reinforcement may be direct, for example 'shade', or associative, that is, deriving from the activity carried on, for example 'eating', or it may simply be familiarity. Most likely some intimate combination of all is involved. Activities may be reinforced by the place in which these activities occur. Individuals may confer social properties on particular places by using them for particular functions, and being reinforced by their suitability, positively or negatively. Just as effectively, the place derives its reinforcing properties in part from the social or task activities carried on there, and these depend in part on the suitability of the place. The whole situation or event begins to emerge as a single unit of function and of context.

Familiarity alone has also been shown to constitute an important reinforcer. In knowing familiar surroundings, people relax and function effectively, and they invest the place with social properties.

The social properties of familiar space are quite different from those of anonymous space, and familiarity is not an all or nothing quality. Familiar spaces seem to evoke attachment and even possessiveness — an area in which people exert some social controls over each other's behaviour, eliminating most disruptive or destructive activities. These social controls do not emerge in anonymous space, which envelopes only anonymous people. Thus streets and passages which are used only as corridors fail to elicit protective social controls over behaviour. The place may first become neglected, littered, and untidy; later vandalism and destructiveness appear, and eventually violence may occur. The elements which facilitate or hinder the emergence of social controls, by specifying who and how many will use the place and for what activities, when, and how often, must be part of the design of an environment.

As familiarity grows with recognition, so does identity, and with it comes a need to acknowledge each other as individuals. Identity seems to be a social property of people, conferred by others, but it may also be fostered by design.

In modern societies, very many environments are designed as contexts for functional activities. The activities may be social intercourse only, as in a conference room, or may be specifically action oriented (actonic), as in a factory floor or kitchen, or there may be some combination of the two, as in a teaching laboratory or game room. Yet the purely actonic situation is usually a myth, for there is always some social context for the activities, and this is generally influenced by design. Sometimes the social features are ignored, and the emphasis is placed on time-and-motion and operations analyses, so that the 'person and the job contact' is central. Yet normally the workers go right ahead and generate the social relationships they need, and then service them by interactions, either continuously while working, or at regular coffee breaks in which productive roles become related to social roles.

People design contexts for a bewildering array of social and task (actonic) activities. The social interactions which must occur may concern strangers in our anonymous world, or any mixture of bonded partners, friends, acquaintances, and strangers together or separately, engaged in any of the incredible array of functional activities associated with high technology societies. Again, function may be remarkably complex, for example bars are as much concerned with meeting partners as with drinking. There is always a social component to the situation, even if it is only maintaining isolation.

In the design of contexts, the parts must complement each other within the whole. As soon as function and its social qualities are built into one part, this automatically changes the qualities of all the other parts. The reinforcement from each component adds a different quality to the person-environment relationship which emerges. In this way, a relationship acquires a number of dimensions or qualities. In people, these are concerned with functions and affect. Imagery or intellectual associations may also emerge, a result of the intellectual activities associated with particular places and times.

Thus, because learning is involved, it is clear that the social properties of places, things, and times exist only within the behavioural organization of individuals, humans and other species alike (McBride & Clancy 1975). The learning process is complex, and all the components are inextricably mixed and interdependent. The nature of the behavioural interaction will be influenced by the design and organization of the physical surroundings and environment. This suggests that therapeutic tasks, and the people participants must be integrated in a process in which skills of all types develop within a sequence of social situations. All events within the therapy situation then become interactive, complementary and a 'context'.

The honey-pot model suggests how a social context for therapy can be established, and how the systematic use of normal attraction forces can facilitate development of the child's social skills (Clancy 1980). There is further detailed examination of the therapeutic relationship, another aspect of the social context, in Chapter 9 and Chapter 14 examines the other major aspect of designing interesting places with therapeutic social properties.

THEORY INTO PRACTICE — THE HONEY-POT MODEL

In Chapter 1 we suggested that children should always be taught skills, e.g., dressing, eating, in the normal social context in which such activities would occur. For example, the therapist might schedule dressing training sessions early in the morning before breakfast — this would require some imaginative timetabling, but it is possible. The important principles are that the child should not only learn the practical skills, but should understand appropriate social behaviour for the activity, and should transfer the practical learning from a special situation to normal everyday life. These principles apply whatever the skills to be developed, re-taught or modified in some way.

Thus the honey-pot model aims to achieve appropriate socialization. The child is presented as a 'honey-pot' (see Fig. 4.1), attracting others, so that his/her personality may develop to foster a rewarding social world for him/her throughout life (Clancy 1980). The goal of the process expressed in the model is to restructure the attention in any social group to include the affected child as a participant (Chance & Larsen 1976). Those facets of the model which are concerned with attracting attention, and rewarding the participants for giving attention, express immediate or short-term objectives. Other facets focus on the development and use of interactive skills and express long-term objectives. It would be unrealistic to expect the child to maintain continuous attention from others. Rather, others must *want* to return to the child, again and again; this constitutes the maintenance goal.

The model reflects an analysis of the normal forces of attraction between people (Bryne et al 1968). Where attention is attracted indirectly by owning attractive things, these need not be expensive or extrinsically valuable. However, they must be highly valued in the child's peer groups. An example is the collection of egg stickers from egg cartons, or marbles, which can be shown, bargained over and swapped. But the choice of the prized objects will depend on such factors as passing crazes, the child's sex, age, and the supply and demand factor.

In the honey-pot model, an attracting environment is defined as one which has the following characteristics:

1. It arouses curiosity and invites further exploration. Whether in a hospital ward or the child's own home, surroundings can be designed to have appeal, not for their own sake, but so that they lead to the child (Clancy 1976a). Status can be attributed to the child through possession of skill and/or belongings.

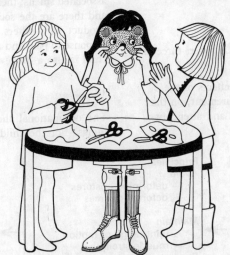

Direct attraction
Child invites other to interact by:
listening to
attending to
orienting to   } other
appeasement of
postures to
looking at
smiling at

Indirect attraction
Child co-operates by:
giving attractive services,
e.g. bat capes
Child shares through:
owning prized things, e.g.
egg stickers, 'swaps'
Child interacts through:
providing attractive
surroundings, e.g. space
that others are drawn to

Combined direct/indirect attraction
Attraction through social facilitation
Doing things that elicit 'join-in'
behaviour, e.g. simple magic tricks

Fig. 4.1 The honey-pot model: how the child attracts others and rewards them (Clancy 1980).

2. There is a combination of familiarity and variety. Aronson et al (1963); Peterson & Kolack (1969) have demonstrated that exploration and learning are maximized when there is a mild degree of discrepancy between newly presented information, attitudes and experiences encountered previously.

Other people's interest may also be held by the giving of attractive services. For example, a child can readily learn to cut simple 'Bat-man' or other super-hero capes from calico, and to dye and decorate them suitably with fabric paint. These capes can then be shared with other children in an infinite number of adventure games.

In all contact with other people the child must use the normal social reinforcers. That is, she/he must listen and attend, and thus reinforce others. Yet, children do not normally develop the socially recognized patterns of 'listener behaviour' until about eleven years of age (Dittman 1972, Llewellyn 1968). Therefore, one of the enabling objectives of therapy ought to be systematic training in 'listener behaviour' in the earlier years. People return to interact with those who appear interested and concerned about them. We normally reinforce others by making it clear that their company gives pleasure and is valued. The behaviours most often used are smiling, nodding, giving eye contact, and paying compliments.

Let us see how the honey-pot model would influence the design of therapy for a child with a physically disabling and disfiguring condition — juvenile rheumatoid arthritis (JRA).

Application to practical therapy

Therapy for the child affected by JRA covers three main action areas, namely:

1. Monitoring and minimizing the effects of the disease process, especially disfigurement, on the child's developing 'self-concept', and attendant social skills.

2. Promoting competent self-management in the physical and social environment.
3. Providing training skills for future vocational and recreational skills.

There are standard therapeutic procedures which are applied to deal with aspects of the physical problems of the disease process and these are summarized in Figure 4.2

Some of these aspects are examined in greater detail.

Pain

There seems to be some difference of opinion about whether children affected by JRA experience the degree of pain described by adult sufferers. In the authors' experience, the children certainly express fear of painful movement, and will at times, guard limbs close to the body and restrict touching by others. Often the child can be enticed into movement, especially the all important extension movements, by the use of attractive play materials and activities that arouse curiosity, leading to interest. Curiosity and interest then become competitors with pain for the child's attention. The mechanism is that information received through the sensory modalities causes the child's attention to be diverted from concern with pain and movement, to engagement in the activity. The activity must be inherently rewarding to the child. For example, when cooking is the chosen activity, there is sensory feedback via handling the ingredients and the associated smells; there is the experience of achievement, and there are the social rewards of sharing the finished product with others. While coming to terms with his response to pain and apprehension about movement, the child is also a 'honey-pot'.

Movement

The occupational therapist helps families select playthings. For the child with JRA, such playthings must

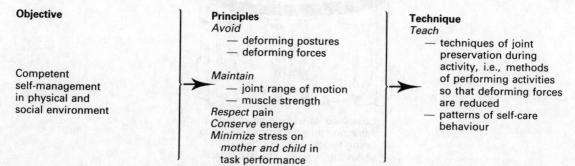

Objective	Principles *Avoid*	Technique *Teach*
	— deforming postures — deforming forces	— techniques of joint preservation during activity, i.e., methods of performing activities so that deforming forces are reduced — patterns of self-care behaviour
Competent self-management in physical and social environment	*Maintain* — joint range of motion — muscle strength *Respect* pain *Conserve* energy *Minimize* stress on mother and child in task performance	

Fig. 4.2 Occupational therapy procedures for a child with juvenile rheumatoid arthritis.

meet movement goals, and be appropriate to the child's general developmental movements. Exercise and movement are most likely to occur if the child regards activity as fun, especially if brothers, sisters and others join in. The 'honey-pot' model is once again translated into action if the games are chosen co-operatively by the child and his siblings and friends. Often, we focus unwarranted attention on the affected child by encouraging other children to join his games 'to help'. An occupational therapist ought to be sensitive and ingenious enough to introduce unobtrusive modifications to most games so that the affected child is not the centre of attention, but remains involved with the others.

Energy conservation

Another aspect of attaining competence in self management is learning to conserve energy by reducing tasks to their minimum components parts (see Watkins & Robinson 1976). The object is to achieve the least tiring and strenuous way of performing a task. Special techniques will be taught to the child in the course of teaching him/her joint preservation techniques.

Dressing is an operation that offers enormous challenges and scope for solutions — to mothers and therapists (see Chapter 13). The mother will be taught ways of dressing and undressing her child, who will in turn take over the task for him/herself later on. Clothing can be modified as well. For preference, clothing should be made from soft, light, synthetic, stretchy fabrics which give and yet retain their shape, e.g., jersey and crimplene or acrylic, polyester, mixes of nylon, and wool or cotton fibres. Such materials are most easily manoeuvred over swollen, sore joints — at first by the mother and later by the child.

Fastenings, including shoes and fly openings on boys' trousers, can be achieved by the use of Velcro, a commercially available pressure-sensitive tape, that can be stitched unobtrusively to clothing. The use of this simple modification hastens the dressing operation for the mother, and promotes more rapid acquisition of independent behaviour by the child. The honey-pot model is still influential. Decorations, such as emblems or appliques may disguise modifications to clothing, and still attract attention — to the child, not the modification. Some examples of modern, attractive, modified clothing designs for children are to be found in the Dutch publication by Cauenbach (1978).

Recreation

As young as four years, it is possible — and wise — to begin planning for the development of long-term rec-reational interests by the affected child. The therapy involves teaching the child and family how to plan interest and recreational activities. Activities should be compatible with the child's abilities and maturation throughout the course of the disease process. Interest and involvement in a pursuit can be established in childhood, and therapy offers an excellent medium for such an introduction to be followed throughout adult life. Again, play must engage the child in active membership of a group where he may share his interests, and so gain increased support and satisfaction. For example, if the activity is ceramic potting — which is excellent therapeutically — then the maturing child could join the relevant community group, e.g., The Potters Association. On the other hand, sporting activities, such as swimming and billiards, can be shared and developed through membership of the YMCA or some similar organization.

As therapists, we should not assume that a child will find his own way to those in the community with similar interests and enthusiasms. The therapeutic plan should provide explicity for the child's introduction to such groups by the occupational therapist. The therapist may then provide support to both the child and the community group leader as modifications are sought, either to the task processes or to tools and machinery used in the activity.

Practical tasks and procedures are integrated into a social context in such a way that the child's 'difference' from peers is minimized. Under these conditions, the child may become competent in tasks, and also develop, for him/herself, reciprocal, satisfying social relationships with others. But whether or not the model is found to be useful, perhaps, the motto that should influence our therapeutic endeavours is, 'develop skills with joy'.

The following examines the design of a therapeutic working environment — the occupational therapy department or facility.

DESIGNING AN OCCUPATIONAL THERAPY FACILITY

The most usual contexts for an occupational therapy facility and service which serve a wide range of child client types are: an urban general children's hospital, a community health centre, and a country or regional hospital. The discussion is organized for the use of a therapist establishing a new department. However, the listings of equipment and materials should also provide useful maintenance guidelines for existing facilities. All occupational therapy facilities for children require a basic core of similar equipment and materials. Specialist centres such as Spastic Centres will require additional specialist equipment, and helpful references and resources are indicated in relevant chapters.

The following is a guide to an appropriate core set of equipment and materials, which should be provided in an occupational therapy department.

Furniture and fittings

Strive for a department space which looks friendly and inviting to both children and adults, including the staff who work there. Clients must be able to relate to the environment. For example, it would be insensitive and counterproductive to furnish a therapy facility in the latest high-tech, chrome and leather fashion, if the clientele group is predominantly families living in rented, poverty stricken, inner urban areas. Also the facility can serve to educate clients and other specialists about the particular roles and functions that the occupational therapist seeks to fulfil. People will make assumptions about roles and functions from what they see, if there is no other information available. Thus, for example, if parents are interviewed in an area in which craft materials and lots of toys are visible, it would be natural for them to deduce that the occupational therapist will 'teach John/Enid how to make things', or 'she will play with John/Enid.' Both activities are luxuries to many client families, and such an uncorrected assumption may influence them to simply not reappear for further therapy. It is worth giving careful thought and planning to the educational aspect of department design. This can be achieved by designing public and private activity zones; through the use of attractive professional posters and literature, such as that produced by American Occupational Therapy Association; and by careful choice of the therapy media displayed in the public working areas.

Space which is organized efficiently should appear uncluttered, and should be organized to facilitate activity preparation, client service delivery, and the business administration of the facility. Plan to eliminate the need for time-consuming space reorganization to cater for particular client groups, such as the hyperactive or easily distracted child. Here are some guidelines:

— Choose primary colours, and plain, unpatterned, washable covers for soft furnishings.
— Choose permanent, washable floor coverings such as vinyl, overlayed by a carpet square. Avoid wall to wall carpet.
— Provide office area equipped for staff use, and suitable for meeting with the client family.
— Provide a store area, preferably a walk-in pantry type room separate from therapy areas. There can never be enough storage. Choose maximum allowable closed and lockable cupboards. Supplement cupboards with movable units that are also lockable.
— Provide a 'wet area' including a kitchen sink, for adequate creative and other activity preparation, and for cleaning, sterilizing and maintaining equipment. A similar, but separate wet area may be necessary if splints and other adaptive items are to be made and serviced.
— Provide at least one wash basin and toilet suitable for children's use — mounted low on a wall.

Basic furnishings for a general paediatric occupational therapy facility
Tables/chairs
Stools on castors
Office equipment, e.g. filing cabinet, desk, typewriter
Stationery
Microcomputer, printer and adjustable-height workstation
Refrigerator
Small stove (a 'plug-in' model is adequate, though a microwave oven is desirable because of its reduced cooking time)
Audio cassette/CD player
Video recording system
Linen

— Provide adjustable-height tables, with heat resistant plain white or neutral coloured laminate tops. Ensure that there is at least one table that will accommodate children's wheelchairs. Round or half-round tables encourage social interaction between children seated at them.
— Provide different styles of chairs which will allow children with special seating requirements to find one most suited to them. Make certain that chairs suit the different possible heights of the tables. Stools fitted with castors allow a therapist greater freedom of movement in an activity situation.
— Provide department linen supplies including protective waterproof children's clothing covers; large sheets of clear or white plastic, useful for covering table tops, especially as a surface for fingerpainting. There should also be a small quantity of bed sheets, towels, blankets, infant diapers or napkins, tea towels. A paper towel dispenser with towel roll is invaluable.
— Provide kitchen utensils including unbreakable eating and other kitchen utensils. Food

preparation and presentation is a useful therapeutic activity with children, and some small electrical appliances such as a sandwich maker, should be considered.

— Provide at least one microcomputer. The choice may be influenced by factors such as an institution's purchasing policy. However, the system to be used in a therapy department must have the capacity to serve administrative functions, and therapy activity functions. That is, there should be wordprocessing, spreadsheet, database functions, and a wide range of games and other software programmes available. After-sales backup service is an important consideration.

— Every department will require stationery; specifically, referral forms, reporting forms, a filing system for internal office use, a client services register. Increasingly, therapists will use a microcomputer to maintain client and office records and statistics. Some helpful references are given at the end of this chapter.

The format of a referral form should be helpful to the medical officer or other specialist who may use it. By informing the referring specialist about the services available through occupational therapy, the form may also fulfil an educational function. An example of how a referral form can be organised to do this in an acute care children's hospital appears at the end of the chapter.

Programme resource materials

Resource material may be divided into two classes: (a) material to be used by the therapist; (b) material to be used by client families.

Therapist's resource materials

Resourse materials form a reference library which supports everyday practice. The collection should include a selection of standard texts on child development, paediatric medicine, and occupational therapy practice; community resource directories such as those distributed by governmental social services agencies and equipment and activity media catalogues.

Resources for families

Such material includes information about special conditions or procedures that will help a family. For example, Western Psychological Services publish an ex-

cellent multimedia film strip kit for parents of intellectually handicapped children. The choice of material to be stocked in an occupational therapy department will be determined by the type of clients referred for therapy. The resources may consist of books to be borrowed or bought by parents, or simpler pamphlets to be given to them, for example, Klein's 1990 *Parent Articles for Early Intervention*. Audiovisual presentations may be used with a family to increase their understanding of their child's special needs, for example, Goudy & Fetzer's 1988 videotape *Infant Motor Development*.

Evaluation materials

Every paediatric occupational therapy facility should maintain a basic set of tests and assessment materials. Recommended types of tests are listed and purchasing details are given in Appendix VI. The information summarized below is a guide to minimum requirements only.

Evaluation materials (see Appendix VI for details)

General development assessments
- A screening and diagnostic test of general developmental maturity
- The Griffith Test of Mental Abilities (approved users)
- Gesell Developmental Appraisal
- Hawaii Early Learning Profile

Motor skill assessment tests
- A general test of motor skill — gross and fine manipulative skill
- A test of reflex behaviour
- An assessment of joint range of motion
- A method of testing of muscle function

Tests of cognitive, and perceptual-motor integration
- An assessment of perceptual-motor skill integration
- An assessment of formal school readiness skills
- A screening test of information processing skills
- Tests of particular aspects of perceptual and sensorimotor integration

Activities of daily living assessments

Play behaviour assessments

Intervention materials

Establishing a new facility is a costly operation. The initial capital outlay will probably extend over two to five institution budgets. The therapy staff must therefore establish priorities for the purchase or acquisition of equipment.

To make or to buy?

Where possible, commercially manufactured equipment and media are preferable to 'home-made' items. In the long run it often proves less expensive to buy the item even though the capital outlay is greater. However, therapists in some centres often make important community links with retired craftsmen and women who produce beautifully crafted items to individual specifi-cation. This is a valuable resource to be tapped when available. The following questions will assist you to decide whether to make or buy.

— How much therapist time would be needed to construct the item? Could this time be more profitably used for client services?
— How will the cost of raw materials, plus cost of therapist's hourly labour compare with the commercial item's cost?
— What is the predictable life (durability) of the home made versus the commercial article?
— How will the appearance or presentation of the home made item compare with the commercial article, that is, influence client motivation?

The usual materials, activities, and equipment used in face-to-face intervention programmes with children have been categorized.

General creative activity materials

Cut and paste kit Blunt scissors, jar of paste, brush, assorted shapes and sizes of coloured paper and sheets of plain paper. Cut out interesting pictures from magazines and organize them in large manila envelopes so that children can make their own scrapbooks.

Drawing/painting requirements Chunky style crayons
Powder colour (e.g., Reeves Tempera colour)
Acrylic mixed paints (in quantity)
Large headed paint brushes
   N.B. Avoid small conventional paint boxes, tubes of paint and small fine brushes. Purchase paper either by roll or large sheet

Fingerpaint

Dough/modelling materials Dough has many uses in therapy with children, ranging from improving muscle strength and finger dexterity, to providing a medium for symbolic play

Pulp papier mache Older children may not be attracted to dough use, but the same objectives can be achieved using modelling pulps

---

Material to modify perceptual-motor dysfunction
Grasp and fine manipulative skill development
● 'Fiddlesticks' game
● Heavy based self righting toy with a musical insert in the base, e.g., 'Jolly Wobler' by 'Kiddicraft' toys
● 'Dandy Dangler' (Kiddicraft toys)
● Construction sets, e.g., 'Baufix', 'Struts', 'Lego'
● Jig-saw puzzles which have grasp knobs of varying size on each piece, e.g., 'ROLF' puzzles from Modern Teaching Aid Range.
Gross motor skill development
● Modern Teaching Aids range, e.g., 'Figura'
● The 'Pathway Programme' from The Teaching Resources range
● Large foam wedges, shapes, and rolls, e.g., Theraflatibles, Therapy Balls, Bolsters
Perceptual skill integration and development
● Programs which have their own accompanying assessment protocol, e.g., The Frosting Programmes
● The Teaching Resources series of programs, notably, The Fairbanks-Robinson programme levels 1 and 2; the Cheeves system; the Dubnoff Programmes
Body image development material
● Jig saws which display a sequential pattern of activity.
● Paper dolls with clothes for dressing.
● Flannel board which emphasize face and body recognition

Sensory integrative therapy materials.
Room, 12 m × 5 m with removeable carpet and overhead mesh grid
T Stools 20 × 25 × 25 cm
hammock
Bolster swing 180 × 20 cm
4 rope swing 100 × 100 cm
Balance boards of varying widths
2 Scooter boards on large castors with castors positioned in pairs
Tunnel — made from large cardboard cylinders, approximately 65 cm in diameter, and carpeted inside
Inner tyre tubes (5) linked with contact cement
Single inner tubes — one suspended from overhead mesh grid
Trampoline
Nystagmus board which should be mounted on a Usi bren swivel .999
Towels and bedsheets
Textured floor rug
Parachute
Quoits
Left and right feet shapes, extra large size in two colours of felt
Empty detergent bottles
Two or more different sized and shaped bean bags for catching/throwing games
Sheepskin

Activities of daily living materials

- Food presentation and feeding training materials, for example:
  Plates with non-slip base and lip
  Non-spill cups — with and without handle
  Knife, fork and spoons of varying sizes, shapes and some with adaptations, e.g., built up grip
- Clothing adaptations, and dressing training materials, for example:
  Shoes with shoe laces, and sandals with buckles
  Equipment promoting button and fastening practice, e.g., dolls clothing; commercial playthings; adult size dressing up play clothes
  Large male and female dolls and appropriate clothing
- Jig-saw puzzles, e.g., 'Cleaning in the house', or 'Getting up' from the Modern Teaching Aids range
- A display of clothing designs including pattern information such as that provided by the Disabled Living Foundation (London) in their manuals
- A supply of frequently used materials, for example Velcro fasteners, for sale to client families
- Grooming and bathing aids, for example:
  Soap mit
  Electric toothbrush
  Hair brush adaptations
  Infant baths, e.g., 'Tubby'
  Training pot — e.g., 'Baby Relax' pot
  Bath seats and safety mats
  Examples of a sling and hoist — wheelchair to bath
- Transport and mobility aids
- Triangle corner seats with work tray
- One mobile prone extension vehicle — such as the Preston Tumble Forms 'Jetmobile'
- Illustrated catalogues of available aids with purchasing information should be available to client families

Non-Directive Play Therapy (Axline 1989)

The set materials comprise:

Creative activity media: paint — oil, water and finger; sand, mud, clay, water and papier mache.

Scissors and paper

Representative media: dolls, dolls' houses and furniture. Glove puppets — man, woman, boy, girl, wicked witch, good fairy. Small figures of animals and familiar humans, for example, policeman, doctor, and family figures. Infant feeding bottles.
Rubber knives, toy guns, boxing gloves and hammer peg board
Building bricks
Toy telephones
Transportation toys, for example cars, boats etc.

A chair for therapist — bean bags are excellent alternatives.

Preparing a child for hospital and surgery

Books There are many specially written books on the market which cater for a variety of ages. For the very young child, choose some books which use words sparingly and engage the child in the process of reading, for example by providing pictures to be coloured.

Play kits for role playing games Collect a range of real items for role playing, for example, kidney dishes, a real stethoscope and sphygmomanometer, thermometers including the newer press on skin variety, bandages, doctors' coats, nurses' caps and badges, broken stop watches, dolls in beds and other items that will be relevant to the children who use the particular facility.

Infant exploration kits (Clancy 1976b). Kits are designed to encourage a cotbound infant to explore and manipulate materials, thereby promoting normal developmental experiences throughout the period of illness. (see Chapter 15)

A kit for 3- to 4-month-old infants
1 swivel overhead arm fitted with cot clamp — painted in a primary colour
Mobiles to be suspended in the midline from overhead arm
1 soft fluffy octopus on elastic
1 noise maker, such as a soft cube containing a bell
1 firm large red ring
1 mirror, large enough to reflect the infant's face and upper half body. The mirror is attached to the cot railing on the side on which the child predominantly displays Asymmetrical Tonic Neck Reflex (ATNR).

Communication aids

Communication aids come in many forms, ranging from cards which are displayed manually e.g. The Bliss Symbol System for deaf people, to computerized voice responsive terminal displays. With the increasing application of microprocessors, the range of sophisticated systems increases, and the cost diminishes. In a time of rapid technology development it is probably not sensible to purchase one supposedly general application system. Rather, close liaison between therapists and bio-engineering specialist groups such as 'Technical Aids For The Disabled', and Independent Living Centre staff will allow for the most up to date and appropriate systems to be prescribed for individual clients. Important evaluation of existing systems is being undertaken by Entwhistle (1984) and Millar & Odor (1984).

> **Splinting Equipment and Materials**
> **Equipment**
> 1 × hydrocollator
> I × household oven
> Cutting knife (Stanley)
> Scissors
> Hole punch
> Heat gun
> Wire bending jig
> Goniometer
> **Materials**
> Low temperature thermoplastics, e.g., San-splint regular, San-splint XR
> High temperature polyethylene 1 mm thickness
> Plastagote 3 mm, 6 mm and 12 mm
> Polycushion 3 mm and 6 mm
> Leather 3 mm
> Suede 3 mm
> Arch supports, metatarsal supports
> Solvent
> Copper wire 2 mm thickness
> Velcro 2.5 cm × 5 cm
> Elastic bands (stationery store)
> Nylon line (fishing line)
> Rivets
> Contact cement glue
> Spring wire
> Vinyl

Splinting materials

In a general paediatric facility a therapist may be asked to supply splints, for example, for a burned child. The following materials represent those generally used for various different types of splints.

Computers.

With the development of modern technology, computers have become a useful tool in daily living and therapy situations. With the rapid expansion and innovations in hardware and software, no attempt has been made to give precise direction. However some useful sources of information about using microcomputers in occupational therapy are Howe (1984), Hume (1984), O'Shea and Self (1983), Rodgers and Gunderson (1984) and *The Bliss Apple Manual.*

SUMMARY

Therapy occurs in a physical environment, often the occupational therapy department, and this environment can facilitate or impede the achievement of goals. Thus it becomes important to design the environment so that it does facilitate the therapy process. Some guidelines have been provided for thinking about environmental design, and the equipping of a general paediatric occupational therapy department.

Also it has been suggested that therapy occurs in a context — the social context which equals the interactions which occur between the child, therapist, family members, and other children present. Furthermore, the media used become invested with social properties which can also be designed and controlled by the therapist. One model has been presented, the honey-pot model, and its application discussed for designing a social context. It is suggested that this model facilitates the integration of practical tasks with social skills in such a manner that all skills are developed 'with joy'. Environmental design in therapy programmes is discussed further in Chapter 14.

REFERENCES

Aronson E, Turner J A, Carlsmith J M 1963 Communicator credibility and communication discrepancy as determinants of opinion change. Journal of Abnormal and Social Psychology 67: 31–36
Axline V M 1989 Play Therapy. Churchill-Livingstone, Edinburgh. First published 1947, Riverside Press, Cambridge
Bryne D, London D, Reeves K 1968 The effects of physical attractiveness, sex and attitudes similarity on interpersonal attraction. Journal of Personality 36: 259–271
Cauenbach 1978 Pas mode aan: kleding tips voor handicaps.
Chance M R A, Larsen R (eds) 1976 The social structure of attention. Wiley, New York
Clancy H 1976a Integrating the environment into therapy. Man–Environment Systems 6: 305–312
Clancy H 1976b Infant exploration kits, designed and made

in the Department of Occupational Therapy, University of Queensland, St Lucia, Australia
Clancy H 1980 Therapy in socializing contexts, the honey-pot model. Australian Occupational Therapy Journal 27: 111–123
Entwhistle N J 1984 Experience of learning. Scottish Academic Press, Edinburgh
Dittmann A T 1972 Developmental factors in conversational behaviour. Journal of Communication 22(4): 404–423
Llewellyn L G 1968 Relationship between vocalizations and head nods as listener responses. Journal of Personality and Social Psychology 9(1): 79–84
McBride G, Clancy H G 1975 Social properties of places and things. In: Rapoport A (ed) The mutual interaction of people and their built environment. Mouton, The Hague

References continue on page 46

REFERRAL TO OCCUPATIONAL THERAPY

Name .... Age .... Department ....

Diagnosis ....

Precautions and/or restrictions ....

REASON FOR REFERRAL: **PSYCHOLOGICAL EXPERIENCES** to meet needs arising from:

A Separation from Home ... ... ( ) Activity Restriction ... ... ( )

   Physical Restraint   ... ... ( ) Painful Experience ... ... ( )

DEVELOPMENTAL GUIDANCE IN

B Appropriate Self-Care ... ... ( ) Socialization ... ... ( )

   Activities of Daily Living Assessment ... ... ( ) Maintaining Present Level ... ... ( )

   Physical Development ... ... ( )

DIAGNOSTIC ASSISTANCE IN

C Observation and Assessment of Performance ... ... ( )

PHYSICAL REMEDIAL MEASURES TO

D Promote Physical Relaxation ... ... ( ) Increase Physical Work Tolerance ... ... ( )

   Increase Co-ordination ... ... ( ) Prosthetic Training   ... ... ( )

   Increase Joint Range of Motion.. ... ... ( ) Encourage Ambulation ... ... ( )

   Increase Muscle Strength ... ... ( ) Improve Respiratory Function ... ... ( )

SPECIFIC PSYCHIATRIC MEASURES TO

E Provide Non-Directive Play Situation ... ... ( ) Provide Supportive Program ... ... ( )

   Other e.g. Develop Intellectual Potential, Self-Confidence, Initiative, etc.

   Please indicate   ... ... ( )

F Parental Instruction .... ( )

Other Forms of Intervention: Remarks

Referring Specialist .... Date................................

Millar S, Odor J P 1984 A proposed bliss banking facility. CAL Centre occasional paper. CAL Centre, Edinburgh

Mosey A C 1981 Configuration of a profession. Raven Press, New York, p 75

Peterson P D, Koulack D 1969 Attitude change as a function of latitudes of acceptance and rejection. Journal of Personality and Social Psychology 11: 309–311

Watkins R A, Robinson D 1976 Joint preservation techniques for patients with rheumatoid arthritis. Rehabilitation Institute of Chicago, Chicago

MICROCOMPUTERS

Howe C 1984 Turning turtle. Department of Artificial Intelligence Research Paper 144, University of Edinburgh

Hume C 1984 A proposed bliss banking facility. CAL Centre 4 Buccleuch Place Edinburgh

O'Shea T Self J 1983 Learning and teaching with computers. Harvester Press, Brighton

Rodgers B L, Gunderson J R 1984 International communications aids: compatibility standards proposals. Trace Centre University of Wisconsin 1500 Highland Ave, Madison WI53704

Scheifelbusch R L 1980 Non-speech language and communication: analysis and intervention. University Park Press, Baltimore

Vanderheim G The Bliss Apple manual. Trace Centre, University of Wisconsin

5. The task context: play as a primary medium

READERS' OBJECTIVES

After reading this chapter, you should be able to:
1. **Discuss whether play is a legitimate therapy technique.**
2. **Describe developmental ages and stages of play activity.**
3. **Be able to select and evaluate play activities which promote therapeutic objectives.**

In Western society we provide toys, games, and equipment to encourage and support children in special activity — play. Occupational therapists use the full range of these familiar tools, mostly in specially designed activity settings, as their bridge between the child client and the therapy objectives. Thus, even when the intervention activity setting is said to be 'free play', it is in fact carefully arranged and manipulated to gain specific outcomes. These outcomes are always associated with learning, achievement and mastery of skills — motor, social, affective and cognitive. Because of the intruded element of arrangement, play in therapy is not quite the same as the naturally occurring phenomenon recognized as 'play' in all social animals, including man. Yet effective use can only be made of play in therapy if it derives from study of the naturally occurring phenomenon. Using the basic research literature about play as a point of reference, this chapter offers some insight into current ideas about play. Guides are presented about selecting, designing and using play activities in therapy.

It is important at the outset of this discussion to deal with the question 'Is play a therapy technique?' because it is concerned with professional accountability. If there is no evidence for the effective use of play then any further discussion about it is redundant. However the confident answer is 'yes', and we will examine the evidence.

Pioneers of educational theory, such as Froebel in Germany, Pestalozzi in Switzerland, and Montessori in Italy made the first proposals for the systematic use of play as part of child rearing and education. Their confidence was based on belief. However, today there is a strong and increasing body of research which substantiates the use of play activity in learning, with an intent to affect child development and maturation in many different areas. Indeed, writer after writer cites a playful environment as an invaluable aid for promoting healthier more mature development, whatever the reason for the intervention (e.g., Fraiberg 1968; Leland & Smith 1965; Li 1981; Sadler 1969; Wehman & Abramson 1976; Whittaker 1980).

There is some research evidence for the positive effect of play, particularly that called 'symbolic play', on children's cognitive, social, and language development. For example, Rosenblatt (1977) demonstrated that it is possible to use symbolic play to improve expressive language use and its generalization. The author concluded that there is an underlying element linking symbolic play and language. Sylva (1977) and Sylva & Lunt (1980) established relationships between symbolic play and problem solving ability. Rosen (1974) concluded that by enhancing symbolic play skills, it was possible to improve children's group interaction, co-operative effort, and effectiveness in role taking tasks and skills. Dansky & Silverman (1975), and Robinson (1977) believe that in free play a child develops the ability to generalize attitudes to a variety of objects, not even necessarily present in the play environment. They believe that such attitudes are central to creative ability and activity.

The studies cited represent only a few, and the reader is urged to read Smith (1986) to gain a comprehensive and scholarly view of the present state of the art in play theorizing and empirical research. For the remainder of the chapter the following aspects of play will be presented and examined:

— Some modern definitions and descriptions.
— The currently agreed classifications and

conventions about ages and stages in play behaviour development.
— Criteria for selecting, designing and using play materials and equipment.

DEFINITIONS OF PLAY

The pioneers in the study of childhood play were mainly psychoanalysts, e.g., Anna Freud, Melanie Klein and Erik Erikson. Thus it is not surprising that early studies were linked to understanding psychodynamic processes associated with disturbed behaviour. Though we recognize play behaviour intuitively, defining it continues to be a most perplexing business. Reilly (1974) perceptively likened the task to 'defining a cobweb'. Some authors have approached the problem by classifying activities called 'play', while others have sought to define play by identifying its functions and observable actions. Still other researchers have attempted to explain it by proposing motivational theories about why social animals, both juvenile and adult, engage in play. In this brief discussion we have decided to take what is perhaps the easy way out, and summarize the current understanding of play under the three groupings of:

1. Definition by classification;
2. Definition by function and outcome; and
3. Definition by motivation.

Detailed evaluative discussions of the full range of theories of play are to be found in Reilly (1974) and Smith (1984, 1986).

Play defined by classification

The most usual classifying distinction made is that between 'work' and 'play'. Adults find it relatively easy to make a distinction between 'work' and 'play' — albeit an arbitrary one. Mark Twain probably states the distinction most succinctly when he said 'work consists of whatever a body is obliged to do, while play consists of whatever a body is not obliged to do.' Therapists may find that parents make such distinctions, and seek reassurance about the relevance of what they see as 'play' for their child in therapy. So it is important to understand possible parental perceptions of play, and to be able to discuss their questions in the light of them.

Play versus work

Sheridan (1977) provided a useful distinction between play, work, and drudgery. 'Play' is the eager engagement in pleasurable physical or mental effort to obtain

emotional satisfaction; work is the voluntary engagement in disciplined physical or mental effort, to obtain material benefit, whilst 'drudgery' is the enforced engagement in distasteful physical or mental effort to obtain the means of survival. Sheridan, however, recognized that all three distinctions may merge — if an activity equals work plus play, she calls it 'play', and if also plus drudgery, then this is 'slog'. Also she notes perceptively that 'slog' is too often witnessed in use with handicapped children where it is thought of as play (her definition).

What is it about activities that leads adults to label them as one or the other? Children don't. Do differences (if they are shown to exist) mean that children are learning something different from play, as opposed to work activities? A British study provided some interesting answers (Open University 1977). Parents were given one list of usual childhood activities and another giving criteria for judging them as work or play. The interpretation arrived at from this study was that adults define children's 'work' as activities which adults do, which often lead to something useful, and which teach a child about adult work and the business of living. Play activities, on the other hand, were seen as those which provide different opportunities by being open-ended and under the child's own direction. These views are peculiarly Western cultural ones, and influenced by our expectations of providing a child with 'toys' and 'games' for 'play'.

The British parents' definitions carry an implication that play and exploration are synonymous. As this is another important classification that has attracted considerable attention and study, it will now be examined.

Play versus exploration

Play and exploration are descriptions often used synonymously (see Thorpe 1963, Welker 1956). Yet some workers suggest that the two concepts are not the same (e.g., Berlyne 1960, Hutt 1966). It is said that exploration and play differ in their goals.

Play versus exploration
The goal of 'play' appears to be, 'what can *I* do with this object?' The goal of exploration, on the other hand, appears to be gaining information, 'what is this object all about', i.e., what are its properties?

Exploration occurs in new, strange situations, and demands that the individual be alert and highly attentive. The underlying assumption is that individuals have a need for optimal arousal, and will learn behaviour which results in pleasant states of arousal. There are those who postulate that this explanation of optimal arousal-seeking applies to 'play'. However, Hutt (1966) maintained that 'play' only occurred in a familiar environment. Her evidence was observation of gradual relaxation of children's mood, evidenced by changes in facial expression, and greater diversity and variability of activities than in exploration.

Berlyne (1960) defined two major forms of exploratory behaviour which appear to be part of the behavioural repertoire of most animal species, including man. These are:

- Extrinsically motivated specific investigative exploration which deals with changes in an organism's environment.
- Intrinsically motivated diversive exploration where there is a search for stimuli without apparent necessity for organism survival.

Hutt concluded that investigative exploration results in the acquisition of information, whereas in play such learning is incidental.

Berlyne (1960) defined the following conditions for eliciting exploratory behaviour; the predictable behavioural response systems:

- Stimuli which elicit exploratory behaviour, namely, 'novelty' and 'complexity'.
- The type of environment in which the stimuli are presented.

Novelty and complexity

An organism responds to new input in accordance with whether or not that input fits its internal representation of past experience (see Mussen et al 1969, 1970). Novelty is not a stimulus characteristic per se; rather it is 'a transactional concept that relates a current stimulus to previous experience with either that stimulus or with one similar to it' (Welker 1971). The degree of novelty inherent in the stimulus situation is defined by how similar or dissimilar the input, or how recently similar input was experienced.

Complexity was defined by Berlyne (1960) as: the amount of variety or diversity in a stimulus pattern; increasing with the number of elements in that pattern and with the degree of dissimilarity among elements, and varying by the extent to which elements may be responded to as a group or class.

The individual's perception of the environmental condition determines whether exploratory behaviour is elicited by novel and complex stimuli. If the condition is perceived as unfavourable, or there is confusing symbolic material, or the individual has no previous experience with which to match the novel condition, then, she/he is thrown into a state termed 'uncertainty' or 'conflict'. If she/he withdraws it may be concluded that the uncertainty produces intolerable distress, anxiety or fear. Defensive response systems have become effective to reduce discomfort.

If, however, the individual deals with the uncertainty or conflict, it is because a state of 'curiosity' has been elicited which then determines a sequence of specific exploratory behaviours. The individual will manoeuvre to achieve the best position from which to learn more about the stimuli, if possible by physical contact with its source. The function of these behaviours is to reduce arousal through sufficient exposure, to facilitate habituation and/or learning, and ultimately to provide adequate information for the construction of internal schema. In future encounters with the same or similar stimulus material the new schema permits the individual to modify or direct behaviour appropriately. She/he could then be expected to respond for example, to aversive stimuli by withdrawal behaviour, to familiar stimuli with disregard or appropriate behaviour, and to novel stimulus conditions with exploratory behaviours of possibly increasing efficiency.

It is inevitable that there will be novel stimuli in the therapy process, so it is important that the environment be designed to elicit exploratory rather than withdrawal responses. Exploration is central to the task context of occupational therapy — whether or not one considers it as synonymous with play, or a component in a play process. Let us now examine another model for defining play.

Play defined by function and outcome

There is a common thread of agreement running through the diverse theoretical propositions. That is the assumption that play, in some way, is the mechanism by which juveniles prepare themselves for their future adult roles and adult responsibilities (see Groos 1901; Huizinga 1949; Klinger 1971). Erikson 1940, the famous developmental theorist said that 'all culture is first played in the form of a game'. The Plowdon Report in the UK (1967) went further in defining what its authors believe play does:

Children gradually develop concepts of causal relationships, the power to discriminate, to make judgements, to analyse and synthesize, to imagine and to formulate. Children become absorbed in their play and the satisfaction of bringing it to a satisfactory conclusion fixes habits of concentration which can be transferred to other learning.

Bruner and colleagues (1976) believe that symbolic play enhances creativity, and thus problem solving behaviour, and that it does so in the following two ways:

1. It is a means of minimising consequences of one's actions, and therefore promotes learning in risky situations.
2. It provides opportunity to try combinations of behaviour which would never be tried under normal pressures.

While Bruner's formulation is expressed in terms of the function of play, it is an interesting example of the overlap between the concepts of play and exploration. Other authors assert that play enables children to realize who they are, and what effects their actions may have on the people around them; that individually, it gives children the opportunity to experience many of life's emotions and to view their position in life in relation to the rest of the world (Opie & Opie 1969). These authors also suggest that play makes children consciously aware of the meaning and value of rules, order, and structure, thus preparing them for the social aspects of life that loom ahead.

Hutt (1966) and others such as Bronfenbrenner (1972), however, caution against adopting too absolute a view that skills learned in childhood play transfer to adult behaviour. Hutt suggests that play activities may prepare an individual for developing and using future skills in the same sense that learning to walk prepares for mastery of the physical environment. Bronfenbrenner observed that Russian children assume 'real' tasks from the age of two years to prepare for adult roles and responsibilities. The type of imitation 'play' which is so much a part of American and other Western cultures, is unknown to Russian children. The Russian concept of 'play' is limited to that type we call 'symbolic play'. Bronfenbrenner believes that much Western play is not useful, and that it distances children from the world of adults, creating an undesirable sub-culture. Finally, let us examine play defined by motivation.

Play defined by motivation

Freud (1940) argued that one motivation for play is to attempt to satisfy drives, or to resolve conflict, in the absence of a realistic opportunity to do so. For example, a child may be angry at a smaller brother or sister, but forbidden to physically hurt that one. Instead, the child may play at punishing a doll, thereby transferring affective responses to a non-harmful situation. The maturational theory has had a significant influence on the use of play in clinical practice, especially with children who display disordered or inappropriate behaviour (Buhler 1935; Erikson 1940; Freud 1965).

Anna Freud (1965), Klein (1945) and Erikson (1940) developed and refined Freud's ideas of the creation of model play situations for the acquisition of skill mastery by a child. Also the psychoanalysts suggested that play acts as a strong defence against unpleasant experiences, by reducing the seriousness of specific experiences.

Developmental theorists, taking their lead from Piaget (1962), conceptualize the motivation for play as an intrinsic need to develop cognitive skills or put another way, intellectual skills. White (1959), on the other hand, believes that play behaviour like other human activity is motivated by an individual's need to produce effects on the environment.

From models and theories we turn to examine some modern descriptions of play which have greatly advanced and altered thinking about the phenomenon. This new knowledge has particular application in the systematic and effective design of therapeutic play activity.

MODERN DESCRIPTIONS OF PLAY

Play activities are generally described as: games of mastery; make-believe games, that is, symbolic play; and games with rules.

The grouping is arbitrary, and we have surprisingly little information about whether these are clearly independent, and recur with sufficient consistency in different groups of children to be valid. The classification derives largely from Piaget's perception of play behaviour and its relationship to a child's maturation.

Play built around mastery of physical feats

The idea that there will be mastery of 'skills' in play activity is a common assumption presented in general textbook discussions. This assumption is quite congruent with a distinction between play and exploration. Bruner (1968) cites examples of skill acquisition through play in young chimps. In the first example, chimps learned to catch termites by watching adults and then practising. In the second example, juvenile Japanese Macaque monkeys learned to wash yams and to separate maize, again by watching their elders.

Singer (1973) defined mastery oriented play as that emphasizing direct relationships to the immediate environment. For example, building a tower of blocks, putting together a jig-saw, riding a tricycle, tumbling and wrestling with others, and running all represent direct concrete experience involving a minimum of make-believe or imagination elements. Piaget suggested that early infant play is concerned with sensorimotor skill mastery. He suggested that the purpose of such play is to exercise newly developed mental or sensorimotor structures, without any attempt to modify them. However it is clear that children continue to engage in games of mastery long after the infancy period.

It has been suggested that there is a class of mastery play that is practice play. Piaget (1962) stated that practice play followed a period of exploration, and presumed learning, and that within practice play there is no new learning (see also Bruner et al 1976). That is to say, after acquiring some new behaviour pattern a child may use all new objects encountered to fit the new pattern, regardless of suitability.

Make-believe or symbolic play

Some writers suggest that symbolic play is a peculiarly Western society middle class phenomenon (Murphy 1962; Whiting 1963). These authors note that children from non-industrialized cultures, and socially poor or deprived children within Western cultures engage in all forms of play except that involving symbolic transformations, that is, the 'as-if' element. Historical records appear to confirm the proposition, for until the Renaissance in Europe the notion of play — probably to be interpreted as symbolic play — did not exist. Children were set to work early in the mature adult occupational roles that they would later adopt for themselves. Certainly symbolic play has assumed increased importance and is promoted in Western cultures, in the early kindergarten settings, in parent play groups, and in intervention with disabled and disturbed children. While there appears to be scant information about handicapped children's use of symbolic play, from other evidence it could be postulated that deficit of some capacities would lead to deficit in, or absence of symbolic play ability. The importance of symbolic play in our own culture appears to be the development of higher levels of abstract conceptual thought processes, and accompanying language use. Piaget (1962) interpreted the purpose of symbolic play to be development of affective capacities. He thought that the content of such play derives from the child's emotional life, and includes issues of compensation, wish fulfillment, and conflict resolution.

The 'as-if' element is an essential component of make-believe play (Klinger 1971). That is, the child modifies the experience/environment based on some experiences carried in the memory, and which undoubtedly involve some use of imagery. The contrast which is made between play involving skill mastery and that involving symbolic transformations can be seen in an example of a boy using a swing in two different ways. The play may be designated 'mastery oriented' when the boy uses a swing to achieve a feeling of exhilaration. The same activity becomes symbolic play when the swing becomes the means for the boy to be an aeroplane in the sky.

Characteristics of make-believe play

Singer (1973) has summarized the characteristics of make-believe play as follows:

- It has social intent, e.g., children having a 'picnic' using play things to represent a real event.
- There are elements of imagery and make believe, for example, chairs become cars for purpose of the play, or again, the doll takes the beating that little brother cannot be given.
- There is some role playing and attempt to simulate adult roles, as in playing at being mothers and fathers.

This form of role playing is distinguished from symbolic play where transformations are made. Indeed, some authors such as Bruner et al (1976) suggest that imitative play should be designated a category of its own, and perhaps be classified somewhere between games of mastery and symbolic play. The crucial difference is thought to be that creative skill development is mediated through symbolic, but not imitative make-believe play.

Factors which elicit symbolic play

Several researchers have suggested some environmental factors which appear to be related to the emergence of symbolic (transformational) play (e.g., Golomb & Bowen 1981). The factors are:

a. The provision of specific play space
b. Time
c. Objects which help the child make a transition to representational play
d. An atmosphere of nurturance by adults.

We see all of these provided in kindergarten and playground environments.

Games with rules

Garvey (1977) has shown how three to five-year-old children, playing in pairs, manage to create and recognize implicit rules and expectancies, even in the most simple games. At the same time the children appeared to distinguish between the structure of make-believe and the real thing.

Summary

The modern views of the phenomenon of play have been discussed. Before proceeding to examine the conventions about ages and stages in play development, let us review the important theoretical ideas presented and their practical application to using play in therapy.

The varied examples of models of play serve to emphasize the complexity of the phenomenon. There is no one model which provides a wholly satisfying general explanation of the range of activities that we label generically 'play'. Nor does this matter, for the models should only serve to help clarify our thinking about play. On the face of the evidence, play can be viewed as the child's attempt to assimilate information and make meaning of the whole environment. There is abundant evidence and agreement that children develop sensorimotor, language, social and problem solving abilities through play, including exploratory activities. Therefore, the use of our society's formalized childhood play activities and media as therapy techniques is clearly substantiated.

It appears sensible to accept a distinction between 'play' and 'exploration' as activities, and to accept that therapy will embrace both. In exploratory activity, there will be learning, and in play there will be practice, and extension of the learning. In all probability play may be revealed as representing a process in operation which is characterized by components of curious investigation and manipulation of the environment to gain information and physical control, transformational manipulation by mental processes to extend and gain internal control, and practice to extend mastery.

Therapists are likely to find that parents distinguish between work and play, especially if their own home environment is impoverished. They may find it difficult to accept that their child is receiving beneficial and useful 'treatment' when they see him/her 'playing', or, as they might see it, wasting time. The basic research about how play is conceptualized should help a therapist to develop simple explanations that may reassure parents.

DEVELOPMENTAL AGES AND STAGES IN PLAY BEHAVIOUR

Parten (1932) was the first to attempt to understand the developmental emergence of play behaviour. Her obser-

vations led her to formulate a developmental time scale, commencing with a period of 'solitary play' from birth to about two years of age. As a result of her work, the generally held view has been that there is a recognizable sequentially emergent pattern which expresses maturational stages. However, recent work suggests that while Parten's categories remain relevant, they are better thought of as descriptive of a child's social participation, rather than as a developmental timescale (Smith 1984). Furthermore, the category of solitary play has been reformulated by Roper & Hinde (1978). These authors observed preschoolers playing and found that they displayed solitary play, where Parten believed it to have disappeared by the age of two. They also found that the amount of solitary play was about equal to that spent in so-called social play. These authors concluded that solitary and social play should be thought of as two separate factors which persist throughout development. This is a very important finding for therapists, for we have been accustomed to interpret observed solitary play in client children older than two years as indicative of immaturity. Others have confirmed Roper and Hinde's conclusion, and redefined solitary play as predominantly made up of constructive learning activities, 'independent task-oriented behaviour which is functional in school situations and indicative of social maturity rather than immaturity' (Moore et al 1974). The descriptions of solitary and social play forms are shown in Table 5.1.

Patterns of social play

Smith (1984) suggests that social play also does not follow a linear sequential model. Parten's (1932) 'parallel play' has been shown to be the least mature form of social participation, though it does not by any means occur universally. Many children display solitary play and group associative and co-operative participation, and never display parallel play. Where seen, parallel play does not appear to decrease with age, remaining a fairly constant phenomenon after about the age of two (Barnes 1971; Rubin et al 1978). Smith interprets these findings as further evidence that parallel play is not a sequential developmental step.

What we seem to be left with is the notion that there are different classes or categories of play behaviour, each having distinctive properties. This notion is compatible with a model of play as a process, for it accepts that the different categories may coexist, and persist over time. We have tended to see 'social behaviour' in adult terms, and thus failure to recognize it in a different form may have blinded us to the existence of social play in the first two years of life. Indeed, Vandell and colleagues (1980)

Table 5.1 Comparative description of solitary and social types of play

Type of play	Description
Solitary	
Early years	Absorbed in own play apart from other children — shows no interest in their activity. Plays with different things. Is often silent, sometimes talks to self.
School years	Engages in independent task-oriented activities, focused on learning about the environment.
Social	
Early months (no conventional name for this time)	Shows interest in other infants and children. Watches, makes social overtures, e.g., offers object. As motor skill develops retrieves objects from others. Shows no preference for company of others, especially children.
Parallel play	
Looking on (1–2 years)	No true sharing or turn taking. Language, if any, is not actually directed to anyone in particular, or play may be silent. Shows interest in other's activity but remains alone. This behaviour is very different from aimless wandering or unfocused attention because the child is quite clearly absorbed in his/her observations. Other children are much more important than playthings, even when children do not converse.
Joining in	2 types:
	1. Tries to join in the group play of others and gain acceptance as a group member. Talks a little, sometimes in imitation.
	2. The second kind arises where group members may be engaged on the same activity (for example, crayoning or sitting at a table doing puzzles) but where the main thing they are interested in is talking to one another. The subject matter of their talk may range far beyond the immediate activity. Relationships within a group are likely to be formed quickly, and as often as not, resumed within a few minutes or hours.
Cooperative play	
Simple	Takes part in shared activity, doing the same things.
	Shares toys, takes turns, works with others. Talk is mostly related to playing. The child has a definite place in the group, which is quite different from that with the emphasis on *individual* activity found in solitary and parallel play, and also from the simple socializing shown in joining-in play. Cooperative play can be the simple sharing of a task — for example three children building bricks together.
Complex	Takes part in complicated make-believe and symbolic transformation games with others, taking agreed parts. Talk is mostly concerned with the parts being played; symbolic games may be carried over from one session to future ones. Characterized by negotiation, agreements, and rule making.

From Open University P911: The first years of life. Copyright © The Open University. Reproduced by permission

found that six-month-old infants demonstrated co-ordinated socially directed behaviours in equal proportion to those of toddlers.

Piaget's model of play development (1962)

Others have conceptualized developmental emergence of play behaviour in different ways. One of the most influential models has been that of Piaget, who proposed that the infant passed through various stages each of which is concerned with developing increasingly com-

plex sensorimotor and cognitive internal schemata. The stages are, the sensorimotor phase, birth to 18 months, itself further divided into six phases; the pre-operational and concrete operational phases, two to four years; and the symbolic phase, first seen in overlap with the sixth sensorimotor phase. Piaget proposed that the schemata develop by two processes: assimilation and accommodation, through the medium of 'play'. Assimilation requires practice, which should lead to mastery seen in the first four sensorimotor phases. Assimilation leads to accommodation or modification particularly in the symbolic phase, culminating in the child's increasingly sophisticated complex adaptation to the environment. Piaget regarded the sound development of sensorimotor schemata in the early years as necessary for later emergence of symbolic make-believe and rule play.

Psychoanalytic model of play development

Peller (1955) offers a pyschoanalytically oriented model of development, expressed in play. At the earliest level the child is seen as playing to achieve a sense of self-image and bodily identity. At the next level, said to occur around two to three years, symbolic play is focused on the 'good versus bad mother' image. The child plays out what she/he perceives to be done to him/her. At the next level, three and a half to five years, the child works to master conflicting oedipal feelings toward parents. Sociodramatic imitative play is seen, with well developed real social relationships played out. The fourth stage marks a shift from symbolic play to peer-centred games of rules, which mirror the schemata of internal rules that the child struggles to master from about age six onward. Though ages have been suggested, with all models it would be wise to regard them as rough descriptive rule-of-thumb guides only, unsupported by data as yet.

Knox (1974) has developed a play scale which identifies types of activities likely to be associated with play behaviour in the various different ages and stages. The Play Scale as updated and modified by Bledsoe & Shepherd (1982) is presented in Appendix IV. Harrison & Kielhofner (1986) have also revised and reported on its use.

Sex differences in play behaviour

The assumption that there will be sex differences in play is a generally held one. From birth, children are treated differently according to their sex. Girls are talked to more softly, and reinforcement of sex roles even appears when choosing something as innocuous as a mobile; boys are given dangling animals or ships and cars, while girls receive pretty, pastel-coloured delicate baubles. However, the assumption of sex differences is supported by considerable evidence. As early as the age of three years the presence of androgens in boys is manifested in their greater display of aggression. They are more prone to rough play, to assertiveness and to competitiveness, while girls show a tendency towards passivity. Girls are equally aggressive towards boys and girls whereas boys display less aggression towards girls than towards boys. Chivalry rules, even in a playgroup.

Yet boys' greater inclinations to explore appear to be directly linked to their greater assertiveness.

Though no more active than girls, boys do tend to be more vigorous in their activities — a result of their larger muscles and greater speed. In the sphere of more delicate activities girls do better, as they have finer control of their hands and fingers. Boys excel when they aim at targets, and their sense of direction and their understanding of spatial relationships are better throughout their whole development. Perhaps because of this, boys play more physical games and their 'territory' stretches farther away from home. Girls, on the other hand, have superior linguistic and oral abilities. They learn to talk earlier than boys, have a wider vocabulary, and they are more articulate. While girls often play together in pairs, boys prefer either their own company or large groups. It appears sensible to accept that children will have play preferences which are influenced by their sex. Parental and therapist concern should not be to stifle the natural preferences, but to aim for a balance which encourages boys and girls to respect each other's gender role. Thus it is necessary to provide a wide range of toys, games, and play activities. The final aspect of play in therapy now becomes the focus of discussion.

SELECTING, DESIGNING, AND EVALUATING PLAY ACTIVITIES FOR THERAPY

There are two aspects of media selection that will be considered, namely:

- Choosing commercial play materials and activities for their usefulness in meeting therapeutic objectives.
- Designing and evaluating custom-made play media for therapy.

Choosing and using commercial play materials and activities

The practical considerations of equipping a children's occupational therapy facility have already been discussed in Chapter 4. The focus now will be on the specific demands that a therapist places on play media, and criteria which should guide the selection. Two important criteria are that play material/games/activities must suit the child's *developmental abilities*, not chronological age, and the chosen media must be intrinsically attractive to the child (Williams & Matesi 1988). In an occupational therapy children's facility, it is often more efficient and helpful if media are categorized and stored in relation to the job they will do, rather than by the type of material. Appendix V contains a list of games and play media, which are useful for both therapists and parents.

Frantzen (1957) attempted to select a range of toys which would promote the development and refinement of fine manipulative hand skill. The usefulness of this work is that it suggests an analytic structure in which toys can be examined in terms of normal growth and development principles, and general therapy objectives. The analysis takes into account the notion that physical development and interest in types of play, ('interest level' in the examples that follow) are equally important factors for determining toy selection. Ordinarily, the normal child starts each stage in the first interest level. With growth and refinement of movement the child passes on to the second and third interest levels. The handicapped child, by comparison, may stay in the first interest level for a much longer time, and then progress to the second or third. Usually an older handicapped child, when first observed, will have progressed beyond

---

Example 5.1: Therapeutic toy selection related to physical development and interest level

Stage of development	Aim of toy	Type of toy to choose
Thumb and finger grasp The child is able to pick up an object by using the tips of all the fingers and the thumb. 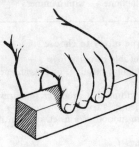	To encourage use of the finger tips to lift an object, rather than with whole hand grasp.	Wide holding toys — e.g. large stacking, take-apart, push, action and construction toys. Lightweight objects or parts of objects because of their shape and size, which can be picked up with thumb and fingers. *Level 1* Kiddicraft, stacking cups, cars or soft animal to push, building blocks. *Level 2* Duplo (Lego) blocks, wide plastic cars, large crayons. *Level 3* Take apart toys, hammer peg board.

Example 5.2: Choosing toys in relation to developmental stages: reach, grasp and release

Stage of development	Aim of toy	Type of toy to choose
Inability to reach Crude reach with no contact: arms move in direction and do not directly contact objects. The child is essentially reaching with the eyes and moving the arms aimlessly. 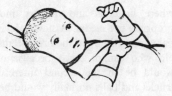	To stimulate and encourage the desire to reach	Dangling or appealing toys Dangling, moving, large, bright, noisy, and desirable toys. Anything that will motivate the child to want to reach. *Level 1* nursery mobile crib dangle bells balloons *Level 2* bright truck beautiful doll shiny bell *Level 3* football shiny saxophone

Example 5.2: Choosing toys in relation to developmental stages: reach, grasp and release (continued)

Stage of development	Aim of toy	Type of toy to choose
Hand fitted; grasp upon stimulation Although the hand is still fisted, the child will voluntarily put his fingers around an object placed near his hand. He still is not reaching directly.	To use the child's ability to hold an object if it is placed in or near his hand.	Rattles or toys with handles Long, thin, noisy, bright toys with either a pliable or hard handle section. Anything small enough to fit into the palm of the hand.
		Level 1 suspended rattle long bean bag rattles
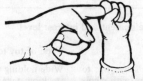		*Level 2* drumsticks toy for thumping bells — handles
		Level 3 flexible dog baton — music xylophone — with hammers

Stage of development	Aim of toy	Type of toy to choose
Reach with hand open The child is able to reach, touch, and push objects with his hand open, although he may still at times hit objects with a fisted hand.	To encourage reaching for and grasping an object	Movable or noisy toys Banging, pushing, or pressing action toys. Anything that produces some result when it is contacted by either a wide arm motion or a fisted or open hand.
		Level 1 chime dangle weighted clown suction rattle
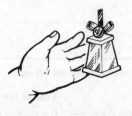		*Level 2* press squeaky book pig — press down chicken — noisy, pull
		Level 3 spiral wire toy punch bag punch — register

the first interest level.

Example 5.1 is a prescription in the Frantzen model for suitable toys for encouraging thumb and finger grasp for three levels of interest.

Example 5.2 shows the stages of acquisition of reach, grasp, and release, the therapeutic objective for choosing toys for each of the developmental stages and some examples of toys to choose.

A normal infant would be in the first interest level,

where balloons and nursery mobiles would be appropriate toy media. A slowly developing six-month-old baby may still be in the first interest level. A three-year-old who cannot reach because of motor dysfunction would be in the second interest level, where dolls, trucks and balls normally would be suitable toys. A ten-year-old cerebral palsied child of average intelligence who cannot control his arms enough to reach would be in the third interest level, where musical instruments,

Example 5.2: Choosing toys in relation to developmental stages: reach, grasp and release (continued)

Stage of development	Aim of toy	Type of toy to choose
Reach and crude grasp The child is able to reach for and grasp objects crudely. However, an object may drop out of his hand, either because the grasp is poor or because he is not able to hold on to it for any length of time.	To encourage reaching for and contacting an object even though the child is not ready to grasp	Grasp or throwable toys Small grasping toys or parts of toys. Anything that can be grasped easily, can be held and then let go, or that involves slight manipulation. *Level 1* chain rattle stuffed dog small plastic blocks *Level 2* men in tub plastic stack small truck *Level 3* grasp instruments suction spin top easy stack blocks

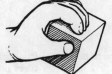

Stages of development	Aim of toy	Type of toy to choose
Reach, grasp, and release The child is able to reach directly, grasp well with the full hand and palm, and release an object at will. He is also beginnig to control the fine opening and closing of his hand.	To develop the ability of the hand to open and close precisely.	Squeeze or placement toys Squeeze, throw, take-apart, stack, or placement toys. Anything that requires repeated grasp and release, that is, repeated closing and opening of the hand. *Level 1* squeaky squeeze toys soft ball rubber squeak blocks *Level 2* spin bowling pyramid stack squeeze handle duck *Level 3* squeeze bulb — ball throw plastic letters score bowl

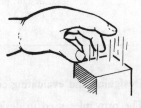

Reproduced by permission from Toys . . . the tools of children, by June Frantzen, published by the National Easter Seal Society, Chicago, Illinois.

footballs and computer games normally would be of interest. One toy can be used in a variety of ways, depending on the need. Balloons represent one interest level when placed in front of an infant to look at. They represent another interest level when given to a four-year-old to blow up, and yet another, when used to explain static electricity to a ten-year-old. Also the balloons can be used to stimulate different hand functions,

by using them as something to reach for, to punch, to catch, or to grasp with the thumb and fingers. Therefore, one should keep in mind when prescribing toys, that activities can be graded and adapted to encourage specific outcomes.

The toys mentioned in Examples 5.3–5.5 are merely a general guide and are offered to show some of the types of toys that have proven useful.

EXAMPLE 5.3 Story strips

Story strips are a very readily available game, which involves story telling by reference to a set of cards, each depicting an event or component of the story.

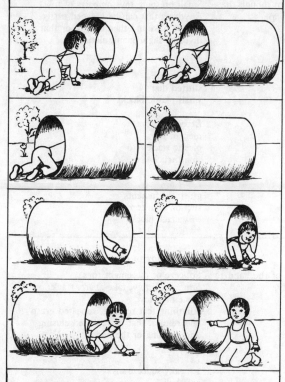

The inherent flexibility of story strips makes them a useful alternative to reading a book. A therapist might use them, for example:

— to develop basic conceptual skills of ordering and sequencing,
— to introduce a child to a practical task such as learning to put on shoes and socks,
— to encourage independent decision making — by choosing the order of pictures,
— or to helping the child to discover the effects of actions and decisions (consequences),
— to achieve any combination of these diverse objectives.

The important point made in Example 5.4 is that with a little thought, imagination and understanding of developmental processes, activities that might be discarded as 'too easy' or 'too difficult' can become interesting and challenging. Such analyses as suggested in all of the examples is time consuming, but essential if occupational therapy is to be more than just 'playing with the children'.

Some ideas are presented about how to approach the task of designing 'custom-made' media to meet specific objectives. The approach also illustrates a practical way of analysing existing play materials.

Example 5.4   Some very simple suggestions for ways that activities can be modified

Activity	Modifications	
	To simplify task	*To increase complexity of task*
Ring stack	Bigger rings	Rings all the same colour. Smaller variation in size of each
5 piece puzzle	Paint matching edges in the same colours	Cover picture on each piece
Screwtop jar	Paint an arrow in direction to be tightened	Provide two similar jars with different threads
Cutting shapes	Mark or score the lines to cut	Provide more complicated design
Threading beads (2.5 cm cubes or balls)	Wax the end of the string. Enlarge holes	Provide smaller beads of various shapes
30 piece puzzle	Do the edge pieces for the child, or 'prefabricate' the major items	Remove the model picture
Tracing pictures	Use thicker outline or simpler design; pin down paper	Trace outline only and get the child to complete the picture

Designing and evaluating custom-made play media

The principles used in designing your own playthings are:

1. There must be a clear identification of the developmental and/or chronological ages for which the plaything is intended.
2. The skills to be developed must be clearly described.
3. The design brief must be based on research literature about normal growth and development, and the particular skills to receive attention.
4. The plaything prototype should be evaluated for its ability to meet original design objectives. Questions to be asked include:
   a.   Did the plaything meet the behavioural

objectives appropriately? (Was it used as intended? If not, why not?).

b. Was the plaything's design attractive to children, safe, and potentially longlasting?

c. Did the children extend its use, beyond that originally intended? If so, why, and what are the implications for extended use of the plaything?

Ideally, all play media used by specialists should be submitted to such analyses, for Quilitch (1975), Sheiman (1979) and others note that there is virtually no basis to claims made about so-called 'educational toys' by their proponents. In fact, Quilitch says that there is 'no believable evidence that educational toys even exist'. Thus therapists should not be misled into purchasing such equipment because of a label. Example 5.5 is an example of a custom designed 'Plaything'.

EXAMPLE 5.5: Variation on Snakes and Ladders (Clark & Longden 1983).

Design description. The adapted 'Snakes and Ladders' game consists of a material 'board' which is single-bed-spread size, a material dice, and several tors. The Snakes and Ladders 'board' is made of 30 cotton patchwork squares all in the basic colours of red, yellow, green and blue, surrounded by a yellow border. It is reversible, lined with polyfibre, backed with bright coloured cotton fabric depicting a story. The 'board' is 112 cm × 172 cm with a wooden end rod to allow it to be hung. Each patchwork square is sewn with a felt number from 1 to 30. 'STOP' and 'GO' indicate starting and finishing places of the game. Cotton lace in a lattice design is sewn onto the material to symbolize ladders; cotton ric rac braiding with large beads for heads at the top of the ric-rac, symbolize snakes.

The dice are also made in patchwork design, with six sides and felt dots to indicate the numbers. A bell in a tin is sewn into the middle of the dice.

Five wooden tors are provided; a round yellow and a white triangular tor; a green square tor sewn with Velcro, to enable a hand to slip between the tor and the Velcro; a blue rectangular tor with a long dowel handle which enables it to be used from a wheel-chair; and a red hexagonal shaped tor with a built-up handle designed for people with poor grasp.

Purpose of Adapted Snakes and Ladders

The purpose of adapting Snakes and Ladders was to provide an attractive and stimulating toy that would enhance and reinforce physical, cognitive and social developmental aspects of children aged six to 11 years. A major design consideration was to enable it to be used by bed-bound children.

Design rationale. Adapted Snakes and Ladders encourages and reinforces physical, cognitive and social components of growth and development.

The toy encourages fine and gross movements, eye-hand co-ordination and sensory input; fine movements such as cylindrical grip, ball grasp, palmar tripod pinch, depending on which tor is used. Incidental fine movements occur by touching and exploring the lace, numbers and beads. Gross movements occur due to the large design of the game, and if played on the floor, lower extremity movements as well as gross upper extremity movements are encouraged. Eye-hand co-ordination is facilitated by movements of the tors, while both hands can be used to throw the dice thus encouraging crossing of the body midline. The game provides tactile input via the materials used, i.e. cotton, felt, beads, ric-rac, lace, wood, foam, velcro and raised numbers. The bright colours are visually stimulating and the bell inside the dice provides auditory input.

Cognitively, the game teaches concepts of 'Stop' and 'Go'. Stop is red, while Go is green and thus teaches and reinforces road safety skills. The numbers 1 to 30 reinforce and encourage number learning. The tors are different shapes and teach concepts of circularity, rectangularity, squareness, triangularity and hexagonality. The coloured patches were sewn in such a manner that the child can learn the additional perceptual concept of diagonal arrangement. Children in the concrete operational age group engage in symbolic play, and understand that lace symbolizes a ladder, while ric-rac symbolizes a snake.

The game can be played by two or more children, thus promoting social interaction. Also the child experiences winning and losing, and can learn to develop tolerance towards others in a group. All of these factors are seen as important for individual growth and for skills and behaviours needed in middle childhood and adolescence.

Therapy application

While Adapted Snakes and Ladders is designed for 'normally' developing children, it has application for use with visually impaired children, paraplegic children and children confined to bed through illness.

Visually impaired children. The bell in the dice assists localization, while the raised felt dots enables the child to interpret the numbers tactually. The Braille Society produced a set of instructions for the game in braille. Buttons could be sewn onto each square in braille formation. This adaptation combined with the deliniation of each square on the 'board' by seams and the tactile input of the lace and ric-rac would enable a blind child to play the game.

Physical impairment. The tor with the built-up handle and the tor with Velcro across would be suitable for a child with poor grasp (e.g. due to nerve injuries, dystrophies etc.). The tor with the long dowel handle also enables the game to be played whilst sitting in a wheelchair.

Bed game. This game would be particularly useful in a hospital setting as it allows a child confined to bed e.g. admitted for observations, rheumatic fever or other non-contagious diseases, to interact with other children.

Teaching aid. The game could be used as a teaching aid in schools, hospitals, and homes to teach such things as numbers, designs, stop, go, and up and down.

Consequently, a physically handicapped but otherwise normally developing child can play this game with other children, and therefore it has benefits as suggested by the 'normalization principle' and the honey-pot model (Clancy 1980).

Evaluation

The game was tested on two boys, Richard aged ten, and Daniel aged seven. In addition, the younger sister, Christina, aged four, was fascinated by the game although she was not old enough to comprehend the rules.

From observations, the game met its design objectives, i.e., encouraging and reinforcing physical, cognitive and social components of development, while being attractive and stimulating in bed. Finally, although Christina was too young to understand the rules of the game, exposure to the game encouraged reaching and manipulating behaviour and the verbal identification of colours. Her mother stated that Christina liked the picture stories on the reverse side of the mat and consequently its objectives of being attractive and stimulating were met.

PLAY ACTIVITY AND THE PHYSICAL ENVIRONMENT

Selecting appropriate play media is one aspect of preparing therapy intervention, but another equally important aspect is designing the play space to gain maximum benefit from the interaction between children, activities and space available. There are many studies now of the ways in which normally developing children interact in play situations. For example, Smith (1974) reported differences in children's social behaviour under three play conditions:

1. In the presence of large climbing and other gross motor activity apparatus.
2. In the presence of fine manipulative type toys only.
3. In the presence of both.

It was found that Condition 1, led to increased active, sociable and creative behaviour. There was significantly more talking between children, physical contact and gross motor activity than in Condition 3. Children who usually played alone or in parallel groups were more likely to engage in co-operative play — an outcome not achieved by simply reducing the amount of play equipment, thereby forcing a greater degree of sharing.

As yet we know little about the special effects of many of the disabling and handicapping conditions of children in therapy on their play behaviour development. Also we do not clearly understand the ways in which much of our therapy acts on children to influence their behaviour and maturation — and this is vital information if we are to be accountable for our professional effectiveness.

Abstract concepts expressed in observable behaviour–environment interaction of children, are best studied with simple useful questions about the activities which can be observed in the designed physical space. For example, 'exploratory play' could be defined operationally in terms of the behaviours to be observed. Predictions could be made about the use of the space, the activities, and other people in the designed context. Information can then be collected and measured in quantifiable terms, e.g., by time lapse photography. The proposal to specify and evaluate environments for children's activities in terms of *activity* measures is indirectly suggested in the work of McGrew (1970). This author set out to develop a taxonomy of motor behaviour patterns to describe the activity of four-year-old preschool children. One hundred and eleven distinct items were developed for five classes of movement, namely, visual fixation, posture, locomotion, manipulation and gestures. McGrew found that the five classes could be rank ordered by frequency of occurrence in the total number of observations. Rank order 1 actions were defined as manipulative. Ranking second was walking, ranking third were actions concerned with picking up the arms, ranking fourth were actions concerned with placing objects, and ranking fifth were actions concerned with turning (i.e., rotation of the trunk, beginning with the face). This represented 46% of all activity observed. Continuing in descending order were actions defined as standing up, running, bending, pouring, and scooping, which represented an additional 12% of all observations. Thus, ten activity types represent 58% of all motor behaviour observed. With the addition of 15 more activity categories (e.g., stepping up or down, reaching, sitting down, pulling, climbing, specialized manipulation, etc.), 25 types of motor behaviour were observed to account for 77% of all children's motor activity.

Studies such as those of McGrew (1979), and Smith (1986) show how hypotheses can be formulated and the data realistically collected in clinical situations. Basic research such as Smith's guide therapists to design and evaluate clinical practice much more precisely, and thus effectively (see also Derman 1974, Francis 1983).

Clearly, the environment can influence play behaviour. The general conditions necessary for effective 'playing', drawn up by White (1959) and modified by Florey (1969) specifically for the guidance of occupational therapists working with children are seen to be that:

— The environment should provide both human and non-human objects. Human objects include both parents and peers.
— The non-human object environment should provide novelty and complexity.

   The best guideline is to provide an environment that offers possibilities for action having both new and familiar elements. Thus for example, the novel situation of the occupational therapy department/clinic should hold some elements that a child may identify as familiar with his own home environment.
— The environment should allow for and provide the opportunity for exploration, repetition, and imitation. Task expectations should be set, but the child must also be allowed to experiment with various ways of meeting these expectations. The therapist should ensure that there are competent role models for a child to imitate.
— The play environment should be free of such stresses as hunger, anxiety, or fear. The play environment should not be associated with isolation, fear, or pain. This factor directs us to be cautious in using and expecting play experiences to divert attention from pain and fear.

Florey has some particularly useful advice about therapeutic 'play', or activity for the child approaching puberty from about ten years old:

1. The environment should provide systematic instruction. This acquaints the child with the tools and symbols of his culture and gives him the opportunity to develop skill.
2. The environment should provide the child with the opportunity to make things and deal with things that have significance in the adult world. At this age, the OT

clinic should provide not dolls, miniature trucks, or blocks, but projects that yield useful items.
3. There should be role models who know things and know how to do things. In occupational therapy we might think of models for craftsmanship and models for sportsmanship.
4. There should be opportunity for association with peers. The peers are the individuals who are most significant to him at this time. This is the age at which the child strives to be the strongest, the best, the wittiest, and the fastest. She/he requires his/her peers in order to measure his own skills and worth.

SUMMARY

From birth we see the child's developing skills expressed through the activities we call play. All systems are engaged, though it appears to us that the focus may shift over time. For example, Piaget (1962) thought that the infant was preoccupied with sensori-motor experience, while the six-year-old focused on language and the inner symbolic life. That may be so, but it may also simply express our tendency to attribute adult explanations to behaviour whose form we do not yet correctly recognize, or fully understand.

The distinction made between work and play appears to be a universal one, though it is defined differently among various societal groups. Play is certainly not an inevitable activity among children. A number of authors have identified the conditions necessary for play in any form to occur, and those conditions for special types of play, such as symbolic play. What is becoming increasingly clear is that play is a primary expression of developing social behaviour. The process is a gradual one, rather like the learning of language — as verbal and behavioural vocabulary grows children are able to express themselves more clearly, and more accurately. Whereas previously we thought that there was a linear progression in the social 'play vocabulary' from one clear-cut stage to another, starting with solitary and culminating in social play, we now realize that this is not the case. Solitary and social play appear to be two phenomena which develop side by side in sophistication, throughout development.

Understanding how play develops as a social activity will help you in the practical business of evaluating behaviour and designing therapy. For example, you may be organizing an early intervention experience for several intellectually handicapped three-year-old toddlers in a group situation. Predictably, the toddlers will seek and require times to play alone, and they will also most probably still be in the stage of parallel, looking on types of play. The activities should allow for each child and mother or other adult 'to do their own thing', alongside each other. Attempts to achieve co-operative group interaction would be predicted to fail — though such play would certainly be an appropriate long range objective.

The prescription of toys and activities for children and families is based on the principles of normal growth and development. Therapists can be innovative and thus use activities and toys in a variety of ways in order to meet a number of objectives. Knowledge of normal growth and development allows therapists to evaluate both commercially available, custom-made toys in terms of age appropriateness, developmental appropriateness, safety and effectiveness in meeting stated objectives. Finally, therapists should be aware of how the environment can impact on play behaviour.

REFERENCES

Barnes D 1971 Language, the learner and the school. Penguin, Harmondsworth

Berlyne D E 1960 Conflict, arousal and curiosity. McGraw-Hill, New York

Bledsoe N P, Shepherd J T 1982 A study of reliability and validity of a preschool play scale. American Journal of Occupational Therapy 36: 783–788

Bronfenbrenner V 1972 Two worlds of childhood: US and USSR. Simon & Schuster, New York

Bruner J 1968 Toward a theory of instruction. Norton, New York

Bruner J S, Jolly A, Sylva K 1976 Play: its role in development and evolution. Basic Books, New York

Buhler C 1935 From birth to maturity: an outline of the psychological development of the child. Routledge & Kegan-Paul, London

Clancy H 1980 Therapy in socializing contexts, the honey-pot model. Australian Occupational Therapy Journal 27; 111–123

Clark M, Longden S 1983 Variation on snakes and ladders. Unpublished manuscript

Dansky J L, Silverman I W 1975 Play — general facilitator of associative fluency. Developmental Psychology 11(1): 104

Derman A 1974 Children's play: design approaches and theoretical issues 1, 2. Man–Environment systems 4: 69–88

Erikson E H 1940 Studies in the interpretation of play. Genetic Psychology Monographs 22: 557–671

Florey L L 1969 Intrinsic motivation: the dynamics of occupational therapy theory. American Journal of Occupational Therapy 23: 319–322

Fraiberg S 1968 The magic years: understanding and handling the problems of early childhood. Methuen, London

Francis M 1983 Negotiating between children and adult design values in open space projects. Childhood City Quarterly 10: (4) 20–31

Frantzen J 1957 Toys — the tools of children. National Society for Crippled Children and Adults, Chicago

Freud A 1965 Normality and pathology in childhood. International University Press, New York

Garvey C 1977 Play. Open Books Publishing, Glasgow

Golomb C Bowen S 1981. Playing games of make-believe: the effectiveness of symbolic play training with children who failed to benefit from early conservation training. Genetic Psychology Monographs 104: 137–159

Groos K 1901 The play of man. Heinemann, London

Harrison H, Kielhofner G 1986 Examining reliability and validity of the preschool play scale with handicapped children. American Journal of Occupational Therapy 40: 167–173

Huizinga J 1949 Homo ludens: a study of the play element in culture. Routledge & Kegan-Paul, New York

Hutt C 1966 Exploration and play. Symposium Royal Zoology Society London 18: 61–81

Hutt C, Hutt S J 1970 Direct observation and measurement of behaviour. Charles C Thomas, Springfield, Illinois

Kendler H H 1963 Basic psychology. Appleton-Century-Crofts, New York

Klein M 1945 The psycho-analysis of children. Hogarth, London

Klinger E 1971 Structure and functions of fantasy. Wiley, New York

Knox 1974 A play scale. In: Reilly M (ed) Play as exploratory learning. Sage Publications, London

Leland D H, Smith D E 1965 Play therapy with mentally subnormal children. Grune & Stratton, New York

Li A K F 1981 Play and the mentally retarded child. Mental Retardation 19(3): 121–126

McGrew W C 1979 In: Hutt C, Hutt S J (eds). Direct observation and measurement of behaviour. Charles C Thomas, Springfield, Illinois

Moore N V, Evertson C M, Brophy J E 1974 Solitary play — some functional considerations. Developmental Psychology 10(6): 830

Murphy L B 1962 The widening world of childhood: path towards mastery. Basic Books, New York

Mussen P, Conger J, Kagan J (eds) 1969 Child development and personality, 3rd edn. Harper & Row, New York

Mussen P, Conger J, Kagan J (eds) 1970 Readings in child development and personality. Harper & Row, New York

Open University Publication 1977 The first years of life. Ward Lock, London

Opie I, Opie P 1969 Children's games in street and playground. Clarendon Press, Oxford

Parten M B 1932 Social participation among preschool children. Journal of Abnormal Psychology 27: 343–369

Peller L E 1955 Libidinal development as reflected in play. Psychoanalysis 3: 3–12

Piaget J 1962 Play, dreams and imitation in childhood. Norton, New York

Plowden B 1967 Children and their primary schools (Plowden Report). HMSO, London

Quilitch H R 1975 Toys may teach — but we don't know what or how. Psychology Today April: 36–37

Reilly M 1974 Play as exploratory learning. Sage Publications, Beverley Hills

Robinson A L 1977 Play an arena for acquisition of rules

for competent behaviour. American Journal of Occupational Therapy 31: 4

Roper R, Hinde R A 1978 Social behaviour in a playgroup — consistency and complexity. Child Development 49(3): 570–579

Rosen C E 1974 Effects of sociodramatic play on problem-solving behaviour among culturally disadvantaged preschool children. Child Development 45(4): 920

Rosenblatt D 1977 Developmental trends in infant play. In: Tizard B and Harvey D (eds) The biology of play. Lippincott, Philadelphia

Rubin K H, Watson K S, Jambour T W 1978 Free-play behaviours in preschool and kindergarten. Child Development 49(2): 534–536

Sadler W 1969 Creative existence: play as a pathway to personal freedom and community. Humanitas 5: 57–79

Sheiman D L 1979 Comparison of raters' and manufacturers' opinions of appropriate ages for selected toy use. Psychological Reports 45: 450

Sheridan M D 1977 Spontaneous play in early childhood from birth to six years. NFER Publishing, Windsor

Singer J L 1973 The child's world of make-believe: experimental studies of imaginative play. Academic Press, New York

Sluckin A 1981 Growing up in the playground: the social development of children. Routledge & Kegan-Paul, London

Smith P K 1974 Aspects of the playgroup environment. In: Cantor D V, Lee T (eds) Psychology and the built environment. Architectural Press, London

Smith P K (ed) 1984 Play in animals and man. Blackwell, Oxford

Smith P K (ed) 1986 Children's play: research developments and practical applications. Gordon & Breach Scientific Publishers, New York

Sylva K 1977 Play and learning. In: Tizard B, Harvey D (eds) Biology of play. Heinemann, London

Sylva K, Lunt I 1982 Child development: a first course. Grant McIntyre, London

Thorpe W H 1963 Learning and instinct in animals. Methuen, London

Vandell D L, Wilson K S, Buchanan N R 1980 Peer interaction in the first year of life: an examination of its structure, content and sensitivity to toys. Child Development 51(2): 481–488

Wehman P, Abramson M 1976 Three theoretical approaches to play. American Journal of Occupational Therapy 30(9): 551

Welker W I 1956 Variability of play and exploratory behaviour in chimpanzees. Journal of Comparative and Physiological Psychology 49: 181–185

Welker W I 1971 Ontogeny of play and exploratory behaviours: a definition of problems and a search for new conceptual solutions. In: Moltz M (ed) Ontogeny of vertebrate behaviour. Academic press, New York

White R 1959 Motivation reconsidered: the concept of competence. Psychological Review 66: 297–333

Whiting B B (ed) 1963 Six cultures: studies of child rearing. Wiley, New York

Whittaker L A 1980 A note on developmental trends in symbolic play on hospitalised profoudhy retarded children. Dance Journal 21(3): 253–261

William S E, Matesi D V 1988 Therapeutic intervention with an adapted toy. American Journal of Occupational Therapy 42(1): 673–676

PART II

THE PROCESS OF THERAPY

The proposition that it is general principles which must be known and understood, carries into discussion of the practical components of the therapy process. In Chapter 6 evaluation of a child and family is discussed in relation to the questions: why evaluate? what should be evaluated? and how should evaluation be implemented?

Chapter 7 presents an approach to intervention which relies heavily on the general system theory of von Bertalanffy. The approach is called 'integrated treatment programming'. Therapy is arranged so that it provides comprehensive intervention and generalization of benefits in the child's developmental experience.

Facing a child who refuses to have anything to do with the carefully planned and organised therapy is enough to provoke a therapist to feelings of desperation,

inadequacy and even anger. This situation reflects a central issue in therapy: that of how to gain a child's co-operation, or in other words, how to motivate the child to therapy tasks and process.

Chapter 9 provides a discussion of some modern theories of motivation which may be helpful in designing the motivational component of therapy, together with some practical guidelines. The use of 're-inforcement', that is positive and negative feedback, by rewards and penalties, will be considered as past of the motivational component.

Chapter 10 in this section deals with the thorny problem of managing children's behaviour and disciplining them in therapy and at home.

The management component

6. General principles of evaluating children

READERS' OBJECTIVES

After reading this chapter, you should be able to:

1. Define and describe what differentiates evaluation from assessment.
2. Describe the different reasons why a child is referred for occupational therapy evaluation.
3. Be able to cite one example of a suitable test or profile for each area of the total evaluation.
4. Describe how to prepare an evaluation situation and present the necessary tasks to the child and family.
5. Discuss how a therapist approaches the task of interpreting evaluation data (information) and reporting findings.

DEFINITIONS AND PURPOSES

An occupational therapist's evaluation of a child assists other specialists make diagnostic decisions. Equally important, the evaluation process establishes a basis for planning intervention — both generally, and specifically in therapy — and it is through evaluative procedures that a therapist monitors the effects of therapy.

Thus evaluation:

— always precedes therapy;
— is repeated at least once throughout the intervention process; and
— concludes the therapy process 'wrapping it up'.

There is still some argument about whether the two words 'evaluation' and 'assessment' are interchangeable. However, both words have distinct meanings, and appear to make the most useful addition to professional language when used in accordance with our guidelines that *evaluation* is the name given to the collective acts of:

1. *Gathering information* about a client;
2. *Analysing* that information; then
3. *Presenting interpretations* arising from the analysis.

> **Terminology**
> *Evaluation* refers to the analysis of *a composite body of information*. There may be, for example, one or more tests; interview information; medical file information; systematic observation data.
> *Assessment* refers to the collection of *one piece of information* in the composite body, for example, estimate of general developmental progress using the Denver Developmental Screening Test.

Figure 6.1 represents a useful model of the relationship of the evaluation component to the total therapy process. This model highlights the dynamic nature of assessment, evaluation and therapy.

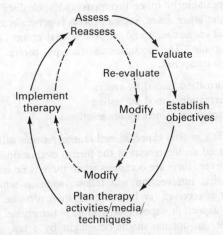

Fig. 6.1 Relationship of the evaluation component to the total therapy process.

Gronlund (1978) also presented a useful model showing how the decision making processes in clinical evaluation relate to other decisions that a therapist makes throughout the intervention process.

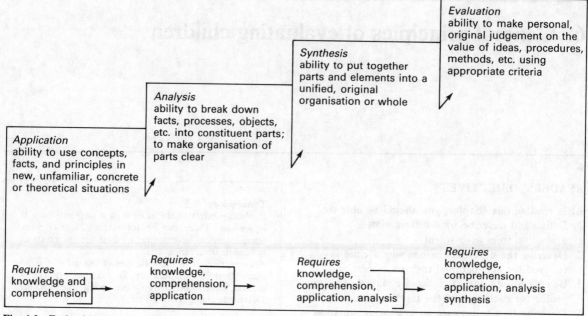

Fig. 6.2 Evaluation processes related to other decision-making processes in therapy (after Gronlund 1978)

TYPES OF EVALUATION AND RECOMMENDED USES

The recommended evaluation process is one in which the therapist uses methods of gaining information that are repeatable by other therapists and specialists elsewhere, at other times. Such a process is generally called a *formal evaluation*, and each professional group has its own profile. The occupational therapy profile with children comprises:

a. Information gained by report
b. Information gained by testing
c. Information gained by observation

There is a general expectation that intervention will follow, based on the results of the formal evaluation.

However, there are occasions when there is no expectation that intervention will follow, such as when a request is received for limited evaluation of some particular aspect or aspects of a child's behaviour. For example, an opinion might be sought by a lawyer to present in a legal case for a damages award to a child injured in a car accident; or again a paediatrician might request special information in order to determine suitable school placement for a child. In such instances it is most usual to employ only the testing component of formal evaluation. This limited form of evaluation is known as *standardized evaluation* and is becoming an increasingly important part of the professional role of a

paediatric occupational therapist. Usually a number of standardized tests are administered and the results are presented and interpreted in a written report. The example of Brigid (Example 6.1) illustrates such a report.

Evaluation which relies solely or very heavily on the therapist making personal judgements is not recommended, even when the evaluator is experienced. Other colleagues would have difficulty in assessing the value of the results gained and their interpretation. Further, another therapist cannot reliably repeat the evaluation at a future time because the testing and other procedures are not available. That is not to deny the usefulness of a period of informal play from which a therapist makes personal observations of the child/family, as a prelude to the systematic evaluation process. Let us examine the components of the formal evaluation process more closely.

THE FORMAL EVALUATION

Gaining information — by report

The child's mother, or primary caretaker, is the most usual informant, and the occupational therapist will seek several types of information. One type of information is historical, which is always retrospective and thus distorted to a degree. Researchers have considered the problems associated with using retrospective infor-

Example 6.1: Brigid
Occupational Therapy Children's Clinic
Evaluation report for *Brigid A*
Date of birth: 11.7.80
Age: 5 years 11 months
Date tested: 12.6.86
Examiner:
Background
Brigid was referred to this Clinic for a second opinion of her general developmental maturity, and detection of any specific problems hindering her ability to learn in the formal classroom situation. Brigid commenced school (grade 1) in January 1986 and her teachers have apparently been concerned about her school performance. She has been tested by the school occupational therapist and guidance officer. Some extra individual work with Brigid has been undertaken by the teaching staff. By report she has found the school experience a stressful one, but this has been resolved to some extent by lessening the normal teaching demands. Brigid has continued with remedial tasks with one teacher, at a reduced pace.
Test results
Two standardized tests were administered:
a. The Griffiths Mental Developmental Scales; and
b. The Meeting Street School Screening Test.

Each is discussed separately, and then a general summary and interpretation of results is given.
The Griffiths Mental Development Scales. This test provides an assessment of a child's developmental maturity, when compared with other children of similar age. The test does not yield an I.Q. score.

The test is divided into 5 sectors, viz, locomotor scale, personal-social, hearing and speech, eye and hand co-ordination, performance scale. Together the scores yield a 'mental age' (MA) and 'general quotient' (GQ). Brigid settled quickly to the test situation, with her mother present throughout. At all times the child appeared interested in the tasks, and relaxed in performance. When given a chance to correct tasks which she failed, Brigid identified her mistakes, corrected them, and expressed satisfaction with her efforts.

Brigid's mental age is calculated as 6 years 2 months when she is 5 years 11 months chronologically. Her G.Q. is 105. This means that she is at least of average general ability *except in the performance sector of the test*. She shows a marked delay, having a mental age of 5 years 2 months and a G.Q. of 87.

The 'performance scale' is concerned with visual-perceptual tasks, spatial relationships and the ability to formulate abstract and symbolic concepts. Normal maturation of these skills is essential before a child can learn to read, write and handle arithmetical problems.
The Meeting Street School Screening Test. This test was devised to detect deficits in a range of information processing skills. Brigid's performance in all aspects of this test was deficient, with the area of 'motor patterning' being most delayed (raw score 12/29). Her

total raw score is 45 and the cut-off point for normal development in the areas tested is 55.

This result confirms that Brigid does have a specific learning problem. The skills affected appear to be those reliant on visual-spatial relationship integrity and motor planning ability — that is, those skills basic to the acquisition of reading and writing competence.

Summary and interpretation

Brigid appears to be a child of at least average abilities. Her general development score is significantly depressed by her score on the 'performance scale' of the Griffiths Mental Development Scales. However there is no doubt, on the results of the two tests administered, that Brigid has a learning disability that is serious.

From my clinical observation, Brigid shows some very minor 'soft signs' suggestive of neurological immaturity. She is awkward in movement, but her underlying problem appears to be one of motor planning rather than motor performance.

The disability appears to be restricted, but unfortunately it would be very apparent in the classroom in the tasks of reading and writing. Her work would predictably appear sloppy and haphazard. Such a child is often vulnerable to the labels 'lazy', 'stupid', and 'doesn't pay attention'. Brigid is fortunate that her teachers have been sensitive to her problems. The particular areas affected respond fairly readily to training to develop the basic skills. I would strongly recommend that Brigid complete one of the standard available special perceptual skills training systems, and my choice would be the Fairbanks Robinson Level 1 programme.

Recommendations

1. Continuation of the present individualized teaching sessions by the school teachers.
2. Completion of an appropriate sensorimotor-perceptual training programme, e.g., the Fairbanks Robinson Perceptual Training Programme Level 1. It would be ideal if this programme could be incorporated into the individual school sessions, with some limited homework.
3. Re-assessment at the completion of the school year, in six months' time.

My recommendation is that the prime objective of intervention in 1986 should be to assist Brigid, within the school setting, to develop the basic skills. It is vital that she come to enjoy the school learning situation and associate it with pleasing challenges, rather than onerous and forbidding tasks. I am happy to offer therapy, however, I believe that it will serve Brigid's interests best for me to provide consultation with her teachers and school therapists.
Signed:
Occupation Therapist

mation (Vestre & Zimmerman 1969; Zunich 1962). However, there are clinical instances — and research ones too — where it is more valuable to draw on the retrospective data than to have none at all (Yarrow et al 1970).

The following guidelines can help an evaluating therapist, namely:

a. Appraise remembered information cautiously
b. Seek sources such as baby books, or photographs to verify memories
c. Think of history as a jig-saw puzzle.

Try to build a factual picture of the child's general development, with emphasis on those areas of particular interest to you, the occupational therapist, e.g., self-care, adaptive and fine motor behaviour, play behaviour, social interactive behaviour.

Seek to discover the concerns which have led the parents, or others, to seek the consultation. A useful guide can be to ask the parents 'what has doctor told you about . . .?' Seek also to discover what the parents (informant) believe the evaluation represents, what they hope to gain from it, what they are willing and able to contribute to it, and what constraints there are on future action.

Facts vs perceptions. A mother's (caretaker) record is of great importance for another reason. By listening carefully both to the content and emotion attached to her account the therapist may gain understanding of the way a mother views her relationship with her child. However, be sensitive when asking parents potentially painful questions. The therapist may also discover how a mother views her child's achievements; what disappoints her, angers her, pleases her. In a word, how she perceives her child. And it can be helpful to ask the mother how she views this child compared with her others. How the family members actually do behave toward each other will be revealed by systematic observation — the third component of the formal evaluation. Takata's (1974) 'Play History' (Example 6.2) presents a history gathering format.

Gaining information by testing

The inclusion of standardized tests as one component of evaluation means that any reader will be able to understand how results were achieved, and interpretations made.

A standardized test is one which is deemed *valid* and *reliable*. A valid test is one which tests what it says it tests and a reliable test is one where test results can be repeated (replicated) by other people on other occasions.

Example 6.2: The play history

1. General Information
   Name: Birthdate: Sex:
   Date: Informant(s):
   Presenting problem:
2. Previous play experiences
   • Solitary play
   • Play with others:
     mother father sisters brothers playmates other family members pets
   • Play with toys and materials (earliest preferences)
   • Gross physical play
   • Pretend and make-believe play
   • Sports and games: group collaboration group competition
   • Creative interests: arts crafts
   • Hobbies, collections, other leisure time activities
   • Recreation/social activities
3. Actual play examination
   • With what does the child play? Toy, materials, pets
   • How does the child play with toys and other materials?
   • What type of play is avoided or liked least?
   • With whom does the child play? Self, parents, brothers, sisters, peers, others
   • How does the child play with others?
   • What body postures does the child use during play?
   • How long does the child play with objects? With people?
   • Where does the child play?
     Home: indoors   outdoors
     Community: park   school   church
     other areas
   • When does the child play?
     Daily schedule for weekday and weekend
4. Play description
5. Play prescription

Validity and reliability are established in the following way. Once constructed, the new test is administered to a large sample of individuals, to arrive at norms for specific behaviour of a specific group. For example, all standardized developmental tests allow for precise comments about children's behaviour at designated ages. So it is possible for a therapist to reliably compare a child client with normal peers. Further, it is possible for a therapist to say with confidence how different the child is from the general population.

Such tests are reported in the literature, and have, therefore, been scrutinized by experts in test construction and the specialty area. The use of a standardized test increases the value of information gained from testing.

Guidelines for the use of tests and assessments
Do's:

- *Always use a standardized test when one exists.*
  This advice cannot be overstressed.
- *When a standardized test is not available, choose an experimental — but published — test.*
- *Always administer and score a chosen test exactly according to the directions given.*
  Once the evaluator deviates from directions, either in equipment used, or method of administration, the test becomes valueless.
- *When presenting the written report, include a copy of the actual test proforma.*
  Others can then see how judgements and interpretations have been made.

Don't's:

- *Don't make your own test.*
  Test construction is a specialist skill and there are now tests available to cover all of the major areas of occupational therapy with children.
- *Don't administer sections of a test if the test criteria state you must administer all test items.*
- *Don't administer tests if you do not meet the test administration criteria* (i.e., certification).
- *Don't comment prematurely to the child's parents, or others*, e.g., 'It looks fine.'
  Wait until the test has been scored, the equations completed, and there has been time for thought about the results. It is very embarrassing to retract, it destroys professional credibility, and it does not facilitate development of the relationship of trust.
- *Don't use test jargon when interpreting test results to parents or others.* State the results in functional terms.

Guidelines for gathering information by observation
Do's

- *Plan what information is required and what behaviour should be observed in order to gain information.*
- *Plan the form of the observation schedule.*
  Using a prepared schedule facilitates the observer's job; it is less likely that important information is missed and the task is a less formidable and tiring one. Also it helps to avoid the problem of missing vital information while writing a running account of everything happening — an impossible task.
- *Collate and summarize the observation as soon as possible after completing it.*
  The evaluating therapist is less likely to forget other qualifying comments about the observation. New lines of enquiry may be opened and preparations made to include them in the evaluation process.

Don't's:

- *Don't gather a large volume of information indiscriminately, with the idea that relevant pieces will be sorted out later.*
  The original objectives of the observation are very easily forgotten, and the exercise is then an expensive useless one.

A test manual should contain all the information necessary to evaluating, scoring and administering a test. It should provide clear answers to the following questions (after Gething 1983):

- Is the aim of the test clearly specified?
- Is the theoretical rationale underlying the test clearly specified?
- Is target population for test clearly specified?
- Does the manual include specific and clear details about administration of test so that the user is able to duplicate the conditions under which norms were established and reliability and validity data were obtained. The manual should specify: ideal testing conditions; equipment needed; detailed procedure; verbal instructions to be spoken by the administrator; speed, timing of the test.
- Does the manual include specific and clear details about *scoring* of the test in order to maximize

scoring efficiency and minimize errors: how the items are to be scored, e.g., scoring key? Are sample answers provided with scores allocated? Is allocation of these scores explained?
- Does the manual include clear details on how to convert *raw* scores to *transformed* scores?
- Are criteria for interpretation provided? Is a quantitative assessment given of precision of scores so that the user can determine the confidence which may be attached to them?

An occupational therapist gains the respect of other professional colleagues, and establishes credibility, through the use of widely recognized valid and reliable tests. Also, other specialists may be trained to use the same tests, and then an agreement should be reached about who will assume responsibility for the test administration. There is never justification for proprietary behaviour about 'owning' a test. Some guidelines are presented in the box to help you choose and use tests in the evaluation process.

Gaining information by observation.

Observation is now a systematized disciplined activity, and the special techniques are discussed in Chapter 8.

A therapist may use observation in the evaluation process to:

1. Verify verbal information
2. Gain information about behaviour for which there is no standardized test, e.g., play interactions.

Observation techniques are particularly useful for gaining information about social interactions, and can yield valuable information about an older child's behaviour in a group, e.g. a peer group in a kindergarten (Medinnus (1976). Some guidelines are presented in the box.

Administering a formal evaluation

Therapists who work in cohesive specialist centres where there is a slow turnover of staff have an advantage over those who must work more independently. Where a team exists to deal with a special problem, such as cerebral palsy, the centre's complete evaluation process can be planned as an integral whole. The family and child move through a co-ordinated set of evaluation experiences and receive a comprehensive integrated report at the conclusion. Intervention services to the family flow from the initial evaluation, and reflect agreements reached by the team about their individual roles and functions. Thus, at re-evaluation some time later, specialists can judge the relative impact of the various forms of intervention. Some general hospitals have developed specialist problem teams, e.g., a burns unit team, and a therapist may find him/herself allocated to more than one specialty team.

Diagnostic and pre-therapy

Where the purpose is to assist in making a diagnosis, or to establish a basis for planning therapy, the general steps are as follows:

Step 1: Prepare for the evaluation
Step 2: Assemble basic data about the child
Step 3: Assess the child
Step 4: Collate the results and arrive at interpretations
Step 5: Present a written report

Preparation

Plan the environment

Organize the physical environment to convey competence, efficiency and caring. The interview space should look as though care is taken to organize and maintain equipment and fittings. Some mothers will have doubts about entrusting their child to the care of

a therapist who can't seem to care even for inanimate objects. Ask beforehand who will attend and have enough adult and child-size chairs.

The clinical environment should be suited to the tasks to be performed, and the usual experience of the majority of clients who use the centre. Clients should neither be overwhelmed by the decor nor insulted by it.

For economic reasons, the initial meeting between therapist and the client family in a hospital or other institutional setting normally occurs in the occupational therapy department. However, the therapist may decide to visit the family at home for the initial meeting. All of the preceding comments apply, but then the therapist is the guest and should observe normal rules of visiting. It is suggested that an apprentice therapist avoids performing initial interviews in the client's home until the skills of evaluation are mastered.

Plan the data required

Dyke & Line (personal communication) have identified the information which is generally regarded as necessary to developing a data base from which therapy can be planned, implemented, and monitored. The information is presented as Example 6.3.

Plan the media

Careful thought should be given to the tests considered most appropriate. A comprehensive guide to tests and assessment that are suitable for the occupational therapy evaluation are presented as Appendix VI. Some more specialised evaluation materials are presented in relevant chapters, e.g., general developmental assessment materials are discussed in Chapter 12 on developmental delay.

Plan behaviour management

The therapist needs to be ready to deal with potential medical and behavioural difficulties. For example, if a child is said to have 'convulsions' then the therapist must know how to handle such an occurrence.

Example 6.4 (page 77) presents an approach to a behavioural problem.

Assembling basic data

How much basic data? Therapists differ in their views of the wisdom of collecting information about the child from other specialist colleagues and reports, before the initial occupational therapist meeting. An argument

Example 6.3: Compiling the data base information needed by an occupational therapist

Information required	*Source examples*	*Desired yield*
Name: Date of Birth: (or age)	Case file	Basic identifying information about
Place of residence:	Referral form	client (i.e. demographic base)
Occupational role:	Other colleagues	Family structure and place of client in
Reason for referral to OT:	Initial interview	it
Time of onset of condition:		
(if appropriate)		
Status in family:		

	Client's history	
1. Developmental (for child)	Parent report	1. Influential pre- and post-natal factors
	Other colleague report	2. Maturation pattern in motor skills, cognitive/perceptual skills, social skills
	Tests, e.g., Griffiths Test	
	Observation	3. Timing and degree of achievement of standard developmental milestones
		4. Family patterns of response to child
and		5. Range of child's experiences with:
		(a) usual community resources, e.g., kindergarten
		(b) specialist agencies, e.g., hospital or private practitioner
Play	e.g., Takata 'Play History'	6. Types of activity during, e.g., exploratory, social, manipulative
		7. Toys and other play objects — range, availability
		8. Play spaces — types and use
2. Occupational	Modified occupational history interviewer's guide Section 1 Supplementary information from client or significant other person.	1. Summary of childhood role experiences, i.e., education; hobbies, sports, interests; friendship patterns.
		2. Pattern of changes in occupational role, e.g., student, income earner, homemaker/part-time income earner
		3. Major events influencing occupational role, e.g., marriage, illness of elderly or close relative, etc.
		4. Factors (people and events) influencing choice of occupational career, e.g., scholarship award; income increase; job satisfaction; etc.
	Summary of job Analysis format (If appropriate to age of child client)	5. Description of tasks associated with occupational role in form of job description covering: physical demands; psychological demands; social demands.
		6. Pattern of achievement in occupations
3. Dysfunction	Medico; file; anecdotal report	1. Medical or other condition(s) influencing occupational role
		2. Management

continued on page 76

Time management

4. Routine	e.g., Modified occupational history interviewer's guide Section 2 24 hour Log Activities configuration	1. Profile of client's pattern of time use of 7-day period either — prior to disabling event; or — to point of taking this history, e.g., for an infant with congenital abnormality, or an adult resident in long stay institution 2. If different from 1 gain profile for *current* time use.
5. Preferential	NPI interest check, Modified occupational history interviewer's guide Section 3 Test	Profile of elected activities — past, present and future planned activities and interests Validation of NPI check list information by testing

Present skill performance

Note: At this point the data collection process widens to include a range of specialist tests and procedures to supplement and validate the history thus granted.

6. Physical motor:	Tests, e.g., observation	1. Measurement, e.g., joint range of movement 2. Muscular and eye-hand co-ordination 3. Muscle strength 4. Degree of mobility; factors influencing
7. Perceptual	Tests, e.g., observation	1. Functioning of one or more areas of sensorium 2. Sensory integration status
8. Cognitive, intellectual	Tests	1. Problem identification ability 2. Problem solving strategies and competence 3. Competence in structuring/managing time 4. Describe presenting affect 5. Describe presenting motivational state
9. Social At this point the data collection forms the basis for problem definition.	Tests, e.g., sociogram Observation	1. Range and type of interactions with people 2. Patterns of communication with others
10. Self care	Tests	1. Self concept; general presentation of self 2. Level of independence in feeding; toileting; dressing; bathing 3. Factors influencing competence in 1 or more of above areas e.g. clothing design
11. Occupational role	Tests Observation	1. Level of competence in tasks associated with OR — to provide validation of information from occupational history

At this point the data collection forms the basis for problem definition.

> **Example 6.4: Sam**
> Sam's (age 5 years) record stated 'slow for age and clings to mother'. The therapist can phone or write to Sam's mother, and suggest that she prepare him by reassuring him of her presence at all times. The therapist would prepare developmental test material for the age range 3 to 6 years, and begin her testing at the lower end. Sam is more likely to relax and co-operate; the therapist is more likely to gain an accurate estimate of developmental maturity.

against is that the therapist's view, and possibly judgement, of the child's presenting problem, behaviour, and needs will be influenced unduly. Arguments in favour of collecting information before assessment are that a therapist can expand on information already available; she/he can verify it in another situation; she/he can seek independent evidence to support or refute the observations and findings of others. There is some strength in both sets of arguments, and the only important guide for a therapist to follow is that all data, whenever gathered, must be regarded impartially and objectively.

Once begun, the initial evaluation process should proceed without delay, because the child continues to develop and mature — and thus change. It is a major difference from adult therapy that the effect of the normal growth and developmental process must be considered to be as influential as the pathological condition(s) and/or situation(s).

The 'I care' message

The therapeutic relationship begins to develop at the first meeting between therapist and child and/or parents. Before the meeting the therapist should have collected enough information about the child (who will be the focus) to give the family the message 'I care'. Avoid making parents repeat information that they may have already given, and which is available in reports. Additional to the obvious demographic fact of name, age, sex and stated reason for the child being examined, the therapist should know who else has already seen the child and what they have done. That skeleton of information can then be filled out in conversation with parents. Any information gained before the opening evaluation meeting should be accepted with reservation, and checked in the course of conversation.

It is equally important to prepare in the same way to meet a child who will not have parents present, e.g. in an acute illness hospital. When the child is hospitalized, information can be checked at the first meeting with

parents after assessment has begun. When the family is non-English speaking, every effort should be made to maximize the chance of obtaining accurate information. It may be desirable to use the services of a professional interpreter.

Example 6.5 highlights the importance of caution and checking.

> **Example 6.5: Jim**
> A young medical officer asked the mother of a 4-year-old autistic boy, Jim, a routine question about his feeding pattern in the first year. He asked a very common form of question, namely, 'Feeding okay?'. The mother's reply was 'yes' and the entry in the child's developmental history chart read 'no problems with feeding'.
> Later an incidental remark led another specialist to seek further information from the mother. This specialist used an open-ended question, with the most astounding results. 'Tell me about Jim's early feeding.' Jim's mother gave a detailed picture of a child who demanded certain foods and routines, and a mother who accommodated with measures that forestalled tempers and made life bearable for her.
> The mother's first answer that feeding was 'okay' was indeed true, for her, but unintentionally misleading.

Conducting the initial meeting or interview

Present self and the evaluation process

Introduction is a usual courtesy (but too often forgotten!). Remember also that parents will be anxious and thus likely to forget information — wear a clearly visible name tag. Ask parents if they know why they are seeing an occupational therapist and have a simple prepared explanation to offer them.

Treat family as guests

Show concern for parents' (informants') comfort, including their positioning in relation to you, the evaluator. If parents are to be included as members of the child's team then this message can be conveyed in many ways, for example, by positioning their chairs in an interactive arrangement (Fig. 6.3).

In the illustrated position parents are free to look at or avoid looking at the evaluator; notes are 'open' not hidden; and the small child and siblings can play close by their mother.

Time initially spent in 'small talk' allows each person to relax into the situation. A cup of tea/coffee/soft drink may further help them to relax and gain confidence —

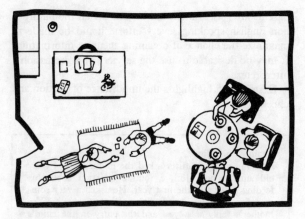

Fig. 6.3 An environment organized to facilitate the evaluation process.

social interactions are always promoted by the presence of food.

Use open ended questions

For example, 'Tell me about . . .', 'I would like to know more about . . .', 'what did you mean when you said . . .'. Leading questions, that is to say, those questions which lead to yes/no answers are of little value, and the example of Jim illustrates how much information may be lost, even when the answer is correctly yes or no. Therapists should use communication skills aimed at eliciting complete and accurate information whilst maintaining the co-operation and goodwill of the client.

Find out what is normal for the client family

Values and customs differ from culture to culture, and subculture. Observe the behaviour that is socially acceptable within the family's culture. For example, in some mid-east cultures the father is the interviewee, though his wife may be present and may provide him with the information. It is important in our multiracial society to determine what is 'normal' within a given family's culture and experience, before making judgements and interpretations affecting the child.

Restrict notetaking

Planning beforehand the information to be collected allows the therapist to structure and control the meeting to some extent. Primarily the initial interview between the therapist and parents opens up avenues of information. The most successful first interview is one which

leads a therapist to ask parents to expand on this or that piece of information, or which leads parents to volunteer information, either then or in later contacts after they have thought about the discussion.

Explain the procedures to be used — simply

It is wise to plan a simple standard statement for each test or procedure which addresses the most important points only. For example, 'The Griffiths Mental Abilities test measures the way Jenny is growing and developing — it is not an intelligence test'. Answer any questions honestly but simply — avoiding technical jargon.

Don't be late and don't conduct the initial meeting in shared space

If possible do not be late for the initial meeting with parents. If that meeting takes place in shared space, both the child and the adults will be distracted and the evaluator's task made more difficult. Parents may interpret the use of shared space as an insult. Arrange with colleagues for the private use of the space.

Don't make parents feel guilty

It is not easy to be a parent! Avoid negative, derogatory and sarcastic comments, the raised eyebrow, the exasperated sigh. Recognize parental need for compassion and support. Banus (1979) suggests a brief statement such as 'We know that this is a problem for many children and it is certainly difficult for the family. For the moment don't concern yourselves with this aspect of the problem. We'll work on it later.'

Don't comment on other colleagues and their techniques

Banus (1979) puts this another way: use discretion when answering the inevitable questions from parents about others that they have already seen. A simple way to fence difficult questions is to turn it back to the questioner, 'What did you have in mind?', 'What do you already know about . . . procedure?' 'What has X already told you about . . .?'

When the child is to be evaluated as an outpatient, the therapist will negotiate the goals and extent of the evaluation with the family at their first meeting. However, where the child is hospitalized and away from the family, the therapist will most likely proceed on her own judgement. The therapist may even begin assessing the child by incorporating some testing into their initial meeting, and the reader is referred to the example of Debbie in Chapter 9.

Assessing the child

Assessing the child is the most time-consuming part of evaluation. Tests are a major source of information (data). A guide to useful tests of different types is presented in Appendix VI. While individual tests have different and specific requirements following practices should always be observed, namely:

1. Include mother

Every effort should be made to include the mother of the infant or young child in the test situation. Ideally the mother should be encouraged to present the test tasks to her child, thus overcoming any resistance to the test situation and promoting a response from the child.

2. Include developmental assessment

A standard developmental assessment should be routinely included in a child's evaluation, at least to the age of seven years. There is always a secondary effect on a child's developmental progress of a pathological condition or situation e.g. spina bifida, Down syndrome, non-accidental injury syndrome. It is important to monitor continuing general developmental progress, and the impact of all intrusions on progress.

3. Avoid excessive testing

Be careful not to overdo testing. Think about what information each of the proposed tests will yield. Then ask yourself if tests are duplicating each other. Don't for example, administer a developmental screening test to a child who is observably delayed. Go straight ahead and administer the full diagnostic developmental assessment.

Example 6.6: Alan
An occupational therapy assessment report
Date of birth: 1.7.1976
Date of assessment: 30.8.79
Alan is the middle child in a family of three: male 6.5 years, male 3 years (Alan), and female 1 year.

Alan came to my attention through his mother Mrs H who is a professional colleague. Subsequently Dr A referred Alan to this Clinic for a full developmental assessment and advice about future management. Mrs H told me that he also suggested that she consult the Assessment Clinic for Intellectually Handicapped, and she arranged that appointment.

Dr A confirmed Alan's diagnosis as 'dygenesis of the corpus callosum', and he defined that as partial but unspecified failure in integration between the two cerebral hemispheres.

Mother's report of developmental history.
Alan was a baby of untoward pregnancy and delivery,

---

but he slept for about 48 hours after birth and refused all attempts to breastfeed him. His facial features were unusual — hairline was at eyebrow level, bridge to nose was not apparent and his nostrils were extremely widespread. A paediatrician queried the possibility of a metabolic disorder; however the baby 'woke up' and behaved perfectly normally thereafter. Some milestones were delayed, e.g., *Sitting*: 8 months (mother feels delay due to low muscle tone). *Crawling*: 1 year. *Walking*: 2 years 1 month but awkward due to low tone. *Fine manipulative skills*: 'at normal time, but awkward', e.g., reached out to mobiles in cot at 5 weeks, held and banged spoon radial palmar grasp at 10 months. *Language*: early cry appropriate, i.e., when needing attention. In quality it was 'a loud bellow'. Babble 'dad dad . . . at 14 months, single clear words at 17 months — 'cat', 'dog', 'light', 'clock'. Two word sentences 'all gone' 17 months. Mrs H feels that his language has regressed since then. *Social behaviour*: an affectionate cuddly little boy' — smiled socially at 4–6 weeks (normal). Attached to family members, shy of strangers.

General summary of occupational therapy assessment
The assessment performed today occupied 1.5 hours; the Griffiths Scale to 2 years was used in conjunction with the Gesell Schedules for 30, 36 and 42 months. Some items from the Albetreccia Test of perceptual function were also presented.

Alan was assessed with his mother present and active in presentation of the test items. The clinic room was free of all objects but the test items and some building blocks, crayons and paper, a telephone, three ladybird picture books on a mat, trampoline and walking board.

General comments

Alan presented as a small lightly built child, thin due to an attack of gastroenteritis. His facial appearance was slightly remarkable – wide set eyes, flaring nostrils, a broad face rather short from hairline to chin. He smiled often at me and his mother, in an engaging manner.

He moved in a loosely co-ordinated awkward manner and appeared 'floppy'. On entering the test room he showed interest in the toys displayed, leaving his mother to explore each. After spending a minute or two with each he sat down and began scribbling in a nonspecific way with large crayons on paper.

Initially, when each of the test items was presented, he appeared curious but resisted most of my attempts to have him use the object or complete the task. All activities were presented with both verbal request and demonstration. It was difficult to judge whether he did not understand the requirement, simply did not wish to engage in the task, or was afraid to fail. Mrs H said that at home Alan spent most of his time playing with his cars.

Throughout the 1.5 hours Alan made frequent vocalizations, and said about four words in recognition of objects on the test cards. All words sounded similar, i.e., 'cat' but his mother was able to distinguish cat, car, key. Alan's Speech was high pitched and high in tone. *It was my strong impression that he did not hear my speech to him.* For example, he did not look up when I spoke, did not watch my face or blink, and made no response when given directions without visual cues. I noted that Mrs H consistently made an effort to catch his eye and used visual cueing whenever she spoke to him. However, she was apparently unaware of her own behaviour when I commented on it. Alan did respond to his own name when his mother called him.

Developmental assessment

Alan's performance on the second year level of the Griffiths Scale was inconsistent between the five areas of behaviour represented on the scale. The area of 'Hearing and Speech' was extremely depressed with only three items passed out of 21. Where he failed in other areas the items were either language related directly, or were adaptive behaviour arising from language experience. Therefore the scale was not scored to arrive at a general developmental quotient.

However, if the language area is excepted, then both on the Griffiths Scale and the Gesell Schedules he appears to be functioning at about the 30 month level when he is chronologically 36 months. The profiles of both tests are attached.

Muscle tone throughout his body is low. Consequently grasp, while being pincer, appears normal.

All movement patterns appear jerky and poorly integrated and even *mildly athetotic*

Bilateral upper limb activity was apparently easy for him, e.g., he could catch and throw a medium sized ball. He had no trouble crossing the midline of his body with either arm. He appeared to be dominantly right handed. Eye dominance not tested.

Gait: Walked on a wide base, putting toe down first followed much later by heel. He could not balance on one foot.

Righting responses: Could not be elicited when Alan was held in prone. He became very vocal in this position, chattering and smiling either in excitement or apprehension.

Attention: He moved very rapidly from one activity to another and it was difficult to hold his attention for more than a few seconds.

Fine motor skills: His experience appeared limited. He could not use scissors but did build a tower of 6 2.5 cm cubes. His mother reported that he is not particularly interested in toys that might facilitate fine motor skills.

RECOMMENDATIONS

1. Hearing test — to be followed up with speech therapy whatever the test result.
2. Examination to determine whether he is mildly athetoid.
3. Inclusion in a systematic development stimulation preschool group where there is a multidisciplinary team, such as exists at the Spastic Centre.
4 Individual therapy with Mrs H included to increase muscle tone, improve attending behaviour, and facilitate independence in dressing and feeding.

I would be very happy to continue work with Alan and his family. However, I believe that they will be better helped by a resource centre, where specialist facilities are available in an integrated team approach including education facilities.

Occupational Therapist

Arriving at interpretations

In some standardized tests the interpretation of the results is straightforward and automatic. For example, should a child score a specified number of items in certain combinations, on the Denver Developmental Screening Test then the test result is 'abnormal', and full diagnostic testing is indicated. There is no need for detailed reporting or further time spent considering the test result. However, such is not the case for most tests, even where a straightforward statistical result is obtained, and the case of Alan provides a useful example.

Variables which can influence results

The evaluating therapist must take time considering what obvious factors (variables) influenced the assessment. The following variables should be carefully considered:

- The observable factors which might have influenced the child's performance
- The range of explanations for the result
- The relationships between the test(s) results, reported information and observation data.

Observable factors. Some examples of observable factors which might have influenced the child's performance are: the time of day in relation to child's normal sleeping; mother's behaviour in the test situation; therapist's experience with the test; amount of testing that child has already experienced.

Explanations for results. Usually evaluation data can be interpreted in more than one way (Example 6.7). Knowing the range of possible explanations, the skill of weighing them against each other and choosing among them will come with experience and practice.

OT test, OT interpretation. The interpretations an occupational therapist will make must reflect a therapeutic frame of reference, different from that of a physical therapist, or other specialist. For example, when an occupational therapist assesses a child's pattern of reflex behaviour, then the interpretations of the test results must go beyond a statement of the presence or absence of a reflex. The test interpretation must explain the relationships between the detected pattern and functional behaviour e.g. feeding for the tested child (see the example of 'Alan' — Example 6.6).

Relationship between test result, reported information, observation data. Taken as a whole the different sets of evaluation information should clarify, confirm and extend the interpretations that a therapist might make. It is quite often the case that one set of information appears to confound another set. Then the therapist must check and recheck until the dissonance between the sets is resolved satisfactorily, if possible. The child must be viewed not only on the basis of his performance in the assessment situations, but also as a component of his family which is a dynamic changing interacting system.

Example 6.7: Katy
Developmental testing revealed that Katy (6 months) could not hold her head erect, nor sit without support, and had generalized trunk and upper limb muscle hypotonia.

The possible explanations (differential diagnosis) were: primary intellectual handicap, CNS pathology, environmental factors.

Mrs Z was a Yugoslav migrant and Katy her first child. To rule out the latter environmental explanation the therapist asked the parents specific questions: namely, 'When Katy is in her cot, how does she lie — on her tummy or back? What parts of the day is she in her cot (*not* 'how long' though that is the desired information)? When she cries how do you quiet her? What parts of the day does she spend sitting (on a floor; in a chair; on a bed)?'

The objective of the questioning was to discover whether Katy is a baby who spends long periods on her back in her cot. As it turned out she did. Mother reported that Katy never cried. However, observation revealed that mother did not alert to Katy's crying and so it went unheeded. The child's failure to manipulate objects and bring them to her mouth and her generalized upper limb hypotonicity were predictable sequelae. Assessment of Katy continued, in order to rule out pathology in the child, and no pathology was detected. Further investigation of mother's handling practices were made. Mrs Z followed her normal cultural practice of placing Katy on her back (in contrast to the American practice of putting children on their tummy). Mrs Z was also found to be deeply unhappy in her new country, and because of language differences, almost totally isolated within society. These findings were enough to explain Katy's delayed developmental behaviour.

Reporting the evaluation results

The evaluation may be presented in two ways:

a. A written report
b. A verbal report

Written reports

A general discussion of how to keep records and present reports is discussed in Chapter 8. However, there are some important elements specific to presenting evalu-

ation reports which logically belong in this chapter and which will assist the therapist to communicate effectively the results to other specialists and families. Some guidelines are given on presenting the initial evaluation report.

Guidelines for presenting a written report
1. Identify the child clearly.
2. State the date, place and reason for the evaluation.
3. Give a *brief* outline of the evaluation process, e.g., tests used, who was present.
4. Present the most important results first, and the useful, but non-essential, detail last.

An evaluation report should be written in clear simple language, understandable by any who reads it. There must be no possibility that the report itself can be misinterpreted either because of information left out, ambiguity, the use of obscure or exotic jargon, or unbalanced presentation of the findings.

It is the evaluating therapist's responsibility to interpret the evaluation procedures and make the findings explicit for the reader. The therapist should not expect that others will understand, or even know of, specialist occupational therapy tests and terminology. The therapist must explain the meaning of findings, as well as the particular interpretations.

The evaluating therapist will always send a formal written report to the person who referred the child. That person would usually be a medical practitioner, a school teacher or another specialist colleague. Should the child's parents have initiated the evaluation, then they receive the report. Usually the therapist seeks their permission to send a copy of the report to the family's doctor for records. It needs to be kept in mind however, that policies regarding who can receive a copy of written reports varies from agency to agency.

Verbal reports

It is likely that a therapist will be required to present a verbal account of her written report to the specialist team, or other colleagues. Some guidelines are presented in the next box.

The listener must absorb a great deal of important information, and anecdotes tend to distract. Nevertheless make the presentation interesting by use of voice change, facial cues, use of eye contact.

The child's parents will also seek a verbal report of the evaluation. In some centres the policy is that only the team leader releases information. In such a case the

---

Guidelines for presenting a verbal report

Do's:

1. Draw attention to *major conclusions* first
2. List recommendation briefly
3. Expand briefly on (1.) and (2.) by noting how conclusions and recommendations have been reached.

Don'ts:

1. Don't read the written form of the report
2. Don't tell amusing anecdotes about the evaluation

---

therapist should direct the parents to the appropriate person. However, more often a therapist will discuss an evaluation report with the child's parents. The evaluating therapist may find it a difficult task, especially if the evaluation has revealed or confirmed pathology in the child. Parents seek a *simple* explanation of what it means in terms of the child's present development, and what the finding means in terms of the predictable future. Much information has to be absorbed, and it may not be welcome or even acceptable. Great caution should be exercised in showing graphs and other baseline assessment information to parents who may not be familiar with such material and may become alarmed unnecessarily.

Parents need to know what help can be offered to them and their child. The therapist should learn to be gentle and supportive of parents as they seek to understand and come to terms with evaluation results. Usually it is helpful if a second appointment is made about one to two weeks after parents first learn evaluation results. Then the family has time to absorb information, formulate their own questions and come to some decisions about their responses. A therapist who listens and responds sensitively to a family at the end point of evaluation, will help them proceed to therapy in a most productive way for their child.

CONCLUSION

There no short cut through the evaluation process, particularly if it is to be a responsible exercise which can provide a reliable basis for assisting diagnosis or planning therapy. The arguments 'We haven't the time', 'Our case load is too big' will not do. A therapist, like other specialists, is a child's advocate. Every precaution must be taken to ensure that wrong decisions are not taken that may affect the child's future growth and development. It is true that evaluation will most likely engage a therapist in many hours of work — often

tedious and exacting. However, there are some practical measures that may be taken to reduce the overall amount of clinical time that must be allotted to evaluations.

Though each child is a unique individual, problems do fall into general classes. The time-consuming task of preparation can be eased by collating appropriate 'kits' of tests and other evaluation requirements. The content of such 'kits' could include history taking and other forms, which would be relevant for dealing with children/families with the range of problems normally referred to the clinical centre. These 'kits' are then

---

Evaluation checklist

1. Prepare for evaluation
- Is purpose of evaluation clearly identified?
- Has information needed been identified?
- Have data collection means been selected e.g. interview profile, tests?
- Has appointment been made to see client child and/or family?
- Has suitable room been booked for use at the appointed time, and the necessary equipment checked for lost/broken parts?

2. Collecting evaluation data
- Is room suitably arranged?
- Have you:
  — introduced self, explained purpose of meeting;
  — recorded demographic information;
  — asked parents what they expect/hope to gain from tests etc?
- If child under seven years, is a standard developmental test included?

3. Interpreting results
- Have all factors likely to influence child's performance been noted? (time of day; environmental distractions; cultural differences/experiences).
- Have relationships been considered between results of tests, reported anecdotal information, and observed behaviour?

4. Reporting findings
- Has a report been prepared for referring specialist; other appropriate persons? Is it free of unexplained jargon? Does it present the most important findings first, followed by qualifying explanations? Are there clear recommendations, with own future role identified?
- Have findings been explained to, and discussed with child's parents — and their response conveyed to referring agent?
- If intervention is to follow, have options been presented to parents about possible goals and methods, related to predictable outcomes?
- Where no intervention, has invitation been extended to parents to return for further support/information/guidance/re-evaluation?

available for use immediately when needed. Another advantage of this practical measure is that lost or broken components, and a diminishing supply of necessary testing forms (profiles) is quickly identified, before there is serious inconvenience to yourself and other therapists sharing the resources.

Develop a recognizable pattern for your evaluation reports. Colleagues will learn to 'know their way around' an occupational therapy report. Your report will be read and valued because it *reliably* eases the team's total work load.

Soon you should find that evaluation is not a chore to be dreaded. Rather, like research, evaluation will become an exciting quest to help find answers to questions which present themselves.

Use a checklist to aid administration of the evaluation process when embarking on a client evaluation. This will develop a disciplined systematic approach.

REFERENCES

Banus B S 1979 The developmental therapist, 2nd edn. Charles B Slack, Springfield

Dyke J, Line J Personal Communication. Student tutorial paper. University of Queensland Department of Occupational Therapy

Gething L 1983 Personal communication

Griffith R 1954 The abilities of babies. University of London Press, London

Gronlund N E 1978 Stating objectives for classroom instruction. Macmillan, New York

Medinnus G R 1976 Child study and observation guide. John Wiley, New York

Takata N 1974 Play as a prescription. In: Reilly M (ed) Play as exploratory learning. Sage Publications, Beverly Hills

Vestre N D, Zimmerman R 1969 Validity of informants of psychiatric patients. Journal of Consulting and Clinical Psychology 33(2): 175–179

Yarrow M R, Campbell J D, Burton R V 1970 Recollections of childhood. Monographs of the Society for Research in Child Development 35(5) No. 138

Zunich M 1962 Relationship between maternal behaviour and attitudes toward children. Journal of Genetic Psychology 100: 155 –165

RECOMMENDED READING

Coley I L 1978 Pediatric assessment of self-care: Ch 13. C V Mosby, St Louis

Ulrey G, Rogers S 1982 Psychological assessment of handicapped infants and young children. Thames-Stratton, New York

7. General principles of intervention

READERS' OBJECTIVES

After reading this chapter, you should be able to:

1. Define and discuss the characteristics and principles of general systems theory.
2. Be able to represent the process of therapy diagrammatically, relating it to the general systems theory model.
3. Be able to write terminal and enabling therapy objectives for children in behavioural terms.
4. From a given set of objectives, be able to write an integrated therapy programme.

Some form of intervention usually flows from the initial evaluation of a child and family. Effective therapy will present a child and family with challenges, in the form of problems to be solved. But the therapy process must also provide the ways and means for the client family to explore different strategies to arrive at solutions. At the broadest level, specialists aim to integrate their intervention with the life activities of the client. At the detailed programme design level each specialist integrates objectives, media, activity, ways of presenting therapy, and procedures for evaluating the programmes' effectiveness and this process was shown in Figure 6.1. There are three questions which confront a therapist considering programme design. They are:

1. What are the desired outcomes from the intervention?
2. What is the information needed to plan a programme, in relation to outcomes?
3. What is the process and set of strategies most likely to achieve the desired outcomes?

INTEGRATED THERAPY PROGRAMMES

An integrated therapy programme represents a systematic interlocking of various components, such as time use, specialist roles and objectives, into one complex intervention plan. One example of an integrated intervention programme in a residential centre, comprising four apartments for intellectually handicapped and autistic children four to twelve-years-old is presented in Figure 7.1. The overriding objective of the intervention team was that the maximum number of the children's waking hours should be controlled to achieve maximum therapeutic impact, and the day's programme. See Chapter 14 for further discussion of this particular programme.

A theoretical model

Integrated therapy programmes reflect practical application of a theoretical model — the General Systems Theory (Cannon 1932, Von Bertalanffy 1968, West Churchman 1968 Wright 1923). In the systems or cybernetic view, a system is defined as a conglomerate of components which interact with each other. Thus, a family or a hospital is a system, and so is a therapy in-

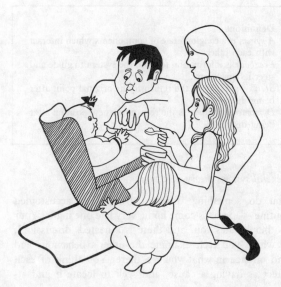

Period	Group activity	Apartment 1	Apartment 2	Apartment 3	Apartment 4
am 8–9	Breakfast Kitchen activities				
9–10		OT	Language	Social skills	School
10–11		School	Social skills	OT	Language
11–12		Social skills	School	Language	OT
pm 12	Lunch Rest time				
1–2	Team meets				
2–3		Language	OT	School	Social skills
3–4	Play				
4–5	Story time — TV 'Sesame Street'				
5–6	Dinner				
6–8	Structured indoor play Bath				
8.00	Bed time				

Fig. 7.1 A fully integrated daily intervention plan for 4–12-year-old children living in an institution in apartment groups of 8–10 children and 2 adults. From Clancy H G 1976 Integrating the environment in therapy. Man–Environment Systems 6: 305–12. Reproduced by permission of the publisher.

tervention programme. The cybernetic model holds that any accidental or designed intervention into an existing system gives rise to disruption and resounding change throughout the whole system as attempts are made to restore the status quo or equilibrium. Before considering therapy examples let us take one everyday experience and compare and contrast the familiar linear cause/effect way of explaining events, with the cybernetic or systems way.

> **Definitions**
> *A system* is a conglomerate of components which interact with each other.
> *Feedback* is information fed into the system to guide and steer its operations.
> *Static equilibrium* is the return to the original point after being disturbed.
> *Dynamic equilibrium* is the return to a new position after being disturbed.

General systems theory in action

You do something different from your accustomed routine — perhaps come home very late one night. Your mother berates you, and there is a heated 'discussion', in which you each examine the other's behaviour and find offence in what you see there. You think of each effect as having a cause, and seek to locate it and at-

tribute blame. Both know that nothing would be settled if you were able to find who was to blame, yet you engage in the exercise — every time — knowing that it is pointless, but not understanding why. The model of blame, responsibility, cause and effect, is one of 'linear thinking'. There are many possible outcomes, but generally there is either 'guilt' and reconciliation, or accumulated bitterness and blame, and a course toward the breaking or loosening of the bond. It seems that everyone starts off as a 'linear thinker', possibly because cause and effect models of events seem very reasonable, and are used all around us as we grow up. Whenever something goes wrong, we look immediately for a cause, someone or something to 'blame' or sometimes to 'cure'.

The systems view of the example event would regard the relationship between you and your mother as one dynamic unit in the *family system*. The relationship is called 'homeostatic', or normally maintained in a steady state. Maintenance involves constant checking for change — a process we are not even consciously aware of, until change is detected.

In another example, wearing unmatched and therefore inappropriate socks may lead your mother to give a vigorous corrective response, called a *negative feedback* — in order to restore the steady state, or equilibrium, in the family system. Negative feedbacks are directed toward the maintenance of stability.

Feedback is defined as information fed into a system to guide and steer its operations. If it is totally effective

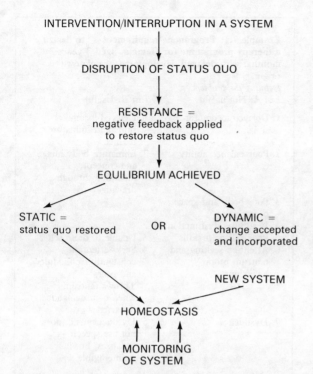

INTERVENTION/INTERRUPTION IN A SYSTEM

DISRUPTION OF STATUS QUO

RESISTANCE =
negative feedback applied
to restore status quo

EQUILIBRIUM ACHIEVED

STATIC =   OR   DYNAMIC =
status quo restored   change accepted
                                 and incorporated

NEW SYSTEM

HOMEOSTASIS

MONITORING
OF SYSTEM

Fig. 7.2 The general systems theory components and their interrelationships.

at first then the original equilibrium is restored — nothing changes in the system, and in our example, you change your odd socks, and don't try that one again! This situation is described as *static equilibrium*, i.e., return to the original point after being disturbed. However, a systems thinking parent would soon see that the authoritarian response was not working, and would reach some negotiated compromise with you about the wearing of the odd socks. In this situation all components of the system — you, your mother, and the rest of the family system — alter in some way. After a tussle, agreement leads to withdrawal of the negative feedback and the new equilibrium reached is termed a *dynamic equilibrium*, i.e., return to a new position after being disturbed. The essential components of systems theory are represented diagrammatically as in Figure 7.2.

The dynamic equilibrium is the one sought from therapy intervention. Yet, it is not uncommon to hear therapists make comments like the following one. 'Well, she/he wears his/her calipers *here*, but my guess is that they get thrown in the cupboard at home between visits to therapy.' Such comments carry an implicit, and sometimes even an explicit message that the child's parents resist the therapy, and are unappreciative. The therapist is using a cause-effect linear thinking ap-

proach, in which the individual model is used — we treat the child and/or symptom or problem — with the best intentions. Sadly, the practical outcome from applying linear thinking is, too often, long drawn-out therapy programmes, with less than maximum effectiveness. Such linear thinking can result in the therapist and the client family becoming alienated, feelings of anger and frustration on both sides and then *overt* conflict; when really all the family is doing is behaving normally as a dynamic unit in a system attempting to maintain a steady state.

The systems model is a helpful one because it allows understanding and prediction about the therapy process, and therefore control over it. Applying systems thinking to the therapy example we would say 'Okay if we want the child to wear calipers, i.e., change his/her behaviour, we must also *simultaneously* work to change the behaviour of the rest of the system — the family — so that it works with, not against the change.' Thus, the value of the systems approach applied as integrated therapy programming appears to be that:

1. It promotes efficient use of resources — therapist, materials, client
2. It promotes effective programme design
3. It facilitates a therapeutic client/therapist relationship based on understanding, empathy and compassion. A systems thinking therapist is genuinely able to programme for 'the whole person'
4. Therapy based on the cybernetic or general systems model leads to role satisfaction for a therapist, and client satisfaction because the effectiveness of intervention becomes obvious quite rapidly.

General systems theory applied to therapy

Weed (1971) applied the general systems theory to medical clinical practice and designed a 'problem oriented record' — the practical expression of a new systems approach to patient case management. Several others have applied Weed's model specifically to occupational therapy practice (for example, Gilaudas 1973, Kielhofner 1978, Line 1969, Olsen 1983, Potts 1972). Figure 7.3 illustrates the occupational therapy system processes that have been identified.

Designing an integrated therapy programme

Deciding what problems to address

Such decisions will be influenced by many factors, such as the time available, the therapist's current case

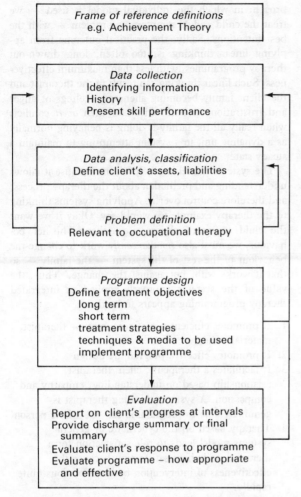

Fig. 7.3 System components of the occupational therapy process, and their relationship (after Dyke & Line, student tutorial paper).

load, and most importantly, the parents, wishes. For example, if the child's mother is most concerned about her child's slowness to be toilet trained, this behaviour should have high priority, even though in the therapist's judgement, the child's peer interaction, and play skills are equally in need of attention.

The outcome will be a set of problems arranged in an order of priority. The priorities must reflect the client's needs, not the therapist's needs. It is from the identified problem list that the therapy intervention strategies will be formulated. Thus, problems must be expressed very precisely, without any hint of ambiguity, and focusing on observed behaviour. Example 7.1 presents a set of problems defined in an unhelpful way, and then redefined helpfully.

Example 7.1: Programme requirement — to design a therapy programme for Gemma, aged 3 years 3 months, with delayed development of unknown origin.
Defining the problem

List A: Not useful	*List B*: Useful
1. Delayed locomotor skills	1. Delayed locomotor skills and immature balance
2. Poor balance ability	2. Immature body image and concept, identified through drawings
3. Poor body and space perception	
4. Vestibular dysfunction	
5. Poor self-help skills	3. Unable to dress self
6. Attention seeking and tantrum prone behaviour	4. Seeks attention constantly from adults and peers. Throws tantrums when own demands thwarted
7. Dysfluency	5. Dysfluency, i.e, does not use speech — vocalizes, but is unintelligible

Problem set A is not considered useful because the wording is imprecise, (e.g., 'self-help skills'), subjective (e.g., 'poor'), and assumptive (e.g., vestibular dysfunction).

Team roles and functions

If specialists do not integrate their roles, and their objectives, it is very easy for aspects of a child's needs to be inadvertently overlooked; duplication and waste of effort can also occur. Here is an example of what may happen when specialists fail to negotiate their roles and functions. Both Miss Best the occupational therapist and Mrs Jones the Special Education teacher correctly identified that Jane's perceptual visuomotor skills needed to be refined and strengthened. Jane also needed help learning to dress. However, both specialists, working alone, put their energies into promoting sound basic perception skills. Dressing was inadvertently overlooked, whilst there was duplication of effort in the area of acquiring basic perceptual skills.

Writing therapy objectives

Writing objectives can be a most perplexing and frustrating task, and it requires a range of skills. In recognition of their importance, the design of well-framed objectives will be discussed in detail.

Therapists often use 'goal' and 'objective' interchangeably. This is inadvisable because a goal is an end or terminal point, whereas objectives represent the steps to be mastered in order to meet the goal.

The value of stating objectives is that the therapist, other specialists, and the client family know what is being attempted in the intervention. Further, the objectives provide a guide to the selection of media/activities and the resources to be used. objectives also guide the choice of assessments to be used for evaluation purposes.

When constructing objectives the therapist must focus on what the child/family should be able to do at the end of the therapy — or at designated points along the line. Thus, we say that objectives must be expressed 'in behavioural terms'. For example, an objective might be stated thus 'The child has age appropriate fine motor manipulation skills'. However, a more appropriate statement would be 'The child reaches for, grasps and manipulates two objects in the midline e.g. bangs them together'. Expressed in this way the objective can be measured, because it is stated so precisely. There must be no doubt what outcome is desired from the interaction (Krathwohl et al 1964).

The words used to express objectives can either facilitate therapy, actually impede the process, or simply render it useless. Fabb & Harrison (1975) formulated a guide to words and phrases that are commonly used by therapists, and that they consider to be suitable or unsuitable for use.

Precise words or phrases *Use*	Imprecise words or phrases *Avoid*
to write	to know
to identify	to understand
to differentiate	to really understand
to solve	to appreciate
to construct	to fully appreciate
to list	to grasp the significance of
to compare	to be acquainted with
to contrast	to be familiar with
to conduct	to perceive
to demonstrate	to be aware of
to express	to realize
to state	to comprehend
to choose	to remember
to describe	to sympathize with
to demonstrate acceptance of	to enjoy
to elicit response from	to believe

Therapy objectives are usually classified as:

1. Terminal
2. Enabling

Definitions
Terminal objectives are those which represent the desired end points of intervention. These may also be called 'long-term goals'.
Enabling objectives are those which, as the name suggests, help to reach the desired end point. These are often, but erroneously called 'short-term goals'.

Checklist for judging whether objectives are clearly expressed (Miller 1971)

- Is the objective real and understandable?
- Is the objective defined in terms of the behaviour of the learner?
- Is the objective based on the educational needs of the learner?
- Is the objective achievable?
- Is the objective measurable?

Poorly constructed objectives are those:
— which state what the therapist intends to do, rather than what is desired of the child;
— which describe the learning process;
— which describe the media/materials/techniques of therapy;
— which contain more than one outcome.

Two sets of therapy objectives are now presented. In Example 7.2 Gemma's problems identified from Example 7.1, (List B) are related to well expressed and associated objectives.

In Example 7.3, a different range of problems are expressed through terminal and enabling objectives.

Designing therapy to achieve objectives

There are different ways of presenting the procedural

Example 7.2: Terminal and enabling objectives for Gemma flowing from identified problems presented in example 7.1, List B

Problem Number (List B)	Terminal Objective	Enabling Objective
1, 2, 3	A Child demonstrates competent motor skills	Aa Maintains static and dynamic equilibrium
		Ab Demonstrates well co-ordinated quadrupedal movements
		Ac Walks up and down stairs one foot at a time
3	B Demonstrates integrated and age-appropriate body image and concept	Ba Demonstrates accurate location of body parts
		Bb Demonstrates functions of body parts in relation to space
4	C Can dress self independently at 3 year 4 month level	Ca Can put on coat and upper body clothes — no fastening
		Cb Can put on trousers and underclothes — no fastening
		Cc Can put on shoes/socks no laces
5	D Complies with reasonable adult demands	Da Shares toys/activities when requested
		Db Complies with simple directions

Example 7.3: Robert, aged 15 months, Prader-Willi Syndrome
Identified problem: significantly delayed motor development

Terminal objectives	Enabling objectives
A R. creeps effectively prone, forward and backward directions	Aa R. lifts head while supports body by flexing elbows and resting forearms on supporting surface.
prone, forward and backward directions	Ab R. supports body while prone, on extended arms.
	Ac R. demonstrates forward and backward crawling movements.
	Ad R. lifts abdomen from floor, takes weight on flexed knees, and moves.
B Explores and manipulates objects in play involving spatial relations, distance, shape, and conservation perception.	Ba R. can find an object and/or person which appears and disappears from sight.
	Bb R. can match shapes as on simple formboard games.
	Bc R. can stack items of graduated sizes in correct relationship to each other.
	Bd R. manipulates and 'stores' up to 4 small objects in bilateral hand tasks.
C Attempts to use language to communicate own needs.	Ca R. identifies familiar objects by pointing at, first on request, later spontaneously.

component of the therapy intervention. Figure 7.4 presents a problem-solving model of practice which illustrates how all of the components should be integrated to achieve an effective total programme.

Figure 7.5 presents another way to express the procedural component of face to face therapy — to be used by either the therapist, or the child's caregiver.

Scheduling therapy sessions. Therapy given on the 'half-an-hour three times a week' prescriptive basis may be irrelevant — for example, to teach dressing skills. At best, it will be very difficult for the child to generalize the special skills learned in the therapy session to the real life situation, e.g., getting dressed in the morning and undressed in the evening each day.

Time is important in another way. The effects of

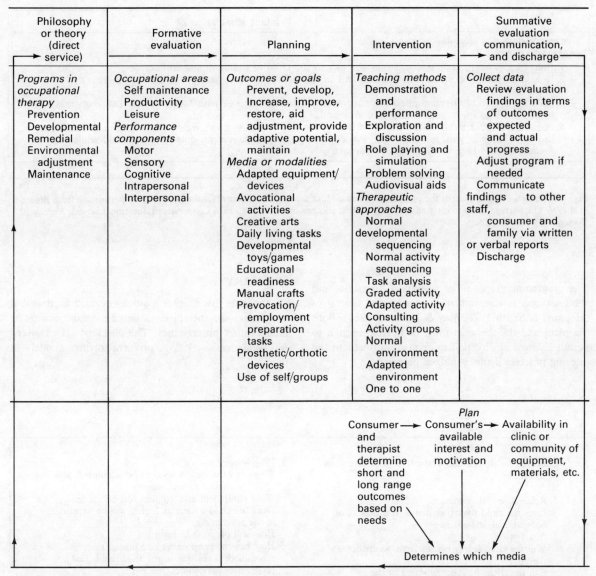

Philosophy or theory (direct service)	Formative evaluation	Planning	Intervention	Summative evaluation communication, and discharge
Programs in occupational therapy Prevention Developmental Remedial Environmental adjustment Maintenance	*Occupational areas* Self maintenance Productivity Leisure *Performance components* Motor Sensory Cognitive Intrapersonal Interpersonal	*Outcomes or goals* Prevent, develop, Increase, improve, restore, aid adjustment, provide adaptive potential, maintain *Media or modalities* Adapted equipment/ devices Avocational activities Creative arts Daily living tasks Developmental toys/games Educational readiness Manual crafts Prevocation/ employment preparation tasks Prosthetic/orthotic devices Use of self/groups	*Teaching methods* Demonstration and performance Exploration and discussion Role playing and simulation Problem solving Audiovisual aids *Therapeutic approaches* Normal developmental sequencing Normal activity sequencing Task analysis Graded activity Adapted activity Consulting Activity groups Normal environment Adapted environment One to one	*Collect data* Review evaluation findings in terms of outcomes expected and actual progress Adjust program if needed Communicate findings to other staff, consumer and family via written or verbal reports Discharge

Plan

Consumer and therapist determine short and long range outcomes based on needs → Consumer's available interest and motivation → Availability in clinic or community of equipment, materials, etc.

Determines which media

Fig. 7.4 A problem-solving model of occupational therapy practice. Reproduced by permission from Reed K L, Sanderson S R 1983 Concepts of occupational therapy. Williams & Wilkins, Baltimore © 1983 The Williams & Wilkins Co, Baltimore.

short periods of isolated special therapy are totally overshadowed when there are long hours spent away, perhaps in ways that positively hinder growth and maturation (Clancy 1976). This can be particularly true in residential institutions where specialists go home at 4.00 or 5.00 pm, and no therapy is offered over weekends. Oswin (1973) perceptively extends this discussion about the importance of time planning in her book *The Empty Hours*.

Evaluating outcomes

In the previous chapter it was suggested that a therapist must always judge programme effectiveness by reference to two aspects:

— the responses of the child and his/her family;
— the therapy process — the appropriateness of identified problems, objectives, media and strategies, and the therapist's own style.

Infant stimulation 27

TITLE: Maintains eye contact 3 seconds
WHAT TO DO:
1. Hold face close to child's face, smile and talk to the child to maintain eye contact.
2. Hold a bright object near your eye and call child's name. Talk animatedly to him to maintain eye contact.
3. Hold child with his head cupped in your hands so that he can see your face and lips. Lean towards him, smile and make some exaggerated sounds.
4. Focus all of your attention on the child during feeding time, i.e. don't watch TV or read a book. When the child looks at you, reinforce with eye contact. Talking or humming quietly to the child while feeding should help to establish eye contact.

Fig. 7.5 Another way to present the procedural component of face-to-face therapy. Card reproduced by permission from Bluma S et al 1976 The Portage guide to early education: checklist and resource cards. © 1976 Cooperative Educational Service Agency 12 Portage, Wisconsin USA.

The programme needs to be reasonable, possible, and show a direct relationship to the formulated objectives (Hopkins & Smith 1978, May & Newman 1980). Both the plan, and the therapist must be flexible enough to permit changes in direction to be made throughout the ongoing process, if this is judged necessary.

SUMMARY

To conclude this chapter a quick checklist is presented to assist a therapist designing and evaluating inter-vention programmes. The checklist reflects Reed & Sanderson's (1983) problem-solving model of therapy.

Checklist for design and evaluation of intervention programmes

1. Referral, initial evaluation
   Does the child have potential or real deficits in occupational performance?
2. Analysis
   Will the child/family benefit from occupational therapy?
   Can the client be accommodated in the occupational therapy schedule?
3. Formative
   What is the child's entering evaluation level of occupational performance?
   Is the child/family receptive to the concept of occupational therapy?
4. Plan
   What are the child's problems in occupational performance (summarized)?
   What principles (outcome) of occupational therapy can be applied?
   What media, method or techniques will be used?
   What short or long range objectives will be established by the person and therapist?
5. Programme
   When can the child's sessions be scheduled, how often, for how long and where?
   What equipment and supplies will be needed?
   Does the child understand what will be happening in the programme?
   How will progress be recorded?
   How can the programme be adjusted to accommodate changes in the child/family and programme environment?
6. Summative evaluation
   What is the change in occupational performance since the programme began?
   Is the change to the desired level or objective?
   Can the programme be changed to increase the chance of reaching the objective?
   Should the programme be stopped, continued or revised?
   Who should be notified of any changes made?
7. Discharge
   Should the child/family be discharged?
   Should referral be made to other resources?
   Has all documentation been completed and communicated?

REFERENCES

Cannon W 1932 The wisdom of the body. Norton, New York

Clancy H G 1976 Integrating the environment in therapy. Man–Environment Systems 6: 305–12

Dyke J, Line J L Student tutorial paper. University of Queensland, Department of Occupational Therapy, Brisbane

Fabb W E, Harrison R F F 1975 Vocational training for family practice — family medicine programme, Royal Australian College of General Practitioners, Melbourne

Gilaudas A 1973 Problem oriented record. Australian New Zealand Journal Psychiatry 7: 138

Hopkins H L, Smith H D 1978 Willard & Spackman's occupational therapy. J B Lippincott, Philadelphia

Kielhofner G 1978 General systems theory: implications for theory and action in occupational therapy. American Journal of Occupational Therapy 3210: 637–645

Kielhofner G 1983 Health through occupation. F A Davis, Philadelphia

Krathwohl D R, Bloom B S, Masia B B 1964 Taxonomy of educational objectives — the classification of educational goals. Handbook II: the affective domain. Longman & Green, New York

Line J M 1969 Case method as a scientific form of clinical thinking. American Journal of Occupational Therapy 23(4): 308–313

May B J, Newman J 1980 Developing competence in problem solving. In Physical Therapy 60(9): 1140–1145

Miller G E 1971 Educational objectives, World Health Organization mimeographed document, Geneva

Oswin M 1973 The empty hours. Penguin, Harmondsworth

Olsen S L 1983 Teaching treatment planning — a problem solving model. In Physical Therapy 63, 4: 526–529

Potts L R 1972 The problem oriented record: implications for occupational therapy. American Journal of Occupational Therapy 26(6): 288–291

von Bertalanffy L 1968 General system theory. George Brazelton, New York

Reed K L, Sanderson S R 1983 Concepts of occupational therapy. Williams & Wilkins, Baltimore

Weed L 1971 Medical records, medical education and patient care. Year Book Publications, Chicago

West Churchman C 1968 The systems approach. Delta Books, New York

Wright S 1923 The theory of path co-efficients. Genetics 8: 239–255

RECOMMENDED READING

The cybernetic or systems view

Boulding K 1956 General systems theory — the selection of science. Management Science 2

Emshoff J R 1971 Analysis of behavioural systems. Macmillan, New York

Gray W, Duhl F, Rizzo N (eds) 1967 General systems theory and psychiatry. Little Brown, Boston

Kantor D 1975 Inside the family. Jossey, San Francisco

Reilly M (ed) 1973 Play as exploratory learning. Sage Publications, Beverley Hills

Weick C 1969 The social psychology of organizing. Addison-Wesley, Reading

Therapy planning, programming

American Occupational Therapy Association 1968 Occupational therapy manual on administration. American Journal of Occupational Therapy, Rockville

American Occupational Therapy Association Task Force on Social Issues 1972 Report of the task force on social issues. American Journal of Occupational Therapy 26: 332–359

American Occupational Therapy Association Task Force on Target Populations 1974 Task force on target populations I & II. American Journal of Occupational Therapy 28(3–4)

American Occupational Therapy Association 1975 An annotated bibliography of journal articles, Occupational Therapy Administration (1965–1974). American Occupational Therapy Association, Rockville

Gagne R A 1970 The conditions of learning. Holt Rinehart, Winston, London

Kaufman R 1976 Identifying and Solving Problems. University Associates, La Jolla, California

Kirchman M M 1975 An assessment of the quality of care. American Journal of Occupational Therapy 29: 54

Kiresuk T J 1973 Goal attainment scaling at a county mental health service. Evaluation 1: 12–18

Llorens L A 1977 Occupational therapy sequential client care recording system. American Journal of Occupational Therapy 31: 367–371

Louria E 1977 Programme planning and instructional media. American Journal of Occupational Therapy, Rockville

Nathan P 1967 Cues, decisions and diagnosis. Academic Press, New York

Schwitzgebel R K, Kolb D A 1974 Changing human behaviour. McGraw-Hill, New York

Welles C 1969 The implications of liability: guidelines for professional practice. American Journal of Occupational Therapy 23 (1)

8. Keeping records and presenting reports

READERS' OBJECTIVES

After reading this chapter, you should be able to:
1. **Describe the most commonly used methods of behaviour observation.**
2. **Describe the difference between description and interpretation of observed behaviour.**
3. **Design observational schedules, record and quantify data.**
4. **Describe and discuss characteristics of different types of occupational therapy reports.**
5. **Prepare and present written and verbal occupational therapy reports.**

KEEPING RECORDS — OBSERVING BEHAVIOUR

In the field of natural sciences it is often possible to apply rigorous, clearly defined tests that will yield precise answers. However, in the social sciences, of which occupational therapy is one, it is most often not possible to apply such tests. The therapist must make considered decisions based on observations of behaviour. There is a danger that where a therapist makes interpretations, without some careful training in the art of observaton, she/he is likely to make responses which are highly coloured by past experiences, expectations, and assumptions. For example, you watch two people in conversation and one is smiling broadly. Your natural comment is likely to be that the smiling person is 'happy and enjoying the conversation'. If you write down your impression in those words, then you have unwittingly influenced the opinion of others reading your report. Your comment represents an *interpretation of data* — that is, the conversation observed, but it is *not data*. The data is an accurate description of exactly *what you saw*, and does not include such words as 'happy' and 'enjoying'.

Observation is a legitimate, indeed respected, scientific method of dealing with data, and ethologists have refined the methods and technologies available today. Nobel laureate Konrad Lorenz (1973) said, 'The current belief that only quantitative procedures are scientific and that the description of structure is superfluous is a deplorable fallacy, dictated by the technomorphic thought habits acquired by our culture when dealing preponderantly with inorganic matter.' Occupational therapists should not feel the need to apologize for our heavy reliance on observational techniques. However, neither should we shun quantitative procedures. The best situation is one in which observation and quantification of the behaviour data collected go hand in hand.

Recording and measuring behaviour are skills that can, indeed must, be learned, and they are not particularly difficult to master, given appropriate resources. Martin & Bateson (1987) have devised a simple, thorough and practical guide to observing and measuring behaviour. These two authors are highly sophisticated observers, with long and respected careers in the field of ethology, which is the study of behaviour.

Research questions from clinical observation

Clinicians often express uncertainty about how routine service delivery can be linked to systematic research. Yet, the therapy context is a natural laboratory, alive with possibilities for identifying research questions for study. Where service delivery is linked to ongoing research there will be dynamic processes, which must lead to refined practice, challenge for clinicians, and increased work satisfaction for those involved in the process.

The successful therapist, in company with the successful researcher, 'is one who can combine a purposeful approach to tackling an initial set of questions with the ability to recognize and respond opportunistically to new questions that arise during the course of studying them'

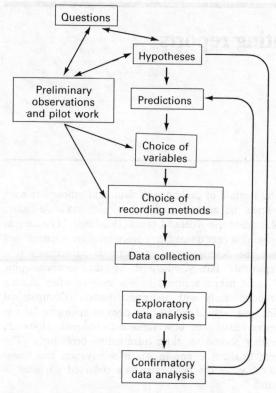

Fig. 8.1 The processes involved in studying behaviour. Reproduced by permission from Martin P, Bateson P 1987 Measuring behaviour: an introductory guide. Cambridge University Press, Cambridge.

(Martin & Bateson 1987). This applies to the clinic, the field, or the laboratory. Martin and Bateson's representation in Figure 8.1 illustrates that the processes in studying behaviour are, in fact, those of the research process.

The observation process

There are two basic types of behaviour description (see Fig. 8.2):

- Empirical description: description of the behaviour in terms of body parts, movements and postures, e.g., baring the teeth.
- Functional description: incorporation of reference to the behaviour's function, proximally or ultimately, e.g., bared-teeth threat (Lehner 1979).

The initial step is to make decisions about what is to be observed and described. To make these decisions, you must identify the questions to which you seek answers, that is to say, why are you observing the child and

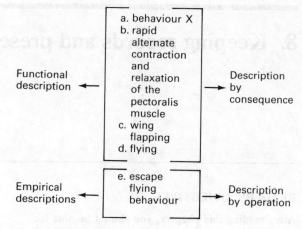

Fig. 8.2 Empirical and functional descriptions of behaviour (Lehner 1979).

family's behaviour at all? You must achieve what Martin and Bateson call 'the right level of analysis'. For example, you may painstakingly collect a large amount of data, only to find that: (a) it doesn't address the appropriate questions and/or (b) it can't be quantified (measured) in a useful way.

Guidelines for designing behaviour observation

1. Define the problem to be investigated — in detail. That is, what are the questions that need answers?
2. Identify the behavioural parameters best suited to answer the questions defined.
3. Select an observational method that gives truly representative information about the identified behaviour parameters.
4. Select quantification methods best suited to the observation.

Thus, whether for normal clinical practice, or for explicit research purposes, it is wise to plan how the observational data will be measured *before* collecting it.

Let us examine how behavioural observations can be quantified before discussing techniques of recording data, as the type of quantification selected will influence the choice of observational technique.

Quantifying observations

It is necessary to quantify behavioural observation so that the information can be analysed objectively. Clinicians may consider that this task is too time-consuming for normal service delivery. However, the option of 'eyeballing' the gathered information does have the inbuilt problem that the interpretations are subjective, and thus the probability is increased that incorrect interpretations will be arrived at, and influence intervention decisions.

Behaviour can be quantified by measuring different parameters, namely:

1. Frequency and/or magnitude — best used for unitary or discrete behaviours, e.g., stretches, urinates.
2. Duration, e.g., how long a child spends building an eight block tower.
3. Social interactions with other people and objects, i.e., who initiates a behaviour, the response of the other(s) in the interaction, who terminates the interaction and how.

Recording methods

Observations may be recorded in many ways, and the most commonly used are:

Time sampling, where behaviours are recorded at uniform, short-time intervals, such as one-minute periods over a total 10-minute span (see Fig. 8.3).

Time sampling is appropriate only for behaviours that occur fairly frequently and are easily observable. For example, the method has been used successfully in the study of mother–infant gaze interaction (Stern 1974), vocal behaviour (Rosenthal 1966) and affective expression (Gaensbauer et al 1979).

All behaviours should be operationally defined (see Example 8.1).
Care needs to be given to the choice of the sampling interval.

Event sampling, where an observer is interested in a particular type of episode or event. For example, a therapist might wish to collect detailed information (data) about a child's behaviour at mealtime.

Example 8.1: Ways to define interactive behaviour operationally
Friendly interaction: Routine conversation. Includes casual talk, asking questions, commenting, bantering.
Helps, shares, comforts: Subject spontaneously offers assistance to another person, gives up materials or space, or offers sympathy or comfort to a child who is upset.
Physical aggression: Refers to physical behaviours intended to hurt another person or make the person feel bad, for example hitting, shoving, kicking, biting, pushing.
Rough and tumble play: Refers to rough physical play which is not intended to hurt or injure. The category includes playful wrestling and other types of rough-housing, for example pushing and tackling.

Naturalistic situations, where an observer records changes occurring in a situation due to factors which are outside the observer's control. Famous studies of naturalistic observation are those of Barker (1963, 1968) in an American mid-west town. Example 8.2 uses a children's playground as a naturalistic situation.

Experimental record, where the observer records an event situation that has been specifically manipulated to elicit predicted responses. The situation is standardized, which means that it is highly repeatable, and therefore the predicted outcomes can be tested by others. Recording a child's response in a standard test situation provides a clinical example.

Diary and anecdote record, where a narrative description of an event is recorded, after the event, and an example is presented in Example 8.3. Many occupational therapy progress notes are, in fact, diary records. Akin to diary records are anecdotal observation. The difference between the two is that in an anecdotal observation, the focus is on a class of behaviour, 'co-operative play', rather than on specific incidents.

Observation period (minutes)

Behaviour	1	2	3	4	5	6	7	8	9	10
Mood Smiling Screaming Frowning Looking into space Huddles Crouches/cringes Laughing Crying										

Fig. 8.3 A 10-minute time sample observation schedule, used for observing a child play in a preschool group context.

Example 8.2: A sample recording schedule used to describe observed behaviour. In this example the context is a group of children in a preschool play situation. Regular activities are specified, as the children spend definite periods in each, and move from one to another as a group.

Before recording descriptions of behaviour, the therapist must find out what goes on in the situation and on the basis of this information, a recording schedule is designed. Thus, descriptive recording schedules are unique to each context.

Behaviour	*Activity Period* Block Play	Morning Tea	Music	Outdoor Playground	Puzzles
1. Play environment i.e., physical context What objects are present? Where? Social — who is present?					
2. Pattern of play activity i.e., What the child does?					
3. Mood Smiling Screaming Frowning Looking into space Huddles Crouches/cringes Laughing Crying					
4. Attention i.e., attends to task — looks up and around frequently in response to noise or other stimuli Obeys adult commands					
5. Movement i.e., bilateral activity dominance quality of movement grasp and manipulation range guadripedal co-ordination					

Example 8.3: Glen, an anecdotal record of a child's imitative behaviour

Glen, a six year old, is on a day's outing with his parents and they stop for a drink. Mum says, 'I think I will have a whiskey and dry'. Dad says, 'I'll have a beer' and then asks Glen what he would like to drink. Glen looks carefully around at posters advertising drinks, pauses and says in all seriousness, 'I'll have a double whiskey'.

When recording anecdotal observations, be careful to identify the basic actions of the key person, what is said, the context, time and activities involved. Whenever possible, use the exact words of the participants to preserve the flavour of the conversation. Also, accurately record the sequence of the episode: give it a beginning, middle and end. Be accurate, objective and complete.

Recording techniques

In the last decade the technology of observational research has made important advances. From paper and pencil recording the field has advanced to voice and film recordings. More recently, researchers have developed computer compatible event recorders. Each method has its advantages and disadvantages, which must be weighed against each other. A brief review is presented of a number of methods available in observational research.

In the following discussion an evaluation will be made of the usefulness of a number of the most common methods used.

Checklists. The checklist is usually a sheet previously prepared for data collection before the actual observations begin. The usual form is composed of columns for categories and rows for unit of time. The observer simply places a check in the row corresponding to the behaviours as they occur. The behaviours are coded in successive columns as the time blocks elapse and a given behaviour is entered only once every block. Generally the observer is fitted with an earplug to provide a sensory cue to indicate the end of each time interval.

Checklists have an extensive history of use as a recording device. Their advantages include the fact that they are relatively unobtrusive, cheap to construct and simple to use. The disadvantages are that only a limited number of behaviours can be recorded at any one time, reliability may be impaired by virtue of the observer having to look away to record, the flow of behaviour may be broken, and unless specifically developed the sequential nature of the behaviour is often difficult to determine from checklists. Hinde (1973) has outlined various details concerning their construction.

Rating scales. Overall opinion is somewhat divided as to the relative merits of rating scales. One of the major weaknesses of rating scales relates to the ambiguity or precise nature of the trait being measured, e.g. what one observer may view as 'aggressive' behaviour, another may not. The global nature of the quality being measured makes the task of rating a difficult one. Another problem of rating scales concerns the assumption that the quality or trait being measured is consistent across time and situation, and such an assumption is not always warranted.

Alternatively, it can be argued that rating scales possess advantages that justify their use in behavioural research. Kerlinger (1973) notes that some of these include their time saving nature, ease of use and wide range of application. Recently a number of writers have argued that rating scales are more useful than discrete behavioural observation for the investigation of certain research problems, e.g., Waters (1978) used rating scales to assess the stability of various mother–infant interactive behaviours over time. He concluded that rating scales were more useful than discrete behaviours for measuring the stability of subjects' behaviour. A similar conclusion was reached by Clarke-Stewart & Hevey (1981) in their study of stability of behaviour in mother–infant interaction from one to two and a half

years. Cairns & Green (1979) in a comparative review of behaviour observations and rating scales noted that, 'for those investigators who aspire to describe individual differences in behavioural style, or distinctive properties of interactions between two or more persons, ratings can be most useful. They help quantify the everyday judgements each of us makes about other persons in classifying them, their behaviours, and their relationships.'

Overall then, in the last few years researchers have come to recognize that despite their potential weaknesses, rating scales do have an important role to play in recording behavioural observations. Some of the advantages and disadvantages of rating scales are as follows:

Kerlinger (1973) noted that the most obvious advantage of rating scales concerns their ease of construction. Rating scales are suitable for the study of a wide range of behaviours, particularly those behaviours which are not easily quantified. Rating scales can be used by people with a minimum of training.

Intrinsically, rating scales are liable to bias error including the halo effect (the rater is influenced by an overall feeling of dislike or like). Constant error may also be present in the form of: (a) error of severity, rating all slow on a quantity, or (b) error of leniency.

Another error is that of central tendency where extreme judgement is avoided.

Event recorders. In the event recorder, ink or heat stylus pens are connected to buttons on a control board. Each button corresponds to a discrete behaviour and when the button is pressed the corresponding pen is displaced, leaving a record on a strip chart which is moving at a calibrated speed to provide a time base. The behaviour is summarized by measuring the length of each deflection and converting the length to time units. Modern computer based event recorders note the time, the button and whether it is pressed or released; this yields the same data.

The primary advantage of event recorders are that they provide a measure of the frequency, duration and sequencing of behaviours as they occur in 'real time'. Unlike checklists, where the time units are imposed on the behaviour stream and the behaviour is recorded only once per time interval, though it may have occurred two or three times, the event recorder measures every occurrence of a particular behaviour as it arises.

The disadvantage is that event recorders are labour intensive. To overcome this problem researchers have adapted the recorders for use with computers, e.g., Anderson & Vietze (1977) have used event recorders in the study of the mother–infant vocal dialogue in the natural home setting where a signal was generated onto a cassette tape. The tape could then be directly interfaced with a computer to facilitate data analysis. Similarly, Simpson (1979) and Stephenson (1979) have developed sophisticated event recorders which are computer compatible.

The system imposes an 'on–off' description onto the data being recorded (Simpson 1979). As such, the method is best used where behaviours under observation have a clear beginning and end, e.g. vocalization or gaze. Behaviours which start gradually, e.g., 'affectionate' or 'warm' emotional expression would be very difficult to record using a keyboard system.

The event recorder also lacks flexibility if the investigator is interested in reviewing the behavioural sequence several times.

Audio tape recorders. Tape recording a voice narrative of ongoing behaviour is another method for recording observations. Usually tape recording does not involve a classification of anticipated behaviours before making the observation, but simply records the flow of behaviour as it unfolds for later analysis. Having recorded the data, the next step is to prepare a transcript, and then divide the transcript into the chosen behavioural categories.

A tape recorded account of observation offers the observer the important advantage of a relatively complete assessment of the ongoing behaviour. On the other hand, it is time consuming to transcribe the data from tape. More serious disadvantages involve the problem of observer reliability and the fact that the interpretation of the data depends on what the observer does record (Ebel 1951).

Videotape recorders. Videotape has enjoyed considerable popularity as a method for recording and storing behavioural data. 'The facility of modern videotape equipment to record and store massive amounts of complex behavioural information with the capacity for an indefinite number of relatively instantaneous replays, would appear to make it an invaluable tool in the study of human interactive behaviour' (Eisler et al 1973). Furthermore, research has shown that assessment of interpersonal behaviour can be made as reliably from videotapes as from live observations (Eisler et al 1973). Newson (1977) has noted in a study of mother–infant interaction, '. . . the problem for the observer is the extraordinary speed with which signals are typically exchanged, so that even with very young infants it seems essential to capture the communication sequence on film or video, allowing the observer to review them repeatedly in context and from the standpoint of each of the participants independently.'

The facility for multiple viewings of the observations is an advantage offered by video recordings. Lamb (1978), Brazelton et al (1979) have noted that where the researcher is interested in viewing and reviewing social interaction that the video tape should be the method used.

The relatively high cost of the equipment is a disadvantage. Technical limitations associated with cameras' restricted fields of view, and the problem that the resolution of detail is inversely related to the area covered by the cameras are other disadvantages.

Summary

At present investigators are still at the threshold in terms of developing methods and techniques for the study of behaviour. A brief overview has been provided of current approaches to recording behavioural observation information. The focus has been on techniques and approaches particularly suited to observing and recording children's behaviour in clinical situations.

Now we will examine the presentation of information through the reporting process.

REPORTING IN THERAPY

Reports are the medium through which we share information. Compiling and presenting a report is a professional skill, to be mastered in the same way as one masters technical therapy procedures.

Effective, clear reporting is dependent on the therapist understanding something of communication processes between people. Reports literally mean 'what is brought back', from the Latin 'reportare'. That is to say, the message sent must have the same meaning to the receiver as it did to the sender. Yet there is an inherent difficulty in reporting information, because the meaning of words varies with individuals, and is shaped by their knowledge of the subject, and their past experience. In practice, the difficulty of communication is particularly evident when one report must serve a mixed audience, made up for example, of other medical and educational specialists and the parents of the child client. It is always best to prepare special reports for each special audience.

Functions of reports

The most obvious function of any clinical report is to inform others about the client's status in therapy. However, another equally important function is to establish a therapist's professional credibility.

Definition
A *clinical report* is an official statement of information
— its sources, an analysis of its importance, and resulting recommendations.

A clinical report conveys messages to the recipient
about aspects of the therapist's competence. For
example, his/her knowledge, ability to think about
problems and *realistic* solutions, sensitivity to client
wishes and responses to the health care situation. The
way in which a therapist organizes and presents a report
affects the way others will accept and interpret what is
said or written. Thus, a report provides an opportunity
for a therapist to promote a relationship based on
respect and trust, both with colleagues and with a child
client's family.

Some generally useful guides to preparing and
presenting clinical reports are presented.

Characteristics of effective reports

A useful, and therefore effective, report can be identified by the following features. The report is:

1. Clearly presented
2. Accurate and objective
3. Logically organized and summarized

Let us consider each of these three features.

Clear presentation

The objective in any report is that it be read, or listened
to attentively, and that it should influence thought and
actions about a client.

A report should always be presented in language that
can be understood by people with differing levels of
knowledge about the matters discussed. The particular
format and style must conform to the administrative requirements of each clinical setting. Typed reports are
always preferable for written documents. Both written
and verbal reports may generally be organized in the following sequence:

— Details of client identification, e.g., name, age,
  reason for referral.
— Summary findings, observations, and
  recommendations. This set of information is the
  most important in the report, and represents
  required reading or listening.
— Explanatory detail — that is, available but
  optional reading or listening.
— Detailed explanation of the recommendations.

Information must be concise and its relevance made
clear, if the report is to capture the attention of busy
people. The spoken report should omit or abbreviate
details of the client identification. Explanatory detail
should only be included in the form of selected brief
examples to support important information.

The layout of report forms should help busy people
read the information rapidly. Important messages, such
as recommendations for future action, should appear
prominently on report forms. One suggested format is
shown in Figure 8.4.

Accuracy and objectivity

Language used must be grammatically correct, free from
ambiguity and obscure jargon. A report always begins
with factual statements. Judgements and recommen-

Child's name:

Address:

Date & place of testing:

General summary of results and interpretation:

Supporting information (that you regard as relevant to the results gained):

Detailed results from specific areas of test (attach the test profile to this report)

Date of birth:
(D.O.B.)

Age at testing:
Yr: in Mo:

Fig. 8.4 A useful layout for an occupational therapy assessment/test report.

dations must be quite clearly linked to the facts. The reporter, like the trained observer, must distinguish 'behaviour' (for example, 'Child smiled and said "that was good"') from 'interpretation of behaviour' (for example, 'child enjoyed the game').

Logical organization

A report should be constructed so that it lightens the task of the reader/listener. Information must be presented logically and systematically, rather than spontaneously and 'psychologically' — as in a novel. Each section of a report should open with a summary of what is to follow. Literary devices, such as underlining and capitalization draw attention to important information.

The majority of clinical, occupational therapy reports will be written. However, there are occasions, such as clinical ward rounds, or client care conferences, when the therapist may expect to speak about a client. Verbal reports have some special characteristics, and some have already been discussed.

Presenting oral reports

- An oral presentation should aim to stimulate interest and discussion.
- Try not to read a report — instead make brief 'skeleton' notes and speak to them.
- State the purpose of the report clearly, and relate all comments to it. Prepare the listener for important conclusion or points to note. For example, you might say, 'My main conclusions are thus . . .'
  A wise general principle to follow in oral presentation is to tell your listener(s), what you are going to say; say it; and finally review what you have told them.
- Use short firm definite sentences and use separate sentences if you must qualify statements. Select essential material only — allow enough time for audience assimilation. It is better to succeed in making a small number of points well, rather than too many points badly. The written report on file is the place for clarifying detail to be placed.
- Use some of the arts of an actor, exaggerating conversational style to gain and hold attention. For example, changing voice tone, using pauses or questions all help to engage your listener.
  Non-verbal behaviour, including the way in which you dress, will also influence the reception of your message.

OCCUPATIONAL THERAPY REPORTS

An occupational therapist will use all of the following forms of clinical report in the course of therapy with a child and family.

1. Client progress notes
2. Official client file report
3. Special purpose report
4. Case study

Client progress notes

Immediately following an assessment or intervention session with a child, the therapist will make some private notes about the child's and family's response. These private notes form the basis for all reporting. The notes in their original form may become the departmental or official file record, or they may be rewritten for special purposes. It is essential that this initial record follow the general guide for useful reports, and above all it must be accurate, complete and objective.

Here is an example of an original progress report, found in a child's official file, which does not meet the criteria of a useful report.

Example 8.4: 'Sabina' — a report which is not useful

Session Date: 23.2.84

Part way through a 'Play Therapy' group program Sabina talked animatedly, and at length, about new exercises she had been doing with an Education Officer at the Home. It was difficult to stop her from jumping from one topic to another, but if asked questions she seemed to slow a little and answer appropriately. Much of her spontaneous speech tended to be rambling and often contained disconnected thought. Talked also about love of trail bikes and what she did in the holidays. Sabina did not seem disturbed at all at the thought of my taking over from C.D. (Therapist). She was interested and enthusiastic when introduced by Chris.

Went through finger exercises, balance exercises, and spinning with Sabina. Then played a game of 'Pick-up-Sticks'. Fine control no problem and there was no evidence of any tremor.

Signed A. Y.

Occupational Therapist

The report of Sabina's therapy session has limited value for the following reasons:

1. The report is conversational, rather than systematically organized, and it fails to draw

attention to the relevance of the information recorded.

2. Information supplied is often insufficient — for example, who is Chris?
3. Interpretations of behaviour are recorded without noting the actual behaviour. There is no possibility for the reader to weigh alternative interpretations.
4. Observations are recorded imprecisely — for example, the statement, 'fine control no problem'.
5. Insufficient information is included.

Example 8.5 is the report rewritten, after discussion with its writer, to illustrate how it could become a more useful record. It will become apparent that some crucial information was lacking in the original version.

Example 8.5: Sabina's report represented
Session date/place: 23.2.84

Therapy room alone with therapist (1 hour)
Activities used: Finger, balance, and spinning exercises (also used in physiotherapy sessions); 'Pick-up-Sticks' game.

When told that A.Y. (self) replaces C.D as therapist from now on, Sabina listened, commented 'Oh good', and made no further reference to the subject. She talked at length throughout the hour long session, 'gabbling' rapidly about various topics — often apparently unconnected — when not engaged in activity. During task performance her speech slowed to be more intelligible, and conversation was always directed to the task.

Sabina chatted about the school holidays spent at home. She spoke with warmth about her foster brother Peter, and their mutual interest in trail bike riding.

Sabina performed all of the required motor skill exercises competently, after initial encouragement to begin each. Fine motor movements and all bilateral upper limb use was well controlled, co-ordinated, and appropriately planned and executed. Similarly, Sabina attended to the 'Pick-up-Sticks' game, and there was no evidence of fine motor control difficulties. She expressed enjoyment of the game, for example, saying 'That was good'.
Signed A Y
Occupational Therapist

This type of progress note might be placed in a private or official file after each session. Alternatively, the therapist may simply record points, which are written into an essay style when the report becomes available to others. Or again, brief sessional notes may be integrated and summarized from time to time to become an official client file report. Client progress notes are almost invariably placed in an official client file, so it is appropriate to discuss that form of report now.

Official client file report

An official file provides a client history, for future reference by specialists. Thus the file should contain occupational therapy evaluation reports, summarized progress reports, special purpose reports such as programme/management advice to a child's school teacher, and a final discharge review report, or case study where appropriate. The official file provides a picture of the child's continuing response to therapy. The therapy objectives should be briefly restated in a summarized progress report, and judgements related to the objectives.

Preparing and presenting an evaluation report has already been discussed in Chapter 6 and that information should be reviewed.

Special purpose reports

Such reports convey selected information, for a clearly stated purpose. For example, a therapist may report to a child's teacher, about evaluation findings. In this case special care must be taken to present the findings in language that will have meaning to a teacher. Care must also be taken to ensure that the findings are interpreted as they are related to the child's performance and behaviour in the schooling situation (see Example 8.6).

Example 8.6: Megan — extract from a report written for Megan's teacher
On a test of general developmental maturity, the Griffiths Mental Development Scales, Megan's mental age is calculated as 6 years 2 months when she is 5 years 11 months chronologically. Thus Megan is at least of average general ability *except in the performance sector of the test*. There she shows a marked delay, having a mental age of 5 years 2 months. The 'performance scale' reflects a child's performance on visual perceptual tasks, specifically those testing spatial relationships, and the ability to formulate abstract and symbolic concepts. Normal maturation of these skills is essential before a child can learn to read, write and handle arithmetical problems. Findings from The Meeting St School Screening Test detect deficits in a range of information processing skills. Megan's performance in all aspects of this test was deficient, with the area of 'motor patterning' being most delayed (raw score 12/29). Her total raw score is 45, and the cut-off point for normal development areas tested is 55.

This result confirms that Megan does have a specific learning problem. The skills affected appear to be those relying on visual-spatial relationship integrity and motor planning ability — that is, those skills basic to the acquisition of reading and writing competence.

Examples of 8.7 and 8.8 are examples of a discharge report written in both an appropriate and inappropriate manner.

Example 8.7: Charles — a report which is not useful

Charles was initially seen on 11.3.81 and assessment was begun.

The *clinical observation* showed mixed dominance, hypotonic muscle tone, irregular eye movements (crossing midline, convergence, quick localization), as well as poor bilateral movements.

SCSIT Out of the tests completed, only figure-ground was in the dysfunctional area.

The last three appointments made after that date, to complete assessment, were not kept. A home visit was made on 9.4.81. At that stage, Mrs G's primary concern was Charles' temper tantrums at home, which were increasing in severity. Also it appeared that his behaviour was becoming more manipulative, with the total family deferring to Charles' 'every wish' in order to avoid a further temper tantrum, which would, it was feared, precipitate a grand mal epileptic fit. Basic management techniques were discussed but Mrs G appeared unprepared to accept them. Also it was found that Charles was not having his midday dosage of medication. This was perhaps contributing to his poor behaviour in afternoon classes. Mrs G was encouraged to send this dosage with Charles to school. Since this home visit, a further appointment has not been kept.

Referral to School Guidance Officer indicated.

Another form of special purpose report is that written for a child's parents, probably to guide them in their management of the child. Again, special care must be taken to avoid using jargon, or to alarm the family by careless reference to findings which may not be fully understood. The general guidelines previously given also apply to special purpose reports.

A clinical case study

A case study represents the systematic examination of a selected phenomenon. The clinical case study is the summary document which reflects synthesis of all material which has been collated throughout the day-to-day process of evaluation and therapy. A case study document is a reference point for specialists dealing with the client in the future. The study may aid understanding of the contribution of past experiences to present function, and so influence action to be taken. A case study contains factual information (data) which constitutes a natural history, for example, of the selected client's reason for referral, and his/her progress through

---

Example 8.8: Charles's report re-presented

Evaluation commenced on 11.3.81
Assessments used were:
The Southern California Sensory Integration Test Battery (SCSIT)
The Guide to Clinical Observations to complement SCSIT

Unfortunately, Charles's family have failed to keep three appointments, and so the evaluation is incomplete.

Summary of results of assessments completed

Clinical Observations revealed:
1) Mixed eye dominance; R hand dominance appears to be established.
2) Irregular eye movements expressed as:
   a. difficulty crossing the midline
   b. converging, and
   c. performing quick localizing movements.
3) Poorly integrated, clumsy, bilateral fine motor manipulative movements.

Southern California Sensory Integration Test Battery:
The following sub-tests were performed and all were within normal limits, *except the figure-ground discrimination test*. Charles was unable to distinguish the test figure stimulus.

(List sub-tests with Charles' results and norms.)

Nine sub-tests remain incomplete, therefore it is not possible to give an accurate evaluation of Charles' general readiness for formal learning.

Home visit interview: 9.4.81 — Mrs G appeared to be seriously concerned about certain aspects of Charles' behaviour at home, namely: 'Temper tantrums', used, as she sees it, to manipulate the family to bend to Charles' wishes. The present method of handling the 'tantrum' is to defer, in order to avoid precipitating a grand mal epilepsy attack. It was suggested that Mrs G and family might try an alternative approach — ignoring the 'tantrum' and leaving the room. However, Mrs G seemed reluctant to try such an approach.

It emerged that Charles did not have his mid-day dose of anticonvulsant (phenobarb). This could certainly explain his reportedly difficult behaviour in afternoon school classes. Mrs G was encouraged to send the medication to the school.

Recommendation: that Charles' class teacher be contacted and her co-operation sought to monitor that he does take his mid-day medication regularly.

A further appointment at this Centre has not been kept and it is felt that Charles' performance and progress may be better monitored through the School Guidance Officer.

Recommendation: that Charles be discharged from this Centre and referred back to the School Guidance Officer.

---

therapy. As well as data, a case study records judgements that have been made about the client. The case study is compiled from records already in existence. Busy people prepare case studies and equally busy people read them. Thus, the document must be succinct and to the point.

A therapist may also prepare a case study when she/he is seeking to increase his/her own understanding of a client. The therapist may, for example, be concerned about a child's special needs in therapy, or about a puzzling or disappointing response to therapy. In this case the therapist's objective would be to use understanding gained, to design yet more appropriate or effective therapy.

Information should be organized and visually presented to give the reader a map of the natural history of events. The relative perceived importance should be emphasized by literary devices — capitals, underlining, use of colour coding, margins.

Here are the headings normally used in a clinical case study, reflecting the therapeutic process:

• Demographic information
• Assessment and interpretation of data gained
• Therapy plan — including objectives and programme design
• Progress notes
• Evaluation of client response to therapy
• Follow-up procedures where appropriate.

SUMMARY

Clinical reporting is a form of consultation with others, for example, your colleagues, and the child's parents. One of the most important aims of reporting must be to reduce confusion. Remember that if there is *any* chance of your being misunderstood, you will be! Try to ensure that the message you send quite clearly does convey your intention or meaning, to the person or people who receive it.

In written communication the *words* must carry the entire message by themselves. But when you speak to others your message is also conveyed ind clarified by your tone of voice, your posture and gestures as well as the words used. It is a good idea to routinely apply some checks on your reports, and a useful guide concludes this chapter.

Checklist for presenting effective reports

1. Is the purpose of the report clear?
2. Is the report suitable for its intended readers?
• Distinguish between primary readers (those who will read) and secondary readers (those who might read).
• How will each use the information?
• Will all readers accept the assumptions — explicit and implied?
• Is the technical level appropriate?
• Is the non-technical language too simple or inappropriate?
3. Does the report achieve its intended purpose?
• Are the conclusions and recommendations clear, emphatic, and sufficiently substantiated?
4. Is everything necessary included?
5. Is everything unnecessary excluded?
6. Is the report developed in a logical appropriate order?
• There are many appropriate logical orders. Is the reader informed of the order chosen?
7. Is the report formatted in an attractive way?
• Will it be easy for the reader Ito follow the structure of the report, and to refer back to information?

REFERENCES

Anderson B J, Vietze P M 1977 Early dialogues: The structure of reciprocal infant–mother vocalisation. In: Cohen S, Comiskey T J (eds) Child development: Contemporary perspectives. Peacock Publishers Itasca, Illinois

Barker R G 1963 Behavior. Appleton-Century-Crofts. New York

Barker R G 1968 Ecological psychology. Stanford University Press, Stanford

Brazelton T B, Yogman M, Als H, Tronick E 1979 Mother-father interactions. In: Lewis M, Rosenblum L A (eds) The child and its family. Plenum, New York

Cairns R B, Green J A 1979 How to assess personality and social patterns: observation or ratings? In: Cairns R B (ed) The analysis of social interactions: method, issues and illustrations. Lawrence Erlbaun Associates, New York

Clarke-Stewart K A, Hevey C M 1981 Longitudinal relations in repeated observations of mother–child interaction from 1 to 2½ years. Developmental Psychology 17: 127–145

Ebel R L 1951 Estimation of the reliability of ratings. Psychometrika 16: 407–424

Eisler R M, Hersen M, Agras W S 1973 Videotape: a method for the controlled observation of non-verbal interpersonal behaviour. Behaviour Therapy 4: 420–425

Gaensbauer T J, Mrazek D, Emde R N 1979 Patterning of emotional response in a play room laboratory situation. Infant Behaviour and Development 2: 163–178

Hinde R A 1973 On the design of check-lists. Primates 14: 393–406

Kerlinger F N 1973 Foundations of behavioural research. Holt Rinehart & Winston, London

Lamb M E 1978 The effects of social context on dyadic social interaction. In: Lamb M E, Suomi S J, Stevenson G R (eds) Social interaction analysis: methodological issues. University of Wisconsin Press, Madison

Lehner P N 1979 Handbook of ethological methods Garland STPM Press, New York

Lorenz K 1973 The fashionable fallacy of dispensing with description. Naturwissenschaften 60: 1–9

Martin P, Bateson P 1987 Measuring behaviour: an introductory guide. Cambridge University Press, Cambridge

Newson J 1977 An intersubjective aproach to the systematic description of mother–infant interaction. In: Schaffer H R (ed) Studies in mother–infant interaction. Academic Press, New York

Rosenthal R 1966 Experimenter effects in behavioural research. Appleton-Century-Crofts, New York

Simpson M J A 1979 Problems of recording behavioural data by keyboard. In: Lamb M, Suomi S J, Stephenson G R (eds) Social interaction analysis: Methodological issues, University of Wisconsin Press, Wisconsin

Stephepson G R 1979 Plexyn: A computer-compatible grammar for coding complex social interactions. In: Lamb M, Suomi S J, Stephenson G R (eds) Social interaction analysis: Methodological issues, University of Wisconsin Press, Wisconsin

Stern D N 1974 Mother and infant at play: the dyadic interaction involving facial, vocal and gaze behaviours. In: Lewis M, Rosenblum L A (eds) The effect of the infant on its care-giver, John Wiley, New York

Waters E 1978 The reliability and stability of individual differences in infant–mother attachment. Child Development 49: 483–494

RECOMMENDED READING

Cantley J D 1979 The study of behaviour. The Institute of Biology's Studies in Biology, No 3

Cooper B M 1975 Writing technical reports. Penguin, Harmondsworth

Damerst W A 1972 Clear technical reports. Harcourt Brace Jovanovich, New York

Dunbar R I M 1978 Some aspects of research design and their implications in the observational study of behaviour. Behaviour 58: 78–98

Fagen R M, Goldman R 1977 Behavioural catalogue analysis methods. Animal Behaviour 25: 261–274

Heatherington M 1971 'Outside-in'. Scott-Foresiman, Glenview, Illinois

Hopkins H L, Smith H D 1978 Willard and Spackman's occupational therapy. Lippincott, Philadelphia, pp 682–685

Hutt S J, Hutt C 1970 Direct observation and measurement of behaviour. Charles C Thomas, Springfield

Jensen P, Algers B, Ekesbo I 1986 Methods of sampling and analysis of data in farm animal ethology. Birkhauser Verlag, Basle

Medinnus G R 1976 Child study and observation guide. John Wiley, New York

Slater P J B 1973 Describing sequence of behaviour. In: Bateson P P G, Klopfer P H (eds) Perspectives in ethology, pp 131–153, Plenum Press, New York

Strunk W, White E B 1972 The elements of style. Macmillan, New York

Weed L L 1970 Medical records, medical education and patient care. Year Book Medical Publications, Chicago

Willems E P, Raush H (eds) 1969 Naturalistic viewpoints in psychological research. Holt Rinehart & Winston, New York

Managing behavioural interactions in therapy

9. Attracting the child and family to therapy — the dilemma of motivation

READERS' OBJECTIVES

After reading this chapter, you should be able to:
1. Describe and discuss three models of motivation which can be applied to therapy.
2. Describe types of reinforcement schedules.
3. Differentiate between negative reinforcement, extinction and punishment.
4. Describe how motivational factors can be designed into the environment, social, and task contexts of therapy.
5. Describe and discuss factors that enhance communication between parents and specialists dealing with them.

WHY IS MOTIVATION IMPORTANT?

It would be perfectly adequate to characterize the therapeutic motivation issue as that of attraction to the therapy process, and avoid the use of the motivation concept. But the concept is part of our culture, and does have real heuristic value for attempting to understand how behaviour is energized. Thus, in this discussion the term 'motivation' will be retained and defined as an interactive process.

> **Definition**
> *Motivation*: the desire or energy a client brings to carrying through a course of action, and to the therapist's role in stimulating such client energy.

Unlike an adult client, a child rarely if ever, seeks therapy services. Thus, from the child's viewpoint, there is no good reason why she/he should 'co-operate', i.e., work together with the therapist *to the same end*. The therapist should expect to assume responsibility for the child's attraction to, and participation in the process.

Any view which holds the child primarily responsible for becoming attracted to, and 'co-operative' in therapy, punishes the child.

It is useful to think of the motivational, or attraction component as a process leading to an end goal of spontaneous co-operation by the child/family in the therapy. At first it is necessary for the therapist to provide inducements to the therapy, and these constitute extrinsic motivators. An effectively guided process will result in spontaneous co-operation. The child/family are then said to be intrinsically motivated, i.e., they generate their own desire to be involved. Extrinsic and intrinsic motivation are useful theoretical ideas which organize discussion, but before we discuss them let us examine some general ideas about the concept of motivation.

Models of motivation, applied to therapy

Motivation is a generic word, used to express inferences made about visible behaviour, in relationship to postulated internal state(s) of the observed individual. There are many views of motivation. Traditional discussions embodied constructs of 'need' and 'drive' (see Allport 1937, 1961), but these theories have been found to be

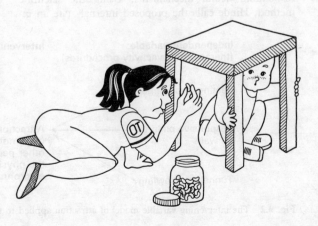

unsatisfying explanations. Modern theorists have grappled further with the problems of defining and explaining the inferred processes underlying motivated states of behaviour. Three modern theories have been selected for this discussion, as they represent current views and can be applied to therapy design.

The three models are useful for occupational therapists because they increase understanding of how the attraction (or motivational) component of therapy can be designed and controlled. Thus, like other aspects of therapy (such as the choice of task), 'attraction' techniques can be evaluated for their contribution to therapy effectiveness.

The first model is that of Hinde (1974) and it represents an attempt to describe motivational processes by reference to scientific methods. Hinde is concerned to achieve understanding of the pragmatic process which gives rise to behaviour we call 'motivated', at the same time avoiding constructs such as 'need' and 'drive'.

The second model is that of the learning theorists (Ferster & Skinner 1957, Premack 1965, e.g., Skinner 1953). This model represents an attempt to show how behaviour may be shaped and changed — that is, how 'motivational processes' may be influenced. This model is concerned with the pragmatics of behaviour change and its proponents discard the use of the word 'motivation', though clearly the concept is dealt with.

The third model of White (1964) provides an interesting and useful attempt to delineate the adaptive function of 'motivation' in man. Let us now examine the three models more closely.

Model 1: Motivation as an intervening variable

Hinde (1974) seeks to explain relationships between external events, behaviour responses, and a proposed internal state without implying its nature, or corresponding neural mechanisms. Using the scientific method, Hinde calls the proposed internal state an *in-*

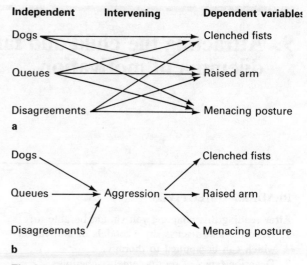

a

b

Fig. 9.1   (a) The relation between three independent variables and three dependent variables. (b) The relation between three independent variables, one (inferred) intervening variable, and three dependent variables. Reproduced by permission from Hinde R 1974 Biological bases of human behaviour. McGraw-Hill, New York

tervening variable. A synonymous term that is frequently used for this concept is 'confounding variable', i.e., the individual differences which cannot be controlled by the researcher or the therapist. The intervening variable can be recognized by reference to external events, which are called *independent variables*, and observable behavioural responses in the situations, called *dependent variables*.

Hinde cites an example where a person's behavioural responses to dogs, queues, and disagreements are observably similar. From the observed behaviour set an intervening variable (or motivational state), can be inferred and named as, for example, 'aggression'. The process is represented in Figure 9.1.

The dependent variables shown in Figure 9.2 provide

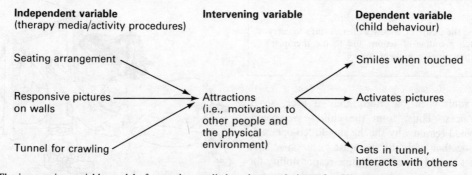

Fig. 9.2   The intervening variable model of attraction applied to therapy design (after Hinde 1984).

the therapist with measures of the child's attraction to the therapy tasks. Here is a simple practical example. The data were derived from a study by Clancy (1976) of young, socially isolated, autistic children. The environmental objective was to structure the children's attention to promote:

1. Interactive social sequences with minimum effort required of the child, and enhanced likelihood of a socially rewarding interaction with an adult caretaker;

2. Generally elevated attention level by the client to both non-social surroundings and to people; and

3. Participation by the child in functional activities (meals, dressing) through enhanced attention levels.

Model 2: Motivation and the operant model

From Skinner's (1953) classical learning theory there arose practical systems of operant procedures and behaviour modification — both frequently used by occupational therapists. Though the learning theorists discarded 'motivation' as an unnecessary concept, the basic question underlying the science of operant conditioning is a motivational one. Namely, 'what makes an organism behave as it does?' (see Azrin & Holtz 1966, Premack 1965).

The 'internal force' explanation for observed behaviour is replaced by one which focuses on the power of external environmental factors to shape or manipulate an individual's behaviour. Much of the literature about operant and behaviour modification procedures focuses on contrived laboratory-type situations. However, the model was presented as a general one for understanding human behaviour.

A major difference in position between learning theorists and others is that the learning theorists deny the need to postulate any intervening variable, or motivational state. Instead, it is argued that the social environment can always be ordered to elicit precisely predicted responses in all individuals. While this is often true in laboratory situations, the argument is increasingly regarded as being without general application.

The value of the operant model for the occupational therapist is that its principles and rules provide useful, systematic guide to designing the conditions (Hinde's independent variables) needed to elicit the child/family's attraction to therapy. There is a detailed explanation of the operant and behaviour modification systems in Chapter 10.

Model 3 — Motivation as an adaptive force

White (1964) proposed that behaviour could be explained most satisfactorily in terms of an individual's desire to use and develop capacities in order to produce effects on the environment. Such effects, when successful, would contribute to adaptation between the individual and his environment. For this to be so, White argued that an individual must be capable of recognizing his own behaviour in terms of developing competence. White, like others, used the concept of 'reinforcement'. However, his usage was different from the other theorists discussed in that he saw the prime reinforcer as the individual's perception of his own behavioural effectiveness. White coined the notion that 'competence is its own reward'. The point is well illustrated by examples of young children learning new motor skills. For instance, when a toddler takes the first unassisted steps after countless attempts, she/he beams with pleasure regardless of the presence of others to acclaim the achievement. However, White notes that the social reinforcement of others will enhance the child's pleasure, and future walking efforts.

Thus, according to White, a child is more likely to be attracted to tasks that challenge, within appropriate developmental capacities. This model of competence providing its own rewards is compatible with the occupational therapy philosophy of developing an individual's competencies. White's model provides useful guidelines for structuring therapy tasks, and setting intermediate (enabling) and long-term objectives.

Summary

From the many theories of motivation three were chosen because they provide different conceptual frameworks which can be interpreted in the clinical therapy process. These theories also introduce the research concepts of variables — independent, intervening and dependent variables. That is to say, the clinical therapy context is also a research setting where independent variables are manipulated by a therapist and outcomes, i.e., dependent variables, can be systematically observed and evaluated. Eliciting the intervening variable, in this case attraction to therapy, provides the therapist with an exciting challenge. Perhaps the difference between a good and/or excellent therapist is that the latter succeeds in engaging a reluctant child in therapy.

REINFORCEMENT

Reinforcement, like 'attraction', can also be thought of as an intervening variable. Reinforcement is anything which, by following behaviour, influences the probability of that behaviour occurring again. By definition, something is only a reinforcer if it changes behaviour. To be effective, the reinforcer must also be seen by the person whose behaviour is to change, as a reward or a punishment. Frequently we assume that because we value something, others will value it similarly, but this is not necessarily the case.

Reinforcement versus influence

Gold (1975) makes an interesting distinction between *reinforcement* and *influence*. Gold defines influence as 'just about everything that happens between a trainer and a learner (i.e. a therapist and client)'. The idea suggests that a therapist may affect the therapeutic process in a general way (influence), and direct it in a highly specific way through the feedback made available to child and family (reinforcement). Before discussing reinforcement let us examine *influence* a little more.

Gold specifies two forms:

1. Content influence — referring to the knowledge/information component of a learning situation.

2. Process influence — referring to the feelings that the trainer/therapist may have about the learning situation.

Gold suggests that a therapist should focus attention on the content component of a task situation. The reasons given are that

● The learning situation is then 'clear, uncluttered' by personal interaction issues
● More useful task information can be communicated
● Such a focus allows for mutual respect and dignity to develop between therapist and client.

It is suggested that counterproductive interactions can develop through 'process influence'. For example, a therapist can, intentionally or not, establish a power relationship in which the client is subservient. Focus on such process influences is distracting from the task in hand, and this interferes with effective therapy. Let us examine reinforcers and their use.

Classes of reinforcers

All reinforcers are either *natural* or *artificial*. Natural reinforcers are those which logically proceed from a situation in everyday life. Artificial reinforcers are those which are not normally associated with a situation, but are employed as temporary inducements for the user to establish control.

Both natural and artificial reinforcers may be classified as follows:

1. Those which strengthen and promote behaviour — positive reinforcers.
2. Those which decelerate or stop behaviour — negative reinforcers and punishment.

Positive

Watson & Lowrey (1973) define three main kinds of strengthening reinforcers as *positive reinforcers*: food; toys, games or activities; and human interaction (praise, attention). White (1960) adds 'competence', saying that it is enough reward or reinforcement for an individual to realize that she/he can do something.

Positive reinforcement is the presentation of a pleasing stimulus contingent on a response by the client to some specified demand (see Example 9.1)

Example 9.1: Positive reinforcement			
Initiator	*Behaviour*	*Reinforcement*	*Result*
Adult says sit down	Child sits	'Thank you for sitting', and adult gives hug, pat, or kiss.	Child sits down more readily next time she/he is asked.

From J Carr 1980 Helping your handicapped child, Penguin. Text copyright © Janet Carr. Reproduced by permission of Penguin Books Ltd.

Example 9.2: Positive reinforcement in therapy: toilet training
For a toilet training programme of five intellectually handicapped boys, Giles & Wolfe (1975) reported that the effective positive reinforcers included: baby foods, a ride in a wheelchair, a shower, a ball, allowing the child to return to bed.

Negative

There are several ways in which reinforcers are used to reduce or eliminate undesired behaviour:

— by the use of negative reinforcement;
— by withholding reinforcement in extinction procedures;
— by the use of punishment.

Negative reinforcement is the presentation of an unpleasant or undesired stimulus, which the child may avoid by performing the desired behaviour.

> **Example 9.3: Negative reinforcement in therapy — toilet training**
> In the toilet training programme reported by Giles & Wolfe (1975), the negative reinforcer was 'sitting on the toilet' which ceased as soon as the child voided.

Another example of negative reinforcement is the giving of an undesired stimulus to the point of saturation, so that the child (or client) will reject that stimulus.

Extinction procedures. Reinforcement may also simply be withheld — the case when extinction procedures are used. It means ignoring the child when she/he does something we do not want him/her to do (see Example 9.4).

> **Example 9.4: Negative reinforcement in therapy — Kate**
> Kate whines and pesters her mother for attention all day long (undesired irritating behaviour). Kate's mother was advised to cease her practice of reprimanding for whining and pestering (i.e., reinforcing undesired behaviour). Rather, she was advised to give attention in abundance for all sorts of helpful and attractive behaviour throughout the day, ignoring the whining. After a few days, Kate had stopped whining and divided her time happily between helping her mother, and playing independently.

The principle is that an hypothesized deprivation state is satiated. In Kate's instance (Example 9.4), it was hypothesized that she perceived herself as not getting enough attention from her mother. A child who is deprived of attention will not only work very hard to get it, but will use any means that brings a response. Kate's mother, by her reprimands, was positively reinforcing an undesirable way of obtaining attention.

Kate's example also emphasized how important it is to communicate clearly and specifically what behaviour is being reinforced. However, Watson & Lowrey (1973) point out two disadvantages:

- The effects of extinction are gradual and the initial effects of extinction are to make the undesirable behaviour occur more often before it begins to deteriorate; and
- Parents and others do not *always* control all reinforcement the child may get for engaging in undesirable behaviour.

For successful use of extinction, adults must *always* ignore the undesirable behaviour being modified. The use of extinction is confined to eliminating undesirable be-

haviours. A careful initial appraisal is essential to determine possible motivations for the behaviour — such as Kate's attention-seeking whining — before extinction is selected as the procedure of choice.

Punishment. By contrast, punishment refers to the application of an unpleasant stimulus immediately following an undesirable behaviour. The stimulus may be a physical act, such as a slap or, more extremely, electric shock (Lovaas 1969). Or the stimulus may be withdrawal of attention, of a desired activity, or of an article.

Punishment should always be used with great caution and in association with positive reinforcement of an identified alternative behaviour (see Example 9.5).

> **Example 9.5: John — Punishment in therapy**
> Two-year-old John's screaming is undesired and a short, sharp slap is administered each time he screams. But when John babbles, he may be stroked, spoken to gently and perhaps given a candy.

Gold (1975) says that the desirable way to commence using any reinforcement is to begin with using a combination of natural, social reinforcers (e.g., smiles) and artificial ones (e.g. sweets) to achieve attraction to the situation/task. Ultimately, artificial reinforcers must be phased out of use and the only reinforcers should be those occurring naturally as appropriate to the situation.

When to use reinforcement

The particular object or social behaviour chosen as the reinforcer is one factor that will determine how effective the modification of the behaviour will be. Another factor, of equal importance, is the timing with which the reinforcer is offered or applied to the child.

Timing

An important principle when applying reinforcement is that it should immediately follow the behaviour. In practice, split-second timing is not possible and most workers use a combination of immediate social reinforcement, 'Good girl, you did that well', or 'No, stop that', and a selected artificial reinforcer.

Moreover, it is important to communicate clearly and specifically just what behaviour is being reinforced. For example, Alan puts on his socks unaided. The adult could say, 'That's really good', but it is much more effective to say 'It's really helpful that you put on your own socks.'

Schedules

In the operant behaviour modification model, several time schedules have been devised and these determine when and how often a reinforcement is given. The schedules are:

Intermittent variable/ratio random schedule. The reinforcement follows the desired behaviour, but in a pattern which is unpredictable by the child. The intermittent/variable ratio/random schedule is the most powerful reinforcement schedule, because the child will keep working, in case the next performance brings the reward. Conversely, it becomes painful to continue with undesired behaviour because the unpleasant reinforcer may occur at any time.

Continuous reinforcement. Every occurrence of the desired behaviour, even in a primitive form, is reinforced. The objective is to achieve closer and closer approximations to the actual behaviour sought. The continuous reinforcement schedule has limited power and is most useful at the beginning of a training programme when a therapist is trying to encourage the child to want to perform the behaviour.

If continuous reinforcement is maintained, the child can become satiated by the reinforcer, habituate to it, lose interest in the training, and cease to work for the reinforcer. Usually, once interest and motivation to work is established, the continuous reinforcement schedule is shifted to become fixed ratio or interval, and finally an intermittent or variable ratio schedule is employed.

Fixed ratio schedules. Every predetermined Nth response receives reinforcement.

Fixed interval schedules. A child is reinforced after a predetermined time period — for instance, every 3 minutes — for the desired behaviour occurring in that time.

The theory thus far discussed leads to the development of a working model for the design of the motivational process in therapy.

MOTIVATIONAL PROCESSES IN THERAPY

Attraction as an intervening variable becomes a key integrating factor when designing the therapy contexts. The issue of attraction further resolves itself into two questions, namely:

1. What will attract this child's/family's attention to the therapy so that they will want to continue and contribute to the process?
2. How should the process be organized to ensure continuing attention?

Some conditions can be specified as leading to an effective attraction process. These conditions are:

a. The child must perceive immediate gains from the situation e.g. access to attractive games or company, or escape from real or perceived punishment. There is an inevitable degree of extrinsic motivation in this step.
b. The child must experience and recognize achievement in the situation.
c. The child must value the achievement(s).

There are some behaviours which allow a therapist to judge whether a child is becoming intrinsically motivated to therapy. For example, the child spontaneously:

- Contributes to planning the tasks — 'next time let's . . .', or, 'after we've finished let's . . .'
- Appears on time, eagerly, for therapy sessions and is reluctant to leave
- Perseveres with disliked but essential aspects of the programme
- Shares generously with others — compliments, ideas and assistance, tools and materials
- Explores unknown tasks, even in the face of doubt about own capacities.

The 'what' question demands individual knowledge of each client, e.g., likes, dislikes, priorities; the 'how' question can be addressed more generally. In Section 2 contexts of therapy were discussed, and these will provide the focus for the present discussion about motivational/attraction processes at work.

The environment

A number of workers have reported programmes in which living environments have been arranged to achieve specific behaviour from those using the space. Two are discussed in detail in Chapter 14 (Clancy 1976; Richer 1971). In the latter programme, living room furniture and fittings were arranged to interrupt the stereotyped behaviour of autistic children. The objective was to encourage or attract the children to attend to their space, to other children and to the nurse caretakers in a socially interactive way. In such studies, the face-to-face interaction of the therapist and child is of little consequence as a therapy modality. The motivational component lies in the sensitive manipulation of physical features of the therapy space, and this may be defined in a number of ways. For example, 'space' may refer to a child's immediate surroundings, as when a child is confined to bed in a hospital ward. Or 'space' may refer to the occupational therapy department while the child is there. Yet again 'space' may be a residential institution where a child lives. Whichever definition applies, the suggested model of attraction/motivation to therapy still offers general principles of design which can be used by the therapist to facilitate the therapy process.

The task

The therapy task itself may provide the prime motivational focus. Naturally though, the therapist will present the task, and so the social interaction must still contribute to and benefit from attracting the child to the task (see Examples 9.6 and 9.7).

Example 9.6: Jack
Five-month-old Jack, identified as a Down syndrome infant, spent much time in his cot. The occupational therapist selected playthings which, by their very design, could be left attached to the cot, and encourage Jack's attention.

Example 9.7: Jenny
Four-year-old Jenny refused all efforts in physiotherapy to re-commence walking after an extended time in a plaster cast and traction. The occupational therapist, with Jenny's help, produced a pair of walking sticks decorated with papier mâche juggler's heads, brightly painted, beribboned and streamered, which tinkled with tiny bells on movement. Jenny walked off — the centre of admiring attention wherever she went.

Social interaction

The inevitably occurring social interaction between therapist and child can be designed as an inducement to therapy, in common with the environment and task. In fact, one aspect of professional behaviour is the development and use of personal interactive skills. Two situations will be discussed. The first is the face-to-face situation in which the therapist might be considered the prime attractor to the therapy tasks. The second is the social situation in which the therapist engages others, e.g. peers, siblings, parents, to be the primary attraction to therapy tasks. In both situations the therapist's personal, and thus therapeutic, relationship with the client and/or family will be developed from the first encounter. Let us examine the first situation of attracting/motivating a child in the face-to-face therapy encounter.

Motivating the child in face-to-face therapy

The therapist as an attractor. The therapist administering a developmental assessment to a very young child provides an interesting example of a face-to-face situation. At first it is not the test that engages the child, but rather the strange environment, situation, and person. As well as being attractors, they also present barriers to be overcome if the child's attention is to be focused on the task. The therapist must personally present certain tests (tasks), not necessarily very attractive, and a response must be enticed from the child in order to meet the assessment goals. The therapist's interaction with the child may be limited to the time taken to administer a complete developmental assessment; or the relationship may continue to develop because therapeutic intervention is indicated.

In Example 9.8, Miss Best, a final year occupational therapy student midway in a paediatric fieldwork placement, has decided to administer block tasks first because they are judged to be most attractive.

Example 9.8: Miss Best and Debbie
Debbie ($3\frac{1}{2}$ years) had been in hospital for two weeks when Miss Best visited her. Miss Best sat facing Debbie, recently woken from a nap, produced eight red blocks from the standard equipment kit, smiled brightly and said 'Hello Debbie, now we are going to build some towers — these are your blocks, off you go', then she sat and waited . . . and waited!! Debbie hung her head. Miss Best became firm but kindly, 'Now come on Debbie, I want you to build me a tower'. No response. 'Well Debbie, I'll show you how' (builds tower while child peeps at it). 'Now it's your turn.' Still no response. At this point Miss Best began to feel slightly panicky, and slightly cross with Debbie. Miss Best tried once more, this time brusquely, but again without effect. She terminated the encounter, intending to try again at some later time.

The therapist might have taken the view that Debbie is 'an unco-operative child', or, 'cannot do the task'. In this example, the child, rather than the therapist, controlled the therapy process. Had Debbie been a little happier, or more awake, or had some other unknown condition operated, i.e., the intervening variable, the therapist might have been luckier, and thus more apparently effective. However, effectiveness which results from serendipity (happy accidents) cannot be analysed, nor the useful elements predicted and applied again with other children in future situations. There are some useful general principles which can aid management of the social motivational context of an initial therapy encounter with any young child in the range one to eight years. The principles are noted, and then expressed through a revised encounter between Miss Best and Debbie.

1. Approach the child quietly, in a relaxed manner, name yourself, and chat quietly while arranging work materials.
2. Avoid the face-to-face position. Adopt a work position where the therapist and child's head are level.
3. Immediately engage the child by appeal to his/her natural curiosity, using selected media, and minimizing the need for a language response from the child.
4. Employ humour — but with care. Slap-stick type, as in knocking over the tower, is usually successful. Avoid a serious portentous approach, *and* a 'silly', overstimulating one which may cause a child to overact and lead to reprimand.

The encounter between Miss Best and Debbie is replayed in Example 9.9, using the general principles.

Motivation leading to rapport

Attracting a child to therapy, and consolidating the attraction throughout an intervention programme, is also spoken of as 'establishing rapport with the child'. The therapist's objective is that a relationship should develop in which there is trust, mutual respect, and probably liking between therapist and child. Rapport with the child is especially important if accurate responses are to be elicited. To achieve rapport the therapist must seek to understand the individual differences in her clients. For example, one child may perform very poorly under observation because a feeling of being watched raises anxiety levels to a point which suppresses normal capability. With another child, minimal anxiety may heighten motivation, producing enhanced performance.

Example 9.10 shows another way in which the social interaction is used as the primary source of attraction with an older child. The first steps are taken toward establishing a relationship of trust — rapport between child, parent, and therapist.

In learning theory terms the therapist has designed an encounter which attracts the child, and at the same time increases the likelihood of a specified behaviour, e.g., risk taking, occurring again. The probability of future risk taking was enhanced by the therapist's positive reinforcement, expressed as pleasure when Clare suppressed her apprehension sufficiently to venture into the strange therapy situation — 'I'm glad that I can show

---

Example 9.9: Therapist as attractor: Miss Best and Debbie replayed

Miss Best seats herself *parallel* to Debbie, avoiding the direct face-to-face position. She greets Debbie, *names herself*, and spends a minute or two casually commenting on, *but not touching*, toys or belongings surrounding Debbie. She then introduces her assessment task by appealing to the child's curiosity.

Ignoring Debbie's downcast head and silence, she proceeds. 'I have brought some games for you and me . . . shakes bag . . . 'Let's see' . . . delves in and produces a familiar object such as a ball, places it casually near Debbie's hands, then quickly produces another object, and yet another, chatting about each, *but not requiring a response*. Finally Miss Best produces the bag of eight red cubes and tips them out on the bed covers.

Debbie should by now be peeping occasionally at events. Miss Best says 'Watch me build a tower', and proceeds to do so slowly, until finally she says 'Now watch me make it go crashing over' and knocks the tower down with mock exclamations of horror as well as laughter. She repeats this performance several times, or until the child begins to join in the laughter about knocking over the tower. Then she casually says 'Now you help me knock it over this time', takes the child's hand and, bingo, down it goes (to the child's astonishment!). Miss Best enthusiastically encourages the effort, e.g., 'Well done, what a big crash.' On the next round the child is invited to place one block. However, if she refuses, the therapist continues as if it is of no consequence, repeating the invitation and substituting a train/bridge/animal to maintain Debbie's interest.

This introductory interaction should occupy about ten minutes at which point the child should be interested, i.e., no longer averting her gaze but watching each move, smiling and probably offering some comment or at least laughing and exclaiming.

The therapist then returns to the required task of building a tower, appealing this time to the child's competitiveness, e.g., 'Now this time let's see who can build the tallest tower, here you are' (handing bundle of blocks. 'I'll put the first one down and off we go'. At which point it is only a matter of handing more blocks to the child until the therapist determines the test response to her satisfaction. The child may now be said to be co-operative.

---

you both our playroom'. The therapist then continues the encounter according to the directions for non-directive play therapy.

The example of Clare illustrates some further guidelines for organizing the social interaction as a motivational force throughout ongoing therapy. The therapist may:

1. Express friendliness by verbal and non-verbal behaviour — especially by listening to the child.
2. Give simple explanation, appropriately timed, to

Example 9.10: Clare

Clare is eight years old and referred to the occupational therapy service for 'play therapy' on an outpatient basis. Clare is described in the referral letter as 'Now refusing to go to school — where she previously did well — of waking regularly, screaming in response to nightmares; of refusing to allow her mother out of her sight; of reverting to less mature toileting and self-care behaviour.' Clare's behaviour is thought to be linked to a series of recent events connected with her mother's serious illness and sudden hospitalization. After discussion with Clare's psychiatric management team, the occupational therapist decides to use non-directive play therapy (Axline 1989). This form of therapy defines precisely how the therapist shall interact with the child (see Chapter 16). The model of therapy is the individual one. Thus the therapist must achieve willing separation of Clare from her mother. Mrs Darcy is an occupational therapist skilled in non-directive play therapy and proceeds with the initial encounter.

She approaches Clare and her mother in the waiting room, greets them in a friendly interested manner, naming herself . . . 'You must be Clare, and Mrs X. Hello, I'm Mrs Darcy — How are you?' Immediately she seeks to reassure Clare 'You must be wondering what sort of place this is and why you are here. Well, over there . . .', a factual *brief* description of the immediate environment follows. 'This is not a hospital or hospital ward. No one will do anything to you. It is to be your special time to use however you wish. At the end of one hour you will go home again.'

She may then sit and chat, but not question Clare for a few minutes. Alternatively, if, for example, the waiting room is full, the therapist may use that fact to firmly invite child and mother to the playroom. 'It is so noisy here . . . let's all go to the playroom which will be Clare's special place.' If Clare holds back, which is likely, Mrs Darcy, gently acknowledges that 'You are not sure about coming. It is hard when you don't know the place or me . . . (pause) . . . Mum and I are going, you may stay here or come with us. While you are deciding I'll show Mum where the playroom is.' Mrs Darcy invites Mum suggesting that she leave her handbag with Clare — for safekeeping.

Poor Clare! There really can only be one decision, and predictably she hurriedly follows her mother. Mrs Darcy expresses pleasure at her 'decision'. 'I'm glad that I can show you both our playroom.'

explain to the child the reasons for attending therapy.

3. Establish clear rules of conduct which will be acceptable in the therapy situation.
4. Assist the child to keep the established rules. For example, avoid question forms such as 'Would you like to . . .?' when in fact no choice exists.
5. Assist the child to recognize his/her mastery of a 'problem', and developing competence.
6. Acknowledge the child's attempts to meet the

requirements and expectations of therapy, thus promoting confidence and willingness to continue in the therapy process.

7. Regard immaturity and misbehaviour as conveying messages from the child. The therapist thus seeks to understand the meaning of the behaviour, before responding, rather than simply suppressing the behaviour.
8. Where reprimand is unavoidable, give it in a just, fair, and objective manner.

Our discussion about ways to attract a child to therapy, and to maintain that attraction throughout an intervention process, is now concluded. We turn to considering how the child's parents and other family members can be similarly attracted to, and engaged in, the therapy process.

ENGAGING THE CHILD'S FAMILY IN THERAPY

Time and available literature are real constraints on how a therapist may introduce therapy to a child's parents, and thus engage them in the therapy process. O'Brien & Budd (1982) have suggested two practical measures designed to deal with these constraints, namely the development of a 'Parent Orientation Package' and 'Parent Support Groups'.

Parent orientation package. The package could contain relevant simple descriptive information about the child's disability/handicap/medical/surgical condition and attendant medical procedures, occupational therapy goals, and media used with the particular child; the contribution that parents can make to therapy; the usual course of therapy, and possible outcomes for children with the identified handicap/condition (see Klein 1990).

Parent support groups. The second suggestion made by O'Brien is that therapists could run evening parent support/education groups, perhaps at monthly intervals. The purpose of these meetings would be to bring parents together for mutual support, to allow discussion about particular therapy issues, and any other related general issues of relevance to the families.

Helpful ways to communicate with parents

Under normal circumstances people demonstrate 'selective perception, i.e., seeing and hearing only what they wish to (Cartwright 1981; Dick 1979; Johnson 1972; Smiley 1975). This tendency is exacerbated under stressful conditions, with the consequence that information becomes distorted and misinterpreted. Parents are often intimidated by the expertise of professionals and regard them with awe, rather than as approachable people. According to Gorham (1975) parents may have gone to professionals in the past and received too little help, either because of time restrictions, or a lack of knowledge in the area. This may have served to erode their confidence in specialists and professionals (Friedrich & Friedrich 1980; Gorham 1975; Green & Souter 1977).

Brimblecombe (1978) identified certain unmet needs of families of handicapped children, a significant one being inadequate information from professionals. Warfield (1975) reported the results of a survey to determine what specific information parents of intellectually handicapped children considered important. Mothers were asked to rank ten topics in order of relevance to them. Generally, the topic that ranked as the most important was 'What is mental retardation?', followed by 'Understanding your own feelings'. The topic judged by the mothers as least important was 'What testing tells us'. 'Getting the most from professional help' ranked seventh.

There are many factors to consider when attempting to communicate information to parents effectively. The literature suggests that there are characteristics of both parents and therapists that should be considered, as well as specific techniques of information transfer that work more effectively than others.

From various studies O'Brien & Budd (1982) reported that the following features were identified by parents as helpful to them in understanding and accepting the therapeutic process.

Gradual approach to information transfer. According to Johnson (1972) when information is presented slowly, it was less likely to be distorted and more likely to be perceived, understood, retained and recalled correctly. The use of a number of sessions allowed time for the therapists to check the level of the parents' comprehension, and to elaborate points that were unclear, either verbally or through demonstration.

Friendly, informal approach. An informal and friendly approach from therapists is one of the most effective means of establishing rapport with a client (Furnhac et al 1980). When the initial situation is made pleasant, the parents are more likely to take an interest in the information and to follow through with suggested activities and future et al recommendations made (Heward et al 1979). This is fundamental to the effectiveness of therapy for the child, because it is the parent who must carry out therapy activities when the therapist is not present (Feldman et al 1975).

Use of several information channels. Demonstration (verbal, written, and practical) and the provision of written information, reports, and home programmes was appreciated by parents. Most authors including Johnson (1972) and Heward et al (1979) strongly endorse the use of multiple communication channels. Documented evidence, in the form of reports, provides a permanent record of the child's performance, and can be referred to at future dates to monitor progress (Baum 1976). Written home programmes are useful, because they remind parents of appropriate therapeutic activities. Using numerous channels of information transfer is particularly appropriate when attempting to overcome communication barriers, e.g., with migrant or illiterate parents.

Use of clear, concise terms. Parents valued information that they ranked as 'relevant', and 'useful'. Interestingly, O'Brien's & Budd's (1982) parent group ranked 'assessment results' as highly valued — in contrast to findings by Warfield (1975).

The parents studied by O'Brien & Budd often sought clarification about aspects of their child's assessment — and this was interpreted as indicative of a desire to be kept informed. Therapists also felt that they were justified in discussing assessment in depth, because the assessment results, in conjunction with clinical observations and the child's history, formed the basis for planning therapy. It was felt to be vital that parents understood assessment in order to understand treatment.

Use of communication aids. O'Brien & Budd (1982) established that special arrangements are rarely made to help meet the unique needs of illiterate or non-English speaking parents. Moreover, such parents are often found to have other problems which may have an impact on plans for their child's therapy. Thus, it becomes very important to make some special arrangements for parents in the two identified groups.

Invitation to parents to question and discuss. The therapist can convey willingness to listen and engage in a reciprocal relationship, rather than a power relationship.

Some unhelpful practices were identified by parents, for example:

1. Too heavy reliance on verbal communication for information transfer.
2. Too little time allowed for sessions, and thus for interaction between parents and therapist, about the proposed therapy.
3. Limited, or non-use of written information about the area/condition/procedures being discussed.

SUMMARY

Unless a child client is motivated to engage in the therapy process, its effectiveness is limited, and the therapy interaction will be marred by frustration for both child and therapist. Three models have been presented, and some conclusions may be drawn about designing the motivational context of therapy. Briefly these conclusions are:

- That the motivational component may be characterized in terms of *attraction to therapy*.
- Hinde's model (1974) provides a way of systematically designing the motivational component so that it may be evaluated and modified using the normal scientific method, thus giving a therapist maximum control over the process. The therapy media/activity/procedure becomes an *independent variable*; the motivation or attraction component becomes an *intervening variable*; and the child's behavioural responses become *dependent variables*.

- Other models have been discussed for their emphasis on the key role that extrinsic and intrinsic reinforcers may play in determining the effectiveness of any designed motivational component of therapy.

It is important that a therapist develop the skills to establish rapport with a child's parents or caregivers, in order to lay the foundations of a long-term relationship based on trust. This involves the conveyance of warmth, friendliness, empathy and a willingness to listen. Expertise about the topic under discussion is also vital. And reliability as an information source is important. This is related to the perceived character of the therapist as being honest and dependable.

REFERENCES

Allport G W 1937 Personality: a psychological interpretation. Holt Rinehart & Winston, New York

Allport G W 1961 Pattern and growth in personality. Holt Rinehart & Winston, New York

Axline V M 1989, Play therapy. Churchill Livingstone, Edinburgh. First published 1947, Riverside Press, Cambridge

Azrin N H, Holtz W C 1966 Punishment. In: Honig W K (ed) Operant behaviour: areas of research and application. Appleton-Century-Crofts, New York

Baum M C 1976 Management and documentation of occupational therapy services. In: Hopkins H L, Smith H D (eds) Willard and Spackman's Occupational Therapy. J B Lippincott, Philadelphia

Brimblecombe F S W 1978 Suggestions for the future. In: Brimblecombe F (ed) Separation and special care baby units. Heinemann, London

Carr J 1980 Helping your handicapped child. Penguin, Harmondsworth

Cartwright S 1981 Why my child? Rigby Publishers, Adelaide

Clancy H C 1976 Integrating the environment into therapy. Man–Environment Systems 6: 305–12

Dick R 1979 Communication skills — not defensive communication for improving relationships and problem solving. Organisational study units. Department of Management and Psychology, St Lucia

Feldman M A, Byalick R, Rosedale M 1975 Parent involvement programmes — a growing trend in special education. Exceptional Children 41(8): 551–556

Ferster C B, Skinner B F 1957 Schedules of Reinforcement. Prentice-Hall, Englewood Cliffs

Friedrich W N, Friedrich W L 1980 Psychosocial assets of parents of handicapped and non-handicapped children. American Journal of Mental Deficiency 85(5): 551–553

Furnhac A, King J, Pendleton D 1980 Establishing rapport: interactional skills and occupational therapy. British Journal of Occupational Therapy 43(October): 322–325

Giles D K, Wolfe M M 1975 Toilet training

institutionalised, severe retardates: an application of behaviour modification techniques. American Journal of Mental Deficiency 70: 766–780

Gold M W 1975 Try another way. Film Productions of Indianapolis, Indiannapolis

Gorham K A 1975 A lost generation·of parents. Exceptional Children 41(8): 521–525

Green A C H, Souter G A 1977 The family and the young handicapped child: the importance of the right start. Medical Journal of Australia 1: 254–257

Heward W L, Dardig J C, Rossett A 1979 Working with parents of handicapped children. Charles E Merrill Publications, Columbus

Hinde R 1974 Biological bases of human social behaviour. McGraw-Hill, New York

Johnson D W 1972 Reaching out — interpersonal effectiveness and self actualization. Prentice-Hall, New Jersey

Lovaas O I 1969 Behaviour modification: teaching language to psychotic children. (16 mm movie). Appleton-Century-Crofts, New York

O'Brien T P, Budd K S 1982 A comparison method for assessing child compliance during behavioural parent training. Journal of Behavioural Assessment 4(2): 153–164

Premack D 1965 Reinforcement theory. In: Levine D (ed) Nebraska symposium on motivation. University of Nebraska Press, Lincoln

Richer J 1971 The physical environment of the mentally handicapped (IV): A Playroom for autistic children, and its companion therapy project. British Journal of Mental Subnormality 17, 2(33): 1–12

Skinner B F 1953 Science and human behaviour. Macmillan, New York

Smiley C W 1975 Feelings and reactions of parents to their retarded child. British Journal of Occupational Therapy 38(February): 29–31

Warfield G J 1975 Mothers of retarded children review a parent education program. Exceptional Children 41(8): 559–562

Watson E H, Lowrey G 1973 Growth and development of children. Year Book Medical Publishers, Chicago

White R W 1960 Competence and the pychological stages of development. In: Jones M (ed) Nebraska symposium on motivation, University of Nebraska Press, Lincoln, pp 97–138

White R W 1964 Motivation reconsidered: the concept of competence. In: Stendley B (ed) Readings in Child Behaviour and Development (2nd edn), Harcourt Brace & World, pp 164–191

RECOMMENDED READING

Ibbotson J 1977 The handicapped family. British Journal of Occupational Therapy 40(June): 134–135

Karnes M B, Zehrbach R R 1975 Matching families and services. Exceptional Children 41(8): 545–549

Kauffmac N A 1976 Occupational therapy theory, assessment, treatment in educational settings. In: Hopkins H L, Smith H D (eds) Willard and Spackman's occupational therapy. J B Lippincott, Philadelphia

Mackinnon J R 1972 Attitudes of mothers of handicapped children. Canadian Journal of Ocupational Therapy 39(1): 25–33

Marion R L 1978 A generic approach to counselling parents of exceptional children. Exceptional Children 44: 465–466

Paul J L 1981 Understanding and working with parents of children with special needs. Holt Rinehart & Winston, New York

Robinson N M, Robinson H B 1976 The mentally retarded child — a psychological approach. McGraw-Hill, New York

Stewart A 1978 Children with handicapped families, as encountered in a child guidance clinic. British Journal of Occupational Therapy 41(December): 387–389

Wainsbren S E 1980 Parents' reactions after the birth of a developmentally disabled child. American Journal of Mental Deficiency 84(4): 345–351

Wortis H 1972 Parent counselling. Mental Retardation 4: 25–31

Wyne M D, O'Connor P D 1979 Exceptional children: a developmental view. D C Heath, Lexington

10. Daring to discipline

READERS' OBJECTIVES

After reading this chapter, you should be able to:
1. Discuss the possible goals of a child's misbehaviour.
2. Compare and contrast the principles and practical implementation of the behavioral modification and socioteleological models, in occupational therapy.
3. Describe the goals of parent education programs, and application to occupational therapy.
4. Describe predictable outcomes from parent education, based on research evaluative studies.

Historically our society has swung from dealing with children in an authoritarian powerful way, e.g., 'don't argue, do as I say', or 'pick up your clothes', to an extremely permissive approach. People, particularly parents, now seek a more moderate approach. Earlier generations of mothers had the benefits of learning child-rearing skills within their own large family context. Mothers also enjoyed a ready-made social support system, wherein the family network of womenfolk were available to help with the practical tasks of rearing children and to give advice. Nowadays, the family unit tends to be small and highly mobile, and therefore independent of the extended family support system. Sadly, few effective alternative support systems have developed. Specialists, including occupational therapists, have become the source of knowledge and advice in many aspects of rearing children. In an interesting development since the 1970s, specialists have devised a range of formal parenting skills training programmes. For occupational therapists these parent education programmes provide useful intervention materials. They may be used in preventive early intervention programmes, to ensure healthy development of children and family relationships. The programmes are also useful for working with families whose children are receiving occupational therapy.

A therapist working with families must:

- Develop general skills of managing children's behaviour, in order to achieve therapy objectives; and
- Be able to provide parents with information and support when they seek help about disciplining their child.

Both situations require that a paediatric occupational therapist has a point of view. This chapter describes and discusses different philosophies and practical systems of managing children's behaviour, and disciplining them. The discussion about discipline will be brief, practical — presented as 'do's and don'ts' — and directed at the problems which commonly confront parents and therapists. The views expressed represent those which are at present acceptable in most westernized societies. The discussion of 'behaviour management' approaches will be more extensive, and related to underlying theory, which leads to particular practical approaches. Parent education programmes are described and compared; there is a brief discussion of the research studies which evaluate programme effectiveness; and the skills of leading parent education groups are presented.

The first section of the chapter provides a discussion of the differences between behaviour management and discipline.

BEHAVIOUR MANAGEMENT VERSUS DISCIPLINE

The term 'behaviour management' is generally used to refer to a method for changing or maintaining some aspect of a person's behaviour. Change might entail increasing the frequency of a desired behaviour, or decreasing an undesirable behaviour. Behaviour management techniques may also be used to maintain a behaviour that has already been learned, and the relevant theory bases have been discussed in Chapter 9.

Discipline, on the other hand, generally refers to the training process by which 'unacceptable' behaviour is controlled or eliminated. Unfortunately, the connotation is a negative one, implying a power relationship centred on control of one individual (the weaker), by another (the stronger). In fact, the training process is directed toward achieving order, co-operation, sharing — those human characteristics which allow us to live together in harmony, and benefit from our mutual association.

'Discipline' also refers to inner personal characteristics. We talk of 'self-discipline', and often refer to a person as being 'well disciplined'. Here we refer to personal characteristics which are expressed as 'orderly', 'co-operative', or 'altruistic' behaviour. We also imply that the individual has suppressed his/her self-oriented wishes for a more important external goal.

The success of all behaviour management and disciplinary procedures will be obvious in the child's developing ability to behave in an orderly co-operative fashion. It will also be measured in the long term by the array of personal and ethical values that the young person adopts, and lives by in the societal group. This long-term goal of early discipline 'training' is one to discuss with parents, and to encourage them to think about in relation to their own value system. The question for parents and therapists is 'what do you want to teach the child?' There is a popular and thought provoking verse which prompts some answers:

. . . if a child lives with criticism
he learns to condemn
. . . if a child lives with encouragement
he learns confidence

(Dorothy Law Nolte)

Discipline and development. Parents need reassurance about what is normal developmental behaviour — even if calculated to drive the most composed parent to distraction and the sherry bottle! For example, Green (1984) asserts that infants up to about one year, do not require 'disciplining'. The infant is busy attempting to engage his/her parents in a mutually secure and trusting relationship. To attain this goal the infant needs to experience rapid response to expressed needs — she/he cannot be 'spoilt'. However, in the second to third year, the toddler enters a stage of learning control of bodily functions and behaviour. All toddlers are 'typically stubborn, self-centred and negative' (Green 1984). There is also the genetic predisposition of each child to be taken into account. Some will be amenable and more naturally co-operative than other children. Parents should be reassured that even within their own family,

different approaches to the same problem situations may be required for each of their children.

What does 'discipline' involve — for a parent or a therapist? There are some excellent books available to help adults, and *A parent survival kit* by Dingle (1988) is particularly perceptive. The guidelines given here are

---

Some do's in situations where discipline is indicated

- Establish trust and confidence between adult and child
- Consider the stage of development that the child has reached.
- Consider the interests, concerns, abilities, and difficulties of the individual child
- Look for any reason behind the behaviour that suggested a need for disciplinary action.
- Be flexible and prepared to change the method used if it is not successful. Different situations require different methods of control.
- Set reasonable limits for children, based on safety and concern for others, and make decisions definite.
- Make sure that the child understands it is the behaviour that is unacceptable — not she/he.
- Remember that all children are learners, and allow time and opportunity for learning, before assuming that the child is being wilfully 'disobedient'.
- Allow consideration for 'hard times', e.g., when a child has been ill, or has encountered many upsets, or is afraid.
- Be honest, natural, and consistent in your approach.

Some don'ts for the disciplinarian

- Allow a simple situation to develop into a major battle.
- Argue with a child — explanation is a different thing.
- Vacillate — you must take positive action.
- Give a choice when there really is none.
- Delay action, and expect someone else to accept the responsibility.
- Worry about mistakes, and don't be afraid to say 'I'm sorry'. Children are remarkably resilient, and they learn by degrees that adults too have feelings.
- Command — requests always receive a better response.
- Expect behaviour to be changed by one disciplinary episode. Children learn slowly and forget quickly.
- Recall past situations where discipline was needed. Handle the situation as it is, and then forget it, and allow the child to progress to the next step.
- Discipline unless your action is one that will eventually benefit the child.

neither exhaustive, nor exact, but are provided to help you organize your own ideas. They were originally devised for use in a preschool centre for normally developing children and have been modified over the years.

This practical advice about disciplinary 'dos and don'ts' leads to consideration of two well developed and widely used behaviour management systems, which have particular use for occupational therapists.

Behaviour management in therapy

Effective behaviour management entails *identification* of the specific behaviour to be taught, modified, or maintained, and *a plan* to accomplish the desired behaviour change. Behaviour management encompasses social behaviour and task behaviour skills. Two very different models will be presented, and both are relevant to social and task behaviour management. Each model is examined as it can be applied to therapy situations. Model 1 is the 'behaviour modification' model. Model 2 is the so-called 'socioteleological model', based on earlier models of Adler (1958) and Dreikurs & Gray (1968). This model holds that success in interpersonal relationships is essential to success with tasks.

Model 1: Behaviour modification

> **Definition**
> *Behaviour modification* is a clinical approach for changing observable behaviour, based on Skinnerian principles of learning.

The important learning theory and operant principles are:

- That both adaptive and maladaptive behaviour are learned.
- That the results of our actions, or behaviour, determine whether or not we repeat that behaviour. For example, if you offer to help your friend with an assignment, and she/he thanks you warmly and accepts, chances are that you will offer help again. This principle is known as the 'reinforcement principle', and discussed at length in Chapter 9.
- That cues or parts of our environment, human and non-human, determine what you do and when you do them. For example, when you first read an exam paper (the cue or stimulus) you go cold all over, feel ill, and cannot begin to write. This

principle is known as 'the stimulus control principle'.

In the behaviour modification model, reinforcers, both pleasant and unpleasant, are used in a systematic way to either increase the occurrence of a behaviour, or decrease it. Thus, an occupational therapist may use behaviour modification to promote acquisition of skills, such as independent dressing. Alternatively, a therapist may seek to diminish some behaviour, such as stereotyped head banging.

'Behaviour modification' is not to be confused with 'behaviour therapy', which is also a clinical application of learning theory and operant principles (Skinner 1953). Behaviour *modification* represents the process by which any behaviour may be altered, in any chosen direction. Behaviour *therapy* on the other hand, represents a strategic system directed at behaviour regarded as a 'problem' or as pathological. For example, an individual may have a fear of flying (a phobia) and may seek the help of a behaviour therapist, who is usually a psychologist. The focus of the therapy is always to design conditions that will change the undesired or unacceptable behaviour, and thus alleviate the problem without seeking for psychic explanations for it. Specialists should not use the terms behaviour modification and behaviour therapy interchangeably as they are not synonymous.

The 'intent to alter behaviour' attracts criticism of behaviour modification, and indeed of all systems which share that intent. Norman (1976) provides an excellent discussion of the criticisms and misuses of behaviour modification. The criticisms address ethical and philosophical questions, for example, does one have the 'right' to manipulate the behaviour of others? Behaviour modification and therapy probably attract criticism because the procedures are described with clarity and specificity, and are demonstrably successful. There is no one answer to the ethical questions posed. In practice, any therapy assumes intent to alter behaviour, but the client is always protected by the ethical rules of professional conduct.

Why use behaviour modification?

A therapist may use behaviour modification procedures for one of the following reasons:

- To *organize* existing behaviour–environment relationships;
- To *alter* existing behaviour–environment relationships; and
- To *develop* new behaviour–environment relationships.

Whatever the behaviour to be modified, the design of the programme follows a consistent predictable pattern:

1. Identification of the desired terminal behaviour(s), and writing the objectives for achieving the terminal behaviour(s).
2. Establishment of a base line profile of existing behaviour.
3. Selection of the reinforcers and a reinforcement schedule to be used.
4. Selection of the modification technique to establish the new behaviour. The three techniques commonly chosen are shaping, chaining and modelling

The four steps in the programme will be outlined.

Identify desired terminal behaviour(s). While recognizing general principles of learning, in the behaviour modification model, each individual is recognized as unique, and therefore requiring individualized goals. Chosen terminal behaviour must be defined as observable behaviour which is measurable, for example, 'smile' can be defined and measured; 'happiness' is an interpretation of smiling behaviour. Another example of a defined terminal behaviour would be '70 units of work achieved in 50 minutes, earns one cigarette'.

On occasions an occupational therapist may elect to use an interpretative word where it can be adequately defined. For example, 'verbalization' may be defined for purposes of the programme as 'anything spoken distinctly enough for a listener to understand, regardless of how many words were spoken at the time'.

Similarly, objectives must be couched in behavioural terms and must specifically include:

• What the person will do
• The conditions under which behaviour will be performed
• The criteria for quality or success of behaviour.

Here is an example of an objective expressed as behaviour. 'The child will approach his/her therapist more often when the therapist verbally praises approach behaviours.'

Establish a base line of existing behaviour. Behaviour modification programmes are always derived from systematic observation and analysis of a client's behaviour. Norman (1976) emphasizes the importance of pre-programme evaluation. Here is a set of questions that a therapist may use to ensure that the observation and analysis process was adequate.

1. What is the client's range and level of skill, relevant to the proposed modification?

2. What are the varying conditions under which the behaviours occur, and/are inhibited?
3. What reinforcers appear most attractive to the client?
4. What are the conditions of learning that seem most appropriate for the client?

The programme must begin at the established level of skill. Beginning at a level that is too difficult or complex (i.e. not yet achieved) will lead to frustration for the client, and ultimately, programme failure. Similarly, beginning at a level already mastered, and too easy, will introduce unnecessary steps in the programme, and lead to the individual being bored, and unchallenged.

Selecting reinforcers and schedule. The two groups, natural and artificial reinforcers, have already been discussed in Chapter 9. Each may be used alone, or in combination. The schedules will usually be structured to proceed from 'continuous' to 'random'.

Select modification techniques. Three techniques are reviewed: shaping, chaining and modelling.

Shaping — by successive approximation. Shaping refers to the moulding of new and complex behaviour from existing simple responses. Reinforcement is actively presented and withheld, in a set of sequenced steps thus:

a. Step 1. The child's general level of activity is raised by reinforcing any appropriate response. For example, where the desired behaviour is removal of a shirt, the child is initially reinforced for any attempt to handle any of his/her clothing.
b. Step 2. The reinforcement is temporarily withheld, and the child is encouraged to work harder for it. This step represents an 'extinction phase'.
c. Step 3. Before the frequency of behaviour decreases (because the child loses interest) a response close to the desired one is reinforced. This step represents a 'selective reinforcement phase'.
d. Step 4. After the reinforced behaviour is firmly established, the reinforcement is again withheld. This step represents a second 'extinction phase'.
e. Step 5. The reinforcement is reintroduced, but only for behaviour more closely approximated to that defined as terminal.
   Steps 3–5 are repeated until the training is completed.

The particular shaping procedure described is one of 'successive approximation' to a defined terminal or desired behaviour.

Chaining is also a behaviour shaping procedure, especially useful for teaching skills which are made up of a series of small steps. Chaining differs from shaping in that the child does not need to have any existing skill or knowledge of the task to be performed. Dressing skills are very suitable ones to teach by the chaining procedure.

The first step is to define the set of steps involved in the total task to be attempted. Bluma et al (1976) give a simple example of the chain involved in tying shoelaces. The steps identified are: 'Lace, cross laces, make knot, make first loop, pull lace around loop, push loop through opening, pull tight' Copeland et al (1976) have presented an occupational therapy training manual for intellectually retarded children based on the operant procedures, using chaining. Example 10.1 shows such a technique.

Example 10.1 Backward chaining technique used to teach child to put on trousers (Copeland et al 1976)

Done by adult	Done by child
a. Trousers put on over both feet to ankles.	a. Pulls up to waist.
b. One of child's feet put into trouser leg to ankle, other foot put two-thirds of the way in, with foot pointing to floor.	b. Pushes second foot all through, pulls up from ankles to waist.
c. As b), but second foot put half-way in, pointing to floor.	c. Pushes second foot through, pulls to waist.
d. As b), but second foot put quarter way in, pointing to floor.	d. Pushes second foot through, pulls to waist.

Modelling refers to the procedure in which a person watches another perform the desired behaviour and get reinforced for it, and then imitates the performance. Modelling is particularly useful for modifying social interactive behaviour skills.

Evaluation

The final procedure in a behaviour modification programme is the design and implementation of an evaluation of the effectiveness of that programme.

The child's progress. It must be apparent that·there is a relationship between each component in the programme and change in the child's behaviour. If precise and appropriate terminal behaviours and objectives were written, then evaluation of the child's performance will be straightforward.

The designed procedures should also be assessed to confirm that they were, and still remain appropriate to achieving the desired behaviour.

The generalization process should also be assessed. Unless generalization tasks are part of the total programme, short-term gains in desired behaviour may be meaningless. For example, to teach a child to reach out, grasp and handle a play object is only meaningful if the manipulation skills are extended to functional activity use, such as using a spoon at meal times. The translation of increased skills per se into functional ability is a central tenet of occupational therapy.

Summary

Behaviour modification is one of a number of strategies that a therapist may use to change or modify behaviour.

The model specifies a set of general learning principles that account for changes in human behaviour. However, the model does not specify information about any particular behaviour that might be modified. Thus, a therapist must also acquire specialist knowledge about the behaviour to which modification procedures are to be applied.

For example, if a child is to be taught to dress, the therapist should know the developmental steps by which independent dressing is normally acquired. Without the specialist knowledge of the behaviour to be modified, inappropriate expectations of the child (client) may be written into the programme, leading to its failure.

Norman (1976) has presented guidelines for therapists proposing to use behaviour modification, and these points provide a fitting conclusion to this discussion.

- Know about the behavioural area to be modified, e.g., cognitive or social or self-care skills.
- Practise writing terminal behaviour(s) and goals.
- Complete a thorough assessment of the child (client) before planning the programme.
- Design the modification programme in accord with all of the learning principles specified by the behaviour modification model.
- Plan and use a systematic evaluation for the intervention programme.
- Anticipate and systematically plan long-term generalization tasks.
- Begin where the learner is — i.e., the behaviour of the individual is used to determine where a programme shall begin.

Model 2: Discipline that develops responsibility

Goals-of-behaviour. The socioteleological position is that humans are responsible beings, capable of making choices, and thus directing their own destiny. A child's behaviour is seen as goal directed, 'even though children are usually thought to be unaware of their goals (Dinkmeyer & McKay 1976a,b). These authors suggest that an adult can gain a fair idea of a child's goal by looking at the *results* of the behaviour, rather than just at the behaviour. This idea represents an important general principle; it frees the adult (therapist or parent)

from the need to recognize and respond to 'temper', 'disobedience', 'defiance', and so on. That is to say, use of the principle of goal recognition negates the need for a comprehensive set of recipes for dealing with a range of specific behaviours. The socioteleological model outlines four goals of children's misbehaviour, which are attention, power, justice, responsibility. These are represented in Figure 10.1.

Goals to be promoted and encouraged

Child's goal (positive) →	Child's belief (desirable) →	Child's behaviour →	Outcome (Adult's response)
Attention Involvement Contribution	I belong by contributing	helps Volunteers	Lets child know the contribution counts, and is appreciated
Power Autonomy Responsibility for own behaviour	I can decide and be responsible for my behaviour	Shows self-discipline Does own work is resourceful	Encourages child's decision making Lets child experience both positive and negative outcomes Expresses confidence in child
Justice Fairness	I am interested in co-operating	Returns hurt for kindness Ignores belittling comments	Lets child know that his her interest in co-operating is appreciated
Responsibility Withdrawal from conflict Refusal to fight Acceptance of other's opinions	I can decide to withdraw from conflict	Ignores provocation Withdraws from power contest to decide own behaviour	Recognizes child's effort to act maturely

Goals to be discouraged

Child's goal (negative) →	Child's belief (undesirable) →	Child's behaviour →	Outcome (Adult's response)
Attention	I belong only when I am being noticed or served	Whinges and whines 'Shows off' Behaves or dresses inappropriately for situation	Feeling: annoyed Reaction: tendency to remind and coax
Power	I belong only when I am in control or boss, or proving no one can boss me	Bosses others Physically hurts others Defies adults Openly or covertly Destroys property	Feeling: angry, provoked, as if authority is threatened Reaction: fight or give in
Justice Revenge	I belong only by hurting others as I feel hurt I cannot be loved	Is 'rude' Verbally hurtful	Feeling: deeply hurt Reaction: tendency to retaliate and get even
Display of inadequacy	I belong only by convincing others not to expect anything from me I am unable I am helpless	Refuses to try Nags for help Refuses any responsibility	Feeling: despair hopelessness 'I give up' Reaction: tendency to agree with child that nothing can be done

Fig. 10.1 The goals of children's behaviour. Reprinted by permission of American Guidance Service, Publishers' Building, Circle Pines, MN 55014. *Systematic Training for Effective Parenting, Parents Handbook* by Don Dinkmeyer, Sr. and Gary D. McKay. Copyright 1976. All rights reserved.

Dinkmeyer & McKay (1976a,b) take the position that the commonly used reward and punishment method has the following negative outcomes:

— It makes the adult responsible for the child's behaviour.
— It prevents children from learning to make their own decisions, and consequently, from adopting rules for effective behaviour.
— It suggests that acceptable behaviour is expected only in the presence of authority figures.
— It invites resistance by attempting to force children to conform.

Exponents of the socioteleological approach have presented a useful alternative system which uses 'natural and logical consequences' (Dreikurs & Gray 1968).

Natural and logical consequences. Here is an example of the difference between using a reward/punishment approach and the natural and logical consequences approach. Tom and Bob are disturbing the evening meal by exchanging taunts and insults. Father responds in the first example by using the reward/punishment approach. (a) 'If you two don't stop that fighting this instant you'll go straight to bed without dinner.'

In the second example father responds by using the logical consequences approach. (b) 'Tom and Bob, settle down, or leave the table until you're ready to join us pleasantly.'

Principles vs recipes. The basic principles which guide the use of natural and logical consequences are:

— Seek to understand the child's goals, behaviour and emotions.
— Be both kind and firm.
— Allow the child to experience the *consequences* of his/her own decisions. Don't 'overprotect'.
— Be consistent in own actions.
— Separate the deed from the doer.
— Encourage independence.
— Avoid pity.
— Do not be overly concerned about 'what other people think.'
— Determine who owns the problem — you or the child.
— Talk less, act more.
— Refuse to fight, or give in.

Here are the action steps in applying natural and logical consequences.

— Provide choices — an essential component if the approach is to work. The adult must reflect, by tone of voice, respect, acceptance and good will toward the child.
— As you follow through with a consequence, give assurance that there will be an opportunity to change the decision later. Children often try to test limits, but a decision must stand, e.g., Mother says, 'I see that you haven't changed your clothes (the request), so I assume that you have decided to stay inside today (the decision and consequence), and try again tomorrow.'
— If the misbehaviour is repeated, extend the time that must elapse before the child may try again, e.g., 'I see that you are still not ready to settle down, and have decided to leave the room. You may try again tomorrow night.'

Misbehaviour and management in therapy

Tom, the 'Clinger', Melissa, the 'Show-off', and Alice the 'failure', provide three short examples of 'misbehaving' children in typical therapy situations.

Example 10.2: Tom the 'Clinger'

Four-year-old Tom arrives for occupational therapy with his mum. Tom hides behind mother, clutching her dress and sucking his thumb. Mother tries, unsuccessfully, to separate from Tom, but he dissolves into sobs and clutches more tightly. How should the occupational therapist respond?

Whatever the driving force behind Tom's behaviour, the outcomes are that:

1. He gains much attention.
2. His mother's response implies that she is irritated and disappointed.
3. Tom's clinging behaviour is reinforced rather than discouraged, though it is undesired.

The goal of attention for the clinging behaviour can be removed by removing its cause — the need for Tom to separate from his mother. Some readers may be tempted to think 'How impractical — after all the child *must* learn to separate'. The latter statement is true, but reflects a narrow view of the situation. The general action principle requires us to ask ourselves 'is "separation" the first priority of therapy?' The analysis of outcomes suggests that it may not be.

The socioteleological model shows that therapy may be planned so that outcome 1 is retained, i.e., Tom gains attention, *but*, he gains it for positive (maturing or growing) behaviour. Outcome 2 is reversed so that mother's response indicates pleasure and support for Tom's behaviour. Outcome 3 vanishes. The terminal goal of therapy is achieved: Tom and mother separate from each other comfortably and confidently.

Example 10.3: Melissa the 'show-off'
Eleven-year-old Melissa never loses an opportunity to display her extensive vocabulary of four-letter words. The children in the group respond, with mock horror, giggles, and (unsuccessful) attempts to outdo Melissa.

The occupational therapist wants to discourage the language — but how? In this situation the outcomes are:

1. Melissa gains attention.
2. Melissa gains a degree of power.

This example is a classical one of the child who has mis-learned how to attract attention. It is also possible that Melissa is expressing feelings of inadequacy, though this is not necessarily so. The occupational therapist needs a strategy which retains outcomes 1 and 2, *but* redefines the conditions for them. For example, 'power' becomes 'responsibility' by giving Melissa an explicit leadership role, with rights and responsibilities towards the others in the group.

Outcome 1 can be redefined in terms of the reinforcement given. Positive feedback given for *any*, and all, acceptable behaviour, combined with a deliberately non-chalant approach to the ugly language, should result in its diminution or disappearance. In other words, the priority objective is to teach Melissa how much more satisfying it can be to gain attention for mature behaviour, than for troublesome behaviour. Getting rid of the ugly language is an outcome; the goal is responsible behaviour.

Example 10.4: Alice the 'Failure'
Eight-year-old Alice always says 'No, I can't', or 'I don't know — you decide' when faced with a choice, or asked to try something new.

How could the occupational therapist encourage her to feel and act more confidently? In Dreikur & Gray's (1968) terms Alice is saying 'I belong *only* by convincing others not to expect anything from me. I am unable and helpless.' The outcomes of Alice's behaviour are:

1. Adults' expectations are lowered — much help is given. Alice is viewed as 'a poor little thing', or 'an irritating nuisance'.
2. Alice learns to be dependent — she is 'let off the hook' for decisions, *and* their consequences.

The goal of therapy is to teach Alice how to accept responsibility for decisions and actions — confident self-initiated behaviour will follow. Using Dreikur & Gray's model, and the action oriented principle of Dinkmeyer & McKay (1976a,b), the therapist would structure the therapy thus:

- Using appropriate language for her development level, acknowledge to Alice that there are risks attached to decisions, which can be frightening to her.
- Refuse to take responsibility for Alice's decision making, but offer limited options for decision making, all having *safe* outcomes. For example, choosing between the red and the blue paint for fingerpainting.
- Give positive reinforcement for Alice's attempts at decision making, using a continuous approximation schedule.

Summary

The desired outcome of behaviour management using the socioteleological model is that the individual (child) be a responsible, caring, and sharing member of a social community. The approach is applicable to task situations, as well as to social interaction situations. For example, learning to put on a coat would be structured so that the child is led to consider by thought and experiment, what are the steps involved, and what is their logical order. The therapist's role is that of a designer and facilitator. This theoretical model has been developed into a practical system of discipline and behaviour management called *Systematic Training for Effective Parenting* (Dinkmeyer & McKay 1976a,b). This programme is discussed later in the chapter.

HELPING PARENTS AND CHILDREN TO LIVE TOGETHER IN HARMONY

It is accepted that parents are usually the most influential educators of children. Yet parents are expected to assume this role with little assistance, guidance, or training. Dreikurs & Soltz (1964) argued that the influence of social democracy changes the atmosphere of society, and renders obsolete the traditional methods of childrearing. In this scenario, formal parent education offers a possible means for assisting parents to adjust their childrearing methods, in order to share rights, responsibilities, and power. Gordon (1975) argued that parents are 'blamed not trained' and for this reason he supports parent education. Hawkins (1976) also identified a need for parent education, viewing it as a way of reversing underachievement, disruptiveness, truancy and other 'innumerable problems' of children and their families.

Definition
Parent education has been described as the 'learning activity of parents who are attempting to change their method of interaction with their children for the purpose of encouraging positive behaviour in their children' (Croake & Glover 1977).

The term, parent education, refers to the imparting of information about parenting skills and attitudes to a group of people, by an instructor who follows a set curriculum of a particular course.

Programmes are concerned with family relationships, particularly those between parent and child. Several disciplines have contributed to programme development, particularly psychiatry, psychology, nursing and education. The proponents all share a common commitment to the development of improved family relationships, by effective preventive techniques.

There are a number of objectives which can be met as an outcome of parents attending parent education study groups. Some of the objectives are to:

- Understand practical theory of human relationships
- Learn new procedures
- Improve communication . . . all feel they are being heard
- Develop skills of listening, resolving conflicts, exploring alternatives
- Learn to use encouragement
- Become aware of own faulty convictions, self-defeating patterns, and
- Become effective parents.

Parent education programmes

Formal parent education training schemes have developed particularly since the 1970s and have proved popular. Sherrets et al (1980) found that there are at least 65 major programmes in existence. Some of these programmes advocate personal, philosophical and religious views under the auspices of parent education. A word of caution: a therapist should be aware of the philosophical and moral underpinnings and the content of a specific programme before endorsing it or she/he may unwittingly and unethically endorse sectarian views.

Several packaged parenting programmes have been selected for discussion in this chapter; all are concerned with skill acquisition, particularly self-awareness, communication, conflict resolution and/or behaviour modification. The selected programmes reflect three major psychological approaches: the humanistic, behavioural, and socioteleological. The humanistic approach is based on Rogerian psychology and stresses the importance of self worth and communication. The behavioural approach is influenced by Skinner (1953) and emphasizes control through the use of reinforcement (Davis & 1978). The socioteleological model is based on the theories of Adler (1958), and behaviour is viewed as goal oriented (Davies 1978).

A comparison of programmes

The programmes to be described and compared are examples of those currently in popular use (Davies 1978). Each reflects one of the major psychological models: humanistic, behavioural, and socioteleological. Generally, Sherrets et al (1980) identified an enormous variation between all programmes in use; in the populations addressed, their needs, and the learning format employed.

Humanistic model

Between parent and child. In Ginott's (1965) approach, emphasis is given to improving communication skills through techniques such as active listening. Praise is seen as useful, as long as it relates to specific actions, rather than to global characteristics of the child. Ginott acknowledges the use of setting limits on children's behaviour. This programme is presented as a book which parents purchase, read and apply to their own situation, according to their own interpretation.

Parent Effectiveness Training (PET). Thomas Gordon's (1975) programme was the precursor to many other formal packaged programmes. The programme seeks to equalize power between parent and child, and stresses the importance of concepts of 'self worth', and 'effective communication'. Techniques such as 'active listening' and 'I messages' are used. Conflict resolution is approached through a 'no lose' method. Parents receive instructions in a group situation, working through the book *Parent Effectiveness Training* and its exercise work book.

Peoplemaking. Virginia Satir's interest in family therapy lead to the writing of *Peoplemaking* (1972) which, like Ginott's approach, does not require attendance at formal meetings. Davies (1978) outlines four key factors in Satir's approach, namely:

1. Individual feelings of self worth
2. Communication style
3. The rules which develop into the family structure
4. Generalization of behaviour from the family to larger society.

Emphasis is placed on congruence between verbal and non-verbal communication, and parents are encouraged to be leaders and guides to their children, rather than 'bosses' and 'pals' (Davies 1978).

Behaviour modification model

Responsible Parent Training Programme. At present this programme is enjoying a degree of success. Parents meet regularly in groups, and are taught basic concepts such as the effects of environmental change in affecting behavioural change, use of positive reinforcement for desirable behaviour, and the use of punishment for undesirable behaviour. While the child's self-esteem is seen as important, the power base resides clearly with the parent, and in this way the programme differs philosophically from those programmes based on the humanistic model. A review of the literature suggests that programmes using behaviour modification techniques tend to aim at the management of children with specific problems (Davies 1978; Seig 1974)

Socioteleological model

Systematic Training for Effective Parenting (STEP). STEP (Dinkmeyer & McKay 1976a,b) focuses on the goal-directed nature of a child's behaviour, specifically the four goals already discussed in this chapter: attention, power, justice, and responsibility. Family values are also seen as important components for achieving harmony between parents and children. Encouragement of the child is advocated as the most important corrective influence that a parent (or therapist) can use. The reward/punishment approaches of the behaviour modification model are rejected. Instead, natural and logical consequences are used to teach the child outcomes of his/her actions, and thereby a sense of personal control. Dinkmeyer & McKay (1976a,b) seek to equalize the power base between parent and child, and the STEP programme aims to facilitate democratic family relationships. However, the need for practical limits on children's behaviour is explicitly recognized.

Parents join together in small groups, and use is made of attractive cartoon style visual material, and audio tapes. The STEP programme is particularly useful for use in occupational therapy. The programme does not rely heavily on verbal instruction and interaction, and it respects parents of all social classes and educational background. Moreover, the audio tapes are readily available in a number of countries, using local examples, making it easier for parents to identify with their own family situation.

There is considerable overlap between parent education programmes. For example those with humanistic and socioteleological models share the emphasis on self worth and communication skills. However, the programmes differ in their view of parental power and use of reinforcement contingencies, probably reflecting the differences in the theoretical models of each approach. One particular approach cannot satisfy all parental needs, nor is one innately superior to the others. Rather, each package has application potential for various parent groups.

STEP is very attractive visually and requires less verbal and reading skills.

PET leads on to other effectiveness training courses: teaching leadership, business and assertiveness training.

Behavioural programmes have application for children with special needs, e.g., behavioural problems such as conduct disorders.

Satir and Ginott's books would be suitable for parents with proficient reading and verbal skills.

In summary, while the designs and content of the programmes differ, they all share the same general rationale to varying degrees, namely that parents can learn parenting skills through the acquisition of particular knowledge. But, how effective is parent education as a tool for learning effective parenting skills?

Evaluating outcomes of parent education

Parent education has enjoyed an almost unquestioned acceptance by professionals and the general public, characterized by a *belief* in its effectiveness. Certainly the notion that parents can learn skills to enhance better relationships with their children has *intuitive* appeal (Dinkmeyer & Dinkmeyer 1979, Terkelson 1976). Yet empirical research about the effectiveness of parent education has not kept abreast with the expansion of programmes.

Evaluation of parenting programmes has been fraught with difficulties. For example, in this field of research, ethical considerations, often make it extremely difficult to apply stringent scientific control. Consequently, many of the parent education studies have been marred with methodological flaws.

Many authors advocate parent education as a method of promoting quality in parent–child interactions, and as a means of equipping people for interacting with children (Hawkins 1976). However there are continuing arguments against the uncritical acceptance of such programmes. Doherty & Ryder (1980) have expressed several concerns about the possible negative effects that parent education could have on families. For example, they argued that education might increase covert manipulation in the family because parent–child relationships become 'technologized'. Another criticism highlights the possibility that applying the right technique to a specific situation may lead to a simplistic belief that it will solve the problem. The counter argument is that techniques cannot be applied universally — that situations arise where parents must use common sense and bend the rules which packaged programmes advocate. A final and important cause for concern has been that parent education may contribute to family division, particularly when only one parent enrolls in the course. Unfortunately, the arguments cautioning against parent education have, in the main, not been subjected to rigorous research.

Even though studies have yielded conflicting results, it appears that there are some confirmed outcomes. These have been identified as follows:

- Parent education programmes do effect change in attitudes (Berrett 1975, Croake & Burness 1976, Freeman 1975, Sharpley & Poiner 1980).
- Parental behaviour is amenable to change after intervention (Berrett 1975; Croake & Burness 1976).
- Parents' cognitive responses to childrearing situations change after attending parent education (Sharpley & Poiner 1980).

Offering parent education has become an increasingly important role of the paediatric occupational therapist. Programmes may be used with parents whose children are receiving therapy, perhaps for behavioural disorders; with parents whose children may be at risk for developmental delay for environmental reasons; and with parents who simply wish to enhance their parenting skills.

The therapist will often be the leader of parent education groups. Leadership requires training, the development of special skills and practice. The final section of this chapter provides a brief discussion of basic leadership skills which can be used quite generally, but are discussed in relation to leading parent education programme groups.

Leading parent education programmes

The occupational therapist as leader

While most people have some general notion of what is meant by leadership, the term is nonetheless difficult to define; (Byrt 1971; Selznick 1957). Most definitions include the common element of 'someone who exerts more influence than the other members of the group' (Middlebrook 1980).

Effective leaders have good interpersonal skills and can influence people on a number of levels.

Shaw (1976) studied the characteristics of leaders and found the following features to be the main predictors of effective leaders:

- abilities relevant to the group goal, such as high general intelligence, verbal fluency, insight and adaptability;

- interpersonal skills, such as co-operativeness, dependability and social participation, and
- motivation to lead, such as initiative and persistence.

Qualities such as *charisma* are often emphasized by the popular media, and can be important for a leader to possess. However, charisma cannot singularly resolve all difficulties of leadership (Jaques 1983). Effective leadership skills can and must be learned, practised and improved. Some guidelines follow which will enhance a therapist's leadership skills as a parent educator.

Guidelines for promoting leadership, and leader skills (Sharpley & Poiner 1980).

Principles of leadership. When conducting parent education classes or other group sessions it is useful to:

- Interpret behaviour in terms of its goal-directed nature
- Promote co-operation and cohesiveness
- Encourage personal growth of group members
- Provide experiences which allow group members to recognise own assets
- Encourage practice of newly learned skills outside group
- Develop atmosphere of mutual trust and encouragement in group.

Leader skills. A leader in a group situation must be able to:

- Structure the learning experience
- Generalize the discussion
- Link to participants' experience
- Provide feedback to the participants
- Develop tentative hypotheses
- Focus on positive behaviour
- Set tasks and obtain commitments from participants
- Summarize

Effective leaders must project an impression of self-confidence, and a belief that one is adequate to meet the demands of life. Such confidence also gives courage to be imperfect. 'Expert' leaders are perceived by group members as being confident and lively. They are well prepared, focus on the task at hand, and treat group members in a democratic and friendly way (Brammer 1979). It is important to remember that the leader is a role model of behaviour, and should demonstrate those principles which we are advocating. It is impossible to 'seek' a democratic approach if one is authoritarian, and displays a lack of trusk or acceptance at meetings. It is important to demonstrate encouragement and logical consequences.

Group processes. A group, like any other dynamic organization, experiences certain predictable stages of growth and development. It is important for the therapist to recognize these stages, and to facilitate the process so that the group meets its objectives. The predictable stages are:

1. The answer to prayers: There is some degree of euphoria, and the leader is frequently flattered by the participants in this stage.
2. Disillusionment: Negative comments are made by the participants about the programme. This stage is sometimes described as the 'what are we doing here stage' The group leader *must* redefine goals, facilitate feedback, encourage effort and progress. Techniques such as role playing can increase the participants' interest and commitment.
3. Maturity: The group accepts responsibility for its own learning. A high degree of cohesiveness and trust has usually occurred by this stage.

While these belief characteristics may seem like a tall order, it is important for helpers to project positive attitudes to clients. In this regard, leaders are also helpers, and a helpful person inspires trust and confidence (Brammer 1979; Rogers 1961).

Beliefs that characterize effective helpers. (Combs 1969)

1. People are *able*, and have capacity to solve their problems.
2. People are *friendly*, and expect a reciprocal relationship.
3. People are *worthy*, and possess dignity which must be reflected.
4. People are basically *internally* motivated, and creative.
5. People are dependable, and essentially trustworthy, predictable and understandable.
6. People are *helpful* not hindering, and sources of satisfaction and enhancement.

SUMMARY

Perhaps more than any other interaction between adults and children, it is the way in which 'discipline' is applied that causes observers to form judgements about the effectiveness of the adult. This focuses attention on the elements of 'power' and 'control' in the relationship. Student therapists feel a compulsion to prove themselves capable of 'controlling the situation'. Equally, young parents face the same compulsion from the older family members and the public in general. The outcome is likely to be a battle in which ultimately both the adult and the child lose.

In this chapter the focus has been on clarifying the possible goals of behaviour, especially from the child's point of view. Our concern has been to deflect attention from adult action based on fear of seeming to be ineffective in the sight of others. Instead, we have focused on the real goal of all discipline and behaviour management — the development of behaviour which allows children and adults to live together in harmony and to benefit from each other's company. The chapter presents different points of view, all concerned with establishing effective two-way communication.

Discipline is about personal values, and all effective approaches to discipline and behaviour management emphasize the following points.

- Adults listen, in an open relaxed caring manner — without judgements.
- Adults act firmly and decisively, but gently — whatever the child's responses.
- Adults seek the *reason* for the child's behaviour, and respond to that, rather than the expression of behaviour.
- There is order and direction in the environment, but rules are not inflexible.
- Children are allowed to learn from the consequences of their actions.
- Allowances are made for the fact that a child is a learner, and will need much practice before acquiring self-control.
- In conclusion — the child who lives with fairness, learns justice.

Parents too, need nurturing, and some formal programmes for them have been examined.

REFERENCES

Adler A 1958 What life should mean to you. Capricorn Books New York
Berrett R D 1975 Adlerian mother study groups: an evaluation. Journal of Individual Psychology 31: 179–182

Bluma S, Shearer M, Trotman T, Hillard S 1976 Portage guide to early education. Portage Project, Wisconsin
Brammer L M 1979 The helping relationship: process and skills (2nd edn). Prentice-Hall, New Jersey

Byrt W J 1971 People and organisations. McGraw-Hill, Sydney

Combs A 1969 Florida studies in the helping professions. Florida University Press, Gainesville

Copeland M, Ford L, Solon N 1976 Occupational therapy for mentally retarded children. University Park Press, Baltimore

Croake J W, Burness M R 1976 Parent study group effectiveness after four and after six weeks. Journal of Individual Psychology 32: 108–111

Croake J W, Glover K E 1977 A history and evaluation of parent education. The Family Coordinator 26: 151–158

Davies E 1978 An evaluation of packaged parent education programmes. Australian Journal of Social Issues 13: 188–196

Dingle A 1988 A parent survival kit. Collins Dove, Sydney

Dinkmeyer D, Dinkmeyer D Jnr 1979 A comprehensive and systematic approach to parent education. American Journal of Family Therapy 7: 46–50

Dinkmeyer D, McKay G D 1976a Systematic training for effective parenting. American Guidance Service, Circle Pines, Minneapolis

Dinkmeyer D, McKay G D 1976b The parents' handbook: Systematic Training for Effective Parenting. American Guidance Service, Circle Pines, Minneapolis

Doherty W J, Ryder R G 1980 Parent effectiveness training (PET): criticisms and caveats. Journal of Marital and Family Therapy 6: 409–419

Dreikurs R, Gray L 1968 A new approach to discipline. Hawthorne Books, New York

Dreikurs R, Soltz V 1964 Children: the challenge. Dutton New York

Freeman C W 1975 Adlerian mother study groups: effects on attitudes and behaviour. Journal of Individual Psychology 31: 37–50

Ginott H G 1965 Between parent and child. Macmillan, New York

Gordon T 1975 Parent effectiveness training. Peter Wyden, New York

Green C 1984 Toddler taming. Doubleday, Melbourne

Hawkins R P 1976 It's time we taught the young how to be good parents (and don't you wish we'd started a long time ago?). Psychology Today 6: 28–40

Jaques E 1983 A general theory of bureaucracy. Heinemann, London

Klein M D 1990 Parent articles for early intervention. Therapy Skills Builders, Tucson

Middlebrook P N 1980 Social psychology and modern life. Knopf, New York

Norman C W 1976 Behaviour modification: a perspective. American Journal of Occupational Therapy 30(8): 491–497

Rogers C 1961 On becoming a person. Houghton Mifflin, Boston

Satir V 1972 Peoplemaking. Science and Behavior, Palo Alto

Seig K 1974 Applying the behaviour model to the occupational therapy model. American Journal of Occupational Therapy 28(7): 421–428

Selznick P 1957 Leadership in administration: a sociological interpretation. Harper & Row, New York

Sharpley C F, Poiner A M 1980 An exploratory evaluation of the systematic training for effective parenting (STEP) programme. Australian Psychologist 15: 103–109

Shaw M 1976 Group Dynamics: The psychology of small group behaviour (2nd edn) McGraw-Hill, New York

Sherrets S D, Authier K J, Tramontana M G 1980 Parent education: rationale, history and funding sources. Journal of Clinical Child Psychology 9: 35–37

Skinner B F 1953 Science and human behaviour Macmillan, New York

Terkelson C 1976 Making contact: a parent–child communication skill programme. Elementary School Guidance and Counselling 11: 89–99

RECOMMENDED READING

Abrams L D 1974 The use of an extinction procedure in the control of self destructive behaviour in a retarded adolescent. Canadian Journal of Occupational Therapy 41(3): 69–71

Bucher R, Lovaas O I 1968 Operant procedures in behaviour modification with children. University of Iowa Symposium on Learning Approaches to Psychotherapy May: 9–11

Clemes H, Reynold B 1980 How to discipline children without feeling guilty. Enrich, San Jose

Ferguson J, Soloman R 1984 A toddler in the family. University of Queensland Press, Brisbane

Ford L J 1975 Teaching dressing skills to a severely retarded child. American Journal of Occupational Therapy 29(2): 87–92

Frazier F, Matthes W A 1975 Parent education: a comparison of Adlerian and behavioural approaches. Elementary School Guidance and Counselling 10: 31–38

Gardner J M, Brust D J, Watson L S 1970 A scale to measure skills in applying modification techniques to the mentally retarded. American Journal of Mental Deficiency 74: 633–636

Giradeau F L, Spradin J E 1964 Token rewards in a cottage programme. Mental Retardation 2: 345–351

Green C 1980 A practical approach to the common behaviour and management problems of the toddler. Journal of Maternal and Child Health February, 64–71

Lemke H 1974 Self-abusive behaviour. American Journal of Occupational Therapy 28(2): 949–989

Lovaas O I 1969 Behaviour modification: teaching language to psychotic children. (16 mm movie). Appleton-Century-Crofts, New York

Morgenstern M, Cow-Beer H, Morgenstern F 1978 Practical training for the severely handicapped child. Heinemann, London

Paris S G, Cairns R B 1972 An experimental and ethological analysis of social reinforcement with retarded children. Child Development 43(3): 717–729

Reynolds G S 1975 A primer of operant conditioning. Scott-Foresman, Glenview

Warren V L, Cairns R B 1972 Social reinforcement satiation: an outcome of frequency or ambiguity? Journal of Experimental Child Psychology 13(3): 249–259

Whelan E, Speake B 1979 Learning to cope. Souvenir Press, London

PART III

SPECIALIZED APPLICATIONS OF THERAPY

One intention in this book was that its contents should encourage a way of thinking about occupational therapy with children. A decision was made not to present detailed prescriptions, or a cookbook approach for the wide range of potential client types and problems. Rather, the selected areas of practice which will be examined were chosen because they provide particular insights and guidelines which can be generalized. Taken as a whole, the discussions provided in Chapters 11 to 17 embody the range of objectives and approaches which are likely to apply in most, if not all, therapy practice with children.

The intervention component

11. The concept of early intervention

READERS' OBJECTIVES

After reading this chapter, you should be able to:
1. **Describe and discuss the theoretical base for the early intervention approach.**
2. **Critically evaluate the research findings about early intervention effectiveness.**
3. **Present practical guidelines for designing therapeutic objectives and programmes for early intervention.**
4. **Describe the aspects of therapy to be evaluated, and the procedures to use.**

There are many definitions of 'early intervention'. Watts (1980, 1982) described it as 'the provision of therapy/ treatment early in life, before four years and usually within the first thirty-six months of life'. More recently the American Occupational Therapy Association (AOTA) presented a position paper and defined early intervention in the following way: 'Early intervention refers to services for biologically or environmentally vulnerable children from birth through the preschool years. Children may be developmentally delayed, disabled or at risk for developmental dysfunction due to pre- post- or perinatal trauma, genetic abnormalities, or nutritional, sensory, emotional or environmental deprivation' (AOTA 1986). The aim of all early intervention is to enrich a child's environmental experience, expand the child's developmental competence and assist the family to meet the challenges of daily living (AOTA 1986).

The thesis central to early intervention is that the young developing child is highly susceptible to the impact of environmental experience. It is an attractive idea that the earlier in a child's life that one can commence systematic development, stimulation and training, the farther reaching and more effective will be the outcomes for the child. Certainly this stance would appear to be well supported by evaluative research studies.

Before examining the evaluative data and its implications for planning programmes, we will discuss the theoretical bases of early intervention and its history.

The theory-base of early intervention

The central thesis arises from three distinct sets of research (Caldwell 1970), namely:

1. Animal studies on the effects of early experience;
2. Developmental studies of children reared in different environments; and
3. Major conceptual analyses of the role of experience in development.

Animal studies. For more than a century, biologists and other scientists have been studying the question that has come to be called the 'nature–nurture' debate. Workers, such as Darwin (1877), Hebb & Williams (1946), Scott (1967) Harlow & Harlow (1969), Spencer-Booth & Hinde (1971) have studied the effects that different kinds of experience have on the developmental progress of a variety of social animals. The consensus of

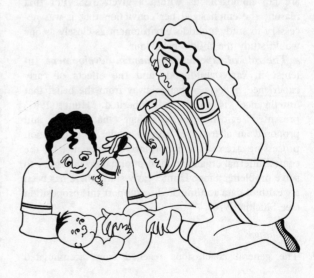

opinion is that early experience is indeed a powerful modifier of emerging behaviour. Timing of various experiences may be of particular importance for non-human animals, where most complex forms of behaviour are mediated by intrinsic processes. Such processes, when fully developed, have been shown to be relatively less sensitive to variations in experience. The situation is not so 'black and white' in human development. Nevertheless, the animal study findings provoked important examination of human learning.

Human studies. There are studies stretching back to 1960 which demonstrate a significant relationship between socioeconomic environment and children's maturation. For example, Bayley (1965), Coleman (1966), and Escalona & Corman (1967) have demonstrated deficits in cognitive performance of children from 'low' socioeconomic status (SES) families — defined by the variables of parental education, occupation, income and residential area. The interesting point is that the deficits become both apparent and most marked between the ages of 18 months to three years.

Caldwell (1967), along with others, sought to identify the features associated with 'low' SES which did not support growth and development. The important features appeared to be: maternal preoccupation with life concerns other than the child; the mother's type and use of language (brief utterances and concrete concerns); teaching style, e.g., 'Do as I say'; and method of controlling the child's behaviour. In summary, while a materially meagre environment undoubtedly contributes to slowed growth and development, it is the nature of the interpersonal transactions, especially those between mother and child, which appear to be most influential.

However, Caldwell proposed that home environments are not homogeneous within a given SES. For that reason, she emphasized her conviction that it was necessary to study a child's environment as closely as one would study the child's behaviour.

The role of experience in human development. Interest in early childhood, and the effects of early experience, reflects a change away from the belief that 'intelligence' is fixed and inherited. Hunt (1961) presented evidence to challenge that belief, and proposed an alternative. Hunt's model of information processing stressed the importance of experience for the central internal organization of information necessary to solve problems. Since Hunt's early study there has been a wealth of data accumulated to support this proposition (see Sluckin 1970).

Conclusions

The general conclusions reached from accumulated evidence is that, for human beings the social and inanimate environment can be presumed to have a powerful impact on a child's developmental process, and resulting maturation. The inference which flowed on was that the environment should, therefore, be manipulated and enriched, to ensure optimum experience, especially early in life.

History of early intervention programmes

The first people to design and use early intervention programmes were teachers and psychologists. The target populations were young children who lived in environments which did not appear to support or promote healthy growth and development. Perhaps the best known of the early programmes is the Head Start Project (Gray & Klaus 1965) in the United States. Head Start was directed at children of low income, usually minority group, families — such as black American — who lived in crowded inner city areas. The objective of Head Start programmes was to enrich the total environmental experience of the children, to promote basic skill acquisition necessary for successful coping in later formal schooling.

There was much interest in the early intervention concept among medical specialists. Since the early 1960s occupational therapists, and others, have increasingly recognized and promoted the logical sense of therapeutic early intervention with infants and young childred with identified delay. Even in those early days, occupational therapists paid attention to the preventive aspects of early intervention, with children thought to be 'at risk' for delay. Interesting and varied examples appear in the work of Howells & Anderson 1960; Anderson & Brown 1962; Clancy & McBride 1969; Llorens 1970, 1971; Moersch 1978; Levitt 1979; and Hanft 1988.

Evaluation findings from early intervention programmes

Therapeutic intervention early in a child's life is an expensive service. For example, the US Federal Budget allocation for educational intervention programmes serving approximately 429 000 children in 1200 communities in 1984 topped one billion dollars (Collins 1983). Such major community investment has, quite rightly, demanded justification, and there have been a number of evaluation studies which are ongoing (Calhoun & Collins 1983; Cicirelli 1969; Mann et al 1977; National Institute of Advanced Studies 1980). Early studies, among them the so-called 'Westinghouse Studies' (1969) were not encouraging to proponents of early intervention, and indeed have been shown be strongly influenced by the political climate of their time. Methodological shortcomings were demonstrated in these studies; however, there is now an impressive body of data which provides clear support for the early intervention model (Collins 1983; Lazar et al 1982; see Schweinhart & Weikart 1980; Slaughter 1983). All of the available research studies demonstrate that particular early experiences affect certain later behaviours. There remains the need for studies which determine how these early experiences result in later change. Such studies should involve the special application of measures of behaviour, between the early experience treatment and the final judgement testing.

The recent evaluation findings provide important guidelines for therapists designing intervention programmes, and so a summary is provided.

Summary of supporting data. Lazar and colleagues (1982) identified 15 studies which examined treated children 12 years after their programmes were completed. The programmes were mainly Head Start ones, though therapeutic programmes for developmentally delayed children were also examined. 21 000 of a possible 41 000 children were located, and all but 3% agreed to participate in the follow-up study. Researchers found that there were significant differences in the treated children, when they were compared with similiar but untreated children. The differences were:

1. Significantly fewer treated children were found in remedial classes ($p = 0.0004$).
2. Significantly more treated children retained normal school grades. Further, performance at Grade 7 was found to predict graduation from High School.
3. Significantly more treated children did graduate from High School.
4. By 17 years of age more treated children had formed and accepted realistic choices about occupational roles.

Collins (1983) noted that gains observed in the treated children focused on their intellectual functioning, with special reference to cognitive skill, and language. However, gains were also observed in socioemotional growth and maturity. The children who seemed to benefit most were the most needy; for example, children from families where the mother had only a primary school education, children with only one parent, and children with 'low' IQ.

Characteristics of effective programmes

Lazar et al (1982) reached the conclusion that there appear to be five characteristics which distinguish the more effective early intervention programmes:

1. Age — the younger the child at the time of the intervention, the better the outcome.
2. Parent participation — the more the parents participated, the greater the impact on the child.
3. Programme orientation — family oriented programmes had more effective outcomes than child oriented programmes.
4. Home visits the higher the proportion of time given to visits to a child's home by the specialist team, the better the outcome.
5. Group size — the lower the ratio of children to staff, the greater the impact on the children.

It did not seem to matter whether a programme was home based, centre based, rural or urban in setting — all were effective to some degree.

An unexpected outcome was that, all programmes significantly changed parents' style of interacting with their children. For example, parents were observed to become attentive to, and rewarding of the child's developing skills. A positive feedback situation developed, and within the family environment continued learning was both supported and valued. Slaughter (1983) found that such altered maternal attention was particularly related to the development of a strong supportive social network, arising from the programmed discussion groups. The social network clearly enabled the mothers to cope with varied life problems, to lose the feeling of being 'embattled', and to relax and enjoy their children.

Intervening — when? for how long?

Palfrey (1982) found that in 10% of children that he studied, some motor and intellectual function problems could not be defined with certainty before the kindergarten years, i.e., age four to five. On the other hand, Palfrey observed that 25 months appeared to be a key age for distinguishing between normal but slowed development, and a pattern of 'problems' which seemed likely to interfere with the child becoming functionally competent. The implication of Palfrey's findings is that some 'problems' observable within the first 25 months will often resolve, without the need for systematic intervention. However, until there is better understanding of problems which may be safely left alone, therapists and other specialists will probably continue to treat all presenting problems.

THE INTERVENTION PROCESS

The team

Early intervention programmes with developmentally delayed children generally reflect an assumption that co-ordinated services from many disciplines are essential when serving the handicapped child and family.

A team may comprise any combination of the following specialists: paediatrician, developmental psychologist, special early childhood teacher, occupational, speech and physiotherapists, and social workers. The success of a team will depend on the ability of each member to cross professional boundaries, to share skills generously, and to avoid territorial behaviour. The precise roles of each team member may vary according to the programme context. For example, in an educational setting such as a special preschool, specialists other than the teachers may act as consultants (Lilley 1975). By contrast, in a primarily medical setting such as centre for developmentally delayed infants and children, the specialists responsible for administering the daily programme are likely to be fairly equally represented.

Occupational therapists are found in early intervention teams in: special agencies such as Spastic Centres and Community Health based centres; the regular and special education school system; and hospitals for children.

The form that intervention takes may also vary. For example, specialists may give 'hands on' service to a child and family, in special group and/or individual sessions. Alternatively, the therapist might recommend that the child participate in a regular kindergarten, but for a longer time than is usual. Then there are variations on basic programme models. In the absence of criteria for judging cost effectiveness of the various programme models for a particular child, the choice is usually made on pragmatic grounds, for example, the availability of services.

Objectives of early intervention

The objective of all early intervention is the reduction of handicapping factors in a child's environment. Programmes have special components designed to meet particular needs of an identified child, or client group.

Rogers et al (1975a, b) have made some suggestions for general therapeutic objectives:

1. To reduce the degree of physical deformity
2. To promote family living as a viable option to institution living for the child
3. To encourage parents to be advocates for their child, to gain special help and management services, for the whole of the child's lifetime.

Early intervention programmes follow the usual pattern known to occupational therapists, namely, that of refer-

ral of the identified child and family, evaluation, and intervention. At the Institute of Mental Retardation And Related Disabilities, University of Michigan USA, following referral a family is visited at home by one or two members of the intervention team (D'Eugenrio & Rogers 1976; Rogers et al 1975a). The visit allows the team representative(s) to explain the project and invite the parents to visit and observe it. There is time to answer parents' questions in their own environment, where they are secure and in control. The specialists also take the opportunity to offer to introduce the new family to other parents already participating in the programme. The evaluation process also commences informally, as the child and parents can be observed interacting in their own natural surroundings.

Designing the occupational therapy component

Roles and objectives

Moersch (1978) has defined the following occupational therapy service roles.

1. To contribute to programme implementation by:
   — providing assessment of the child's abilities and behaviour;
   — giving face to face therapy;
   — providing families with information about developmental patterns, managing, children's behaviour, selection of activities and toys, community resources and support systems.
2. To be an advocate for the child and family in:
   — professional interaction with other special services personnel, e.g., teachers;
   — approaches to government, State and Federal, to protect the rights of the child, and to influence policy.
3. To provide team management:
   — be prepared to co-ordinate the intervention programme.

Usually the occupational therapist works with mothers of identified infants and children to overcome or minimize a range of problems; for example, difficulties associated with handling and positioning the infant for various activities, such as feeding, toileting, and playing. Play activities receive special attention, and mothers are guided in their choice of suitable toys and games. Bearing in mind, however, that the family is the unit of intervention, fathers too, have a role to play (Crowe 1981). Special emphasis is given to encouraging play which promotes the development of a satisfying interaction between mother, father and child, and the normal affectional relationship.

With older children the therapist is concerned to facilitate independent behaviour. The child is guided to assume responsibility for all aspects of self-care, exploratory behaviour, and fine motor manipulative skills. The therapist may provide special assisting aids such as a seat, or eating utensils, or the Bliss Symbol System for a blind child.

Some helpful resources for therapists, parents and families are provided in Appendix VII.

General principles of occupational therapy in early intervention

The occupational therapy contribution to an early intervention programme is generally based on the following principles:

1. The intervention promotes the infant–mother affectional bond.
2. It promotes social interactive skill development by the child.
3. It minimizes movement dysfunction in the child.
4. It encourages the child to be independent in self-care skills.
5. It promotes fine motor manipulative skills.

An intervention programme should reflect the five characteristics which defined effective intervention in the longitudinal studies of Lazar et al 1982 discussed before. Intervention should commence as soon as possible in the child's life, and certainly as soon as possible

after referral. The unit of treatment should be the family, not the child, and parents should have an active role in all aspects of the intervention. Any group sessions should have a high staff to child ratio, and therapy sessions in the child's own home should be a dominant feature of the programme.

In Chapters 12 and 13, the particular occupational therapy needs of developmentally delayed and disabled children, with different diagnoses are examined. However, as all programming reflects the five general principles, these will now be discussed in some detail.

Principles 1 and 2: promoting the infant–mother affectional bond. The first intervention priority, as in the case of a Down syndrome infant, is the promotion of social interaction between the infant and mother. The objective is to develop and reinforce a healthy primary attachment. The special bonded relationship between infant and mother is the normal context in which a child learns all of a culture's socialization skills. Parmelee (1982) has also shown that a robust mother–infant bond is a crucial element in diminishing the effects of a developmental disability. Clancy (1973, 1984), Clancy & McBride (1969, 1975) and Bromwich (1976) have presented theoretically based programmes for promoting mother–infant interaction.

Occupational therapists, and others, assist in promoting satisfying and effective intraction between an infant and mother. Non-verbal skills are the most important and a mother is taught, for example, how to elicit eye contact by playing with her infant. (Gordon 1970, 1973).

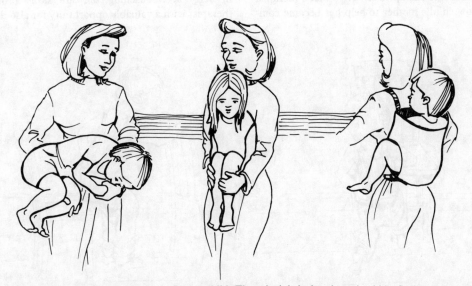

Fig. 11.1 Efficient ways to carry an athetoid (or floppy) child. The principle is that there should be flexion and thus stability of the child's hips. These positions will facilitate more normal head and neck extension.

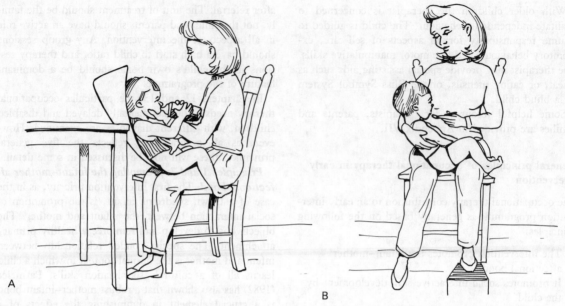

Fig. 11.2   Two different ways to offer food and drink. Again the principle is that the child's hips are slightly flexed and support is given to the child's head. Note that in (B) one of the caretaker's feet rests on a support, thus creating a 'hammock effect' for the child's hips.

Later on, the close affectional bonds developed within the family must be generalized to others, through friendships.

Principle 3: minimizing movement dysfunction in the child. The management of movement disorder is basic to all programme implementation. Presented in Figure 11.1 are some examples of advice that a therapist might give to a child's mother to help her become com-

fortable when handling her child.

Occupational therapists also evaluate environments and furniture to minimize the effect of a movement disorder and a fuller discussion is provided in Chapters 13 and 14.

Principle 4: encouraging the child to be independent in self care. Teaching self-care skills provides the therapist with a valuable opportunity for also developing

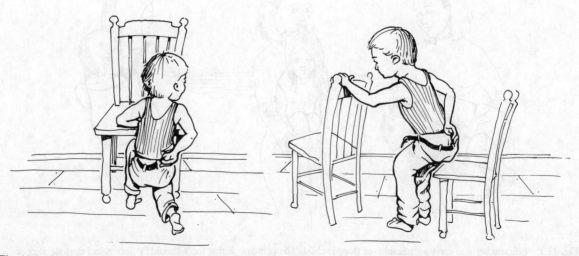

Fig. 11.3   Simple ways to help a child gain confidence in dressing.

a satisfying, relaxed, social interaction between the mother and her child. An example is shown in Figure 11.3. A more complete discussion is to be found in Chapter 13.

Moreover, there are some very helpful training systems available, and a selection is noted in Appendix VII. An example from one such scheme written specifically for parents to use appears in the box.

Principle 5: fine motor, manipulative skill development. Fine manipulative and problem solving skills begin to emerge and develop with reaching, grasping, and manipulating objects in early play experience. The basic manipulative skills then become generalized to other functional activities such as feeding, dressing and toileting.

Examples of occupational therapy contributions to early intervention programmes are to be found in the following publications. AOTA (1986), Bidder & James (1981), Bricker & Bricker (1977), Clunies-Ross (1976), Rogers et al (1975b).

Evaluation of therapy

Outcomes are often difficult to determine and to measure, however we have listed, as a guide, the broad areas that should be evaluated.

1. The child's behavioural response.
2. Changes in parent–child interaction style.
3. Changes in parental behaviour within the family generally.
4. Therapeutic objectives and procedures.

Simmel (1980) argues strongly that effectiveness of the intervention is best judged by the data from a systematic series of rigorous observations and measurement of behaviours of the treated children at regularly spaced time intervals. By so doing the evaluation (therapist and/or team) 'might be able to gain critical information regarding any relationship between the early intervention and any of several behavioral changes'.

For assessment purposes every effort should be made to use standardized tests. Such tests are most reliable when administered about six-monthly, to minimize the 'learning effect' on the child's performance. An evaluation profile of a child should she define those skills in which she/he is proficient, and those skill areas where the child remains developmentally immature. Standardized developmental assessment tests provide valuable objective data about changes in a child's developmental status. Such tests are also very useful as a focus for talking with parents, in order to enhance their understanding of normal development. Through

increased understanding of their child's development, parents may adjust their expectations of him or her.

Probably the most important information to be gained

Part of a dressing programme written for parents — Putting on Pants

Setting the stage

Begin with short pants or underpants with an elastic waistband, since these are easier than long pants.

If pants have a button, snap, or zipper, you should fasten them for your child.

Have him sit to put the pants over his feet, and stand to pull them up.

Stay on each step, giving your child less and less assistance, until he can successfully do the step for four to five teaching sessions without your physical guidance. Then move to the next step. Have your child's rewards ready. List them here:

Programme

1. With your child sitting, you put his pants on both feet, then have him stand up. Pull the pants up to his hips. Then place his hands on the sides of the pants with his thumbs inside the waistband. Say, "Pull your pants up," and guide him with your hands on his to pull the pants up to his waist. Then say, "Good, you pulled your pants up," and give him his special treat.

2. You put your child's pants on up to mid-thighs. Place his hands on the sides of the pants with his thumbs inside the waistband, saying, "Pull your pants up." Guide him with your hands on his to pull the pants up to his hips. Then allow him to finish pulling the pants up to his waist. Say "Good, you pulled your pants up," and give him his special treat.

3. Continue in the above manner, helping your child after you have put his pants on up to his knees, then later his ankles.

4. Sit beside your child and put the pants on one foot for him. Place his hands on the pants and, with your hands on his, say, "Put your pants on." Guide him in putting his pants on the second foot. Have your child stand up and finish putting on his pants without assistance. Praise him and give him the special treat.

5. With your child sitting, place his hands on the pants, saying "Put your pants on." Guide him in putting his pants on the first foot. Remove your hands and he can now finish putting his pants on! When he has mastered this step, the task is his and he will be able to put on his pants without assistance once you hand them to him.

From Baker B L, Brightman A J 1989 Steps to independence. Paul H Brookes Publishing Co, Baltimore.

from serial developmental assessments is an indication of the rate, or velocity, of change in the child's performance. Identifying the velocity of change enables a therapist to judge where intervention efforts are most effectively directed, and when to terminate the special programme.

SUMMARY

The early intervention model is based on the thesis that the young developing human child is highly susceptible to the impact of environmental experience. There are impressive studies supporting this thesis, and these have been reviewed. The therapeutic use of the early intervention model has been fruitful for several reasons, namely:

1. The model encourages the development and use of general principles of intervention, across the boundaries of medical diagnoses.
2. The model encourages greater interaction and

sharing of skills between educationalists and medical and therapy specialists — to the child's and family's advantage.
3. Negative expectations associated with many diagnostic labels are diminished, or avoided, by focusing on solving functional problems, rather than on signs or symptoms.

The occupational therapy programme profile should reflect the characteristics of effective early intervention programmes; intervention should commence as early as possible in an identified child's life; the unit of treatment should be the family, and who should be actively involved in all aspects of the programme; the specialist–child ratio should be high; though many forms of programme are appropriate, the first priority should be promotion of a healthy mother-infant attachment process; other special occupational therapy priorities are to minimize movement disorder, to promote independent self-care behaviour, and fine manipulative skill development.

REFERENCES

American Occupational Therapy Association 1986 Roles and functions and occupational therapy in early childhood intervention. American Journal of Occupational Therapy 40(12): 835–837

Anderson R, Brown N 1962 Occupational therapy in a family psychiatry program. Proceedings 3rd International Congress World Federation Occupational Therapists, Philadelphia

Baker B L, Brightman A J, Heifetz L J, Murphy D M 1977 Advanced self-help skills. Research Press, Champaign

Baker B L, Brightman A J 1989 Steps to independence. Paul H Brookes Publishing Co, Baltimore

Bayley N 1965 Comparison of mental and motor test scores for ages 1–5 months by sex, birth order, race, geographical location and education of parents. Child Development 36: 379–411

Bidder R, James J 1981 Home intervention for developmentally delayed pre-school children–occupational therapy contribution. Occupational Therapy September 44: 282–283

Bricker D R, Bricker W A 1977 A developmentally integrated approach to early intervention. Education and Training of the Mentally Retarded 12(2): 12–17

Bromwich R M 1976 Focus on maternal behaviour in early intervention. American Journal Orthopsychiatry 46(3): 439–446

Caldwell B M 1967 Descriptive evaluations of child development and of developmental settings. Pediatrics 40: 46–54

Caldwell B M 1970 Preschool inventory revized edn. Educational Testing Service, Princeton

Calhoun J A, Collins R C 1983 From one decade to another: a positive view of early childhood programmes. Theory into Practice 20(2): 135–140

Capon J 1975 Basic and 'perceptual' lesson plans for perceptual-motor programs in preschool and elementary grades, 4th edn Perceptual-Motor Plans Level I. Front Row Experience, Alameda, California

Cicirelli V 1969 The impact of Head Start: an evaluation of the effects of Head Start on children's cognitive and affective development. Westinghouse Learning Corporation, Ohio University

Clancy H G 1973 Autistic processes in infants. Unpublished Masters Degree Thesis, University of Queensland, Brisbane

Clancy H G 1984 Detecting the autistic process in infants. Paper presented at a scientific interlocution at the Department of Child Health, University of Queensland, Brisbane

Clancy H G, McBride G 1969 The autistic process and its treatment. Journal of Child Psychology and Psychiatry 10: 223–244

Clancy H G, McBride G 1975 The isolation syndrome. Developmental Medicine and Child Neurology 17: 198–219

Clunies-Ross G 1976 A model for early intervention with developmentally handicapped pre-schoolers' programmes. Australian Journal of Mental Retardation 4(4): 23–27

Coleman J S 1966 Equality of educational opportunity. United States Government Program Office (USGPO), Washington DC

Collins R C 1983 Head Start: an update on program effects. Summer newsletter, Society for Research in Child Development, Univeristy of Chicago Press, Chicago

Crowe T K 1981 Father involvement in early intervention program. Physical and Occupational Therapy in Pediatrics 1(3): 35–47

Darwin C 1877 A biographical sketch of an infant. Mind (2): 286–294

Escalona S K, Corman H H 1967 Piaget's hypotheses concerning the development of sensorimotor intelligence: methodological issues. Paper presented at biennial meeting of the Society for Research in Child Development, New York

D'Eugenio D B, Rogers S J 1976 Developmental screening of handicapped infants: a manual, 2nd edn. University of Michigan, Michigan

Gordon I J 1970 Baby learning through baby play. St Martin's Press, New York

Gordon I J 1973 Infant learning through infant play. St Martin's Press, New York

Gray S W, Klaus R A 1965 An experimental preschool program for culturally deprived children. Child Development 36: 887–898

Hanft B 1988 The changing environment of early intervention services. American Journal of Occupational Therapy 42: 724–731

Harlow H F, Harolw M K 1969 Effects of various mother-infant relationships on rhesus monkey behaviours. In: Foss B M (ed) Determinants of infant behaviour, Vol 4. Methuen, London

Hebb D D, Williams K A 1946 A method of rating animal intelligence. Journal of Genetic Psychology 34: 59–65

Howells J G, Anderson R 1960 Family psychiatry and occupational therapy. Occupational Therapy 23: 11

Hunt J, McV 1961 Intelligence and experience. Ronald Press, New York

Lazar I, Darington R, Murray H, Royce J, Snipper A 1982 The lasting effects of early education: a report from the consortium for longitudinal studies. Monographs of the Society for Research in Child Development 47: 2–3, (Serial No 195)

Levitt S 1979 Treatment of cerebral palsy and motor delay. Blackwells Scientific Publications, Oxford

Lilley D 1975 Early childhood education. Science Research Associates, Chicago

Llorens L A 1970 Facilitating growth and development: the promise of occupational therapy. American Journal of Occupational Therapy 24: 1–9

Llorens L A 1971 Occupational therapy in community child health. American Journal of Occupational Therapy 25: 335–339

Mann A J, Harrell A, Hurt M 1977 A review of Head Start research since 1969 and an annotated bibliography. Social Research Group, The George Washington University

Moersch M S 1975 Early intervention project for handicapped infants and young children. Institute of Mental Retardation and Related Disabilities, Ann Arbor, Michigan

Moersch M S 1978 Developmental disabilities. American Journal of Occupational Therapy 32: 93–99

National Institute for Advanced Studies. Summary report: an analysis of 1979–80 Head start program performance indicators, October 15 1980. Prepared for Administration for Children, Youth and Families, US Department of Health and Human Services, Bethesda, Maryland

Palfrey J 1982 An early education project. Paper presented at conference 'Environmental intervention for infants at risk'. Harvard Medical School, Boston

Parmelee A 1982 What are the functions of follow-up programs for high risk infants? Paper presented at conference 'Environmental intervention for infants at risk'. Harvard Medical School, Boston

Rogerg S J, D'Eugenio D B, Brown S L, Donovan C M, Lynch E W, Moersch M S 1975a Early intervention Development Profile. University of Michigan, Michigan

Rogers S J, D'Eugenio D B, Brown S L, Donovan C M, Lynch E W, Moersch M S 1975b Early intervention project for handicapped infants and young children. Institute of Mental Retardation and Related Disabilities, Ann Arbor, Michigan

Schweinhart L J, Weikart D P 1980 Young children group: the effects of the Perry preschool program on youth through age 15. Monographs of the High/Scope Educational Research Foundation 7

Scott J P 1967 Early experiences and the organization of behaviour. Brooks/Cole, California

Simmel E C 1980 The analysis of the effects of early experiences. A Note from the Behaviour Genetics Laboratory, Department of Psychiatry, Miami University, Oxford, Ohio

Sluckin W 1970 Early learning in man and animal. George Allen & Unwin, London

Slaughter D 1983 Early intervention and its effects on maternal and child development. Monographs of the Society for Research in Child Development 48(4): (Serial No 202)

Spencer-Booth Y, Hinde R A 1971 The effects of 13 days maternal separation on infant rhesus monkeys compared with those of shorter and repeated separations. Animal Behaviour 19: 595–605

Watts B H 1980 Evaluation of early intervention programs for young handicapped children. Paper presented at the August workshop of the Schonell Educational Research Centre, Brisbane

Watts B H (ed) 1982 Early intervention programs for young handicapped children in Australia 1979–80. Australian Government Publishing Service, Canberra

Westinghouse Learning Corporation/Ohio University 1969 The impact of Head Start: An evaluation of the effects of Head Start on children's cognitive and affective development. Office of Economic Opportunity, Washington DC

12. The concept of developmental delay

READERS' OBJECTIVES

After reading this chapter, you should be able to:
1. Demonstrate understanding of the difference between 'developmental delay' and 'developmental disabilities'.
2. Review and compare the factors which may lead to developmental delay in infants and young children.
3. Describe how to assess developmental maturity.
4. Discuss the role of the occupational therapy in developmental assessment and intervention.

PATHWAYS TO DELAYED DEVELOPMENT

A distinction has been made, for purposes of discussion in this book, between the concept of 'developmental delay' and 'developmental disability'. The reason is that delay is a general phenomenon associated with a very wide range of childhood disorders and environmental situations; whereas developmental disability is a generic term for five specifically defined clinical conditions. Chapter 13 provides a description of each condition; there is also a discussion of the impact of these defined conditions on the lives of the affected child and family; and an outline is provided of the principles and objectives of intervention with the children in each diagnostic category.

In this chapter there is a general discussion of the concept of developmental delay, the factors which may precipitate it, methods of assessing developmental progress for diagnosis, and for monitoring the effectiveness of intervention. Approaches to early intervention are discussed in detail in Chapter 11.

A child is described as developmentally delayed when she/he is unable to accomplish the developmental tasks considered appropriate to his/her chronological age. The term came into use in the 1960s when standardized tests made it possible to compare reliably one child's performance with norms established for children of the same chronological age.

Pathways to delayed development may be initiated by factors within a child, such as injury to brain tissue, immaturity, or defective development of the brain and/or special sensory pathways. Alternatively, delay may be initiated by factors external to the child, such as an unfavourable environment. Non-accidental child injury (abuse) is one clinical condition where environmental experience leads to delayed development.

Other environmental circumstances may render any child more vulnerable (at risk) to being developmentally delayed, or to displaying learning and serious behavioural difficulties in later childhood (Court 1981). For example, such circumstances include a family living in financial poverty, which is very often a single parent family where the mother is rearing young children; a migrant family that remains aloof from their adopted culture – and thus socially isolated; a family with one member experiencing serious psychiatric illness, and a child of a very young teenaged mother. Such children are usually born with full normal potential, and any effects of developmental delay are fully reversible if intervention commences in early childhood. This situation is quite distinct from that of the developmentally disabled child, who has inborn motor, intellectual or sensory disturbances which lead to chronic and irreversible disabilities. The effects of developmental delay on such child can be reversed, but only to the limits imposed by the disabling condition. Court (1981) presented a useful classification of childhood disorders that may be associated with developmental delay in early childhood (see box next page).

Holt (1977) postulated three pathways leading to a clinical picture of delayed development, and his model provides a useful 'mind picture' of a rather nebulous concept. In the first pathway, Holt observes that there are some children, boys especially, who do develop according to the usually expected pattern, but much more slowly. There is no evidence of intellectual handicap in

Examples of major handicapping disorders that may present with developmental delay in early childhood
Physical disorders
  cerebral palsy
  infant hemiplegia
  disorders of muscle
Sensory disorders
  deafness
  visual defects
  language disorders
  learning disorders
Intellectual disorders
  mental retardation
  metabolic diseases associated with brain development
  Down syndrome
  cretinism
Social disorders
  maltreatment and child abuse
  deprivation syndromes
Emotional disorders
  behaviour disorders
  learning disorders
Psychiatric disorders
  autism (Court 1981)

such children, and eventually they simply 'catch up'. Holt calls this pathway 'developmental lethargy', and he postulates that the mechanism may be a general slowing of the biological process in the affected child.

The second pathway is that of 'developmental deprivation', and here the child is described as being unable to act on the environment effectively, and/or to learn from interaction with objects and people. Holt postulates two mechanisms:

1. The presence of sensory or physical deficits in the child.
2. Lack of environmental opportunity for learning and exploration.

The third pathway is that of 'developmental distortion and non-assimilation'. Children thus implicated appear normally endowed, yet their behaviour suggests that the desire for growth and maturity has been diverted in some way. The continuous rocking, pacing or destructive behaviour (stereotypes) seen characteristically in intellectually handicapped and autistic children, and in those living in impoverished institution surroundings, are clinical manifestations of 'developmental distortion'.

Factors influencing severity of delay

So far the discussion has focused on factors and pathways which lead to developmental delay. However, there are other factors which determine how severe an impact the delaying condition or situation will have on a child's developmental progress. These factors are:

1. The extent of dysfunction in the child (intrinsic factors).
2. The quality of environmental experience – specifically caregiving interactions, and the nature of social relationships found between the child and others.
3. The availability and use made of special habilitation programmes, such as early intervention programmes.

Dysfunction in the child. Any damage to a child's bodily system will limit both the scope of the child's actual performance, and his/her capacity for exploring and learning from the environment (Erickson 1976; Gabel & Erickson 1980; Holt 1977). For example, the child with cerebral palsy has dysfunctional motor skills. She/he is physically limited in moving around, exploring and finding out how things work by manipulating objects. She/he is also restricted in the degree to which motor skills can be developed and refined — for example, walking, feeding, putting together construction sets. Yet these two very different dimensions of performance and exploratory experience will only be represented as one dimension in a formal assessment of developmental maturity. The child will be judged against peers as 'delayed in motor skills'. Specialists must carefully identify the contribution to a clinical picture of delayed development made by past restrictions, imposed from within the child (intrinsic factors), and restrictions imposed on learning experiences. The latter is much more amenable to intervention strategies than is the former, which may be more amenable to compensatory strategies.

The distinction is an important one for programme planning. Where a child clearly lacks experience, it may, for example, be sufficient to provide planned play and other experiences. However, where ability is also limited, a variety of special procedures and even adapted equipment may be required to promote the child's skill development. For example, the child with a motor dysfunction may need to be seated in a special supportive chair before the planned playtime can be of interest and therapeutic use.

Environmental experience. Parmelee (1982) considers that the most important factor in modifying the effects of a delaying condition on a child's developmental progress is a strong mother–infant attachment, or bond. The key qualities in a 'healthy' attachment process appear to be that mother's handling of her infant is both *consistent*, and therefore *predictable*, and that there is *reciprocity* in their interactions.

A number of workers have studied the way in which an infant's behaviour shapes the responses of adults. The normal situation is that an infant attracts adults by the early behaviours such as crying or 'windy smiles'. However, in the early days of life before a delaying condition is detected the affected baby's behaviour may have the effect of 'pushing others away' from him/her.

Fraiberg (1964) reported an experiment (Example 12.1) in which a mother was asked to approach her blind infant lying in its cot, and behavioural interaction was recorded by the researchers.

Example 12.1: A mother's response
Prior to the mother entering the nursery, the infant lay playing with its feet, generally moving around and quietly babbling. However, as the mother's footsteps approached the cot, the infant became still and quiet. When she reached the cot she saw an unmoving, unsmiling baby. After looking at baby for a minute she moved away and commented to the researcher that baby seemed contented, and so she decided not to disturb him.

  In this example the mother had wrongly, but understandably, interpreted her baby's behaviour as unfriendly — perhaps even rejecting. More likely, the infant had quietened in order to focus on the approaching footsteps and to make sense of them. However, the consequence of the baby's behaviour, was to reduce the number and quality of experiences of being picked up, spoken to, and played with by his mother. The attachment process was influenced so that both slowly but inevitably drew away from each other.

A different example is seen in the event that an infant is born prematurely and is cared for apart from its mother (Goldberg 1978; Kennel & Klaus 1976). A different situation is that where a mother becomes ill, for example with clinical depression, so that she is preoccupied and inconsistently attendant to her infant.

Any family system will become distorted when one member interacts in an unusual manner (O'Neil et al 1977). For example, when an infant is known to have a handicaping condition at birth, or has caused concern for some reason, parents may devote a disproportionate amount of time, energy, and thought to him/her. Siblings may find that it is difficult to gain the time and attention from their parents that had been theirs before the birth of the affected infant. Also, the relationship between husband and wife may change subtly, if the wife becomes preoccupied with the infant's care, and her concerns about her infant.

Thus, the infant may exert a direct effect on behavioural interactions with others by giving cues which do not promote healthy growth and development. The infant may also exert an indirect effect on others, especially to reshape relationships within a family so that they become stressful, and less satisfying to the family members. A vicious circle is then established, and attention in the therapy programme must be directed at changing the family pattern of interacting — the family must be the unit of treatment.

Available intervention. Lazar et al (1982) have confirmed that the earlier an intervention programme can begin for an infant at risk of developmental delay, the more effective is the outcome. Thus, it follows that where no such services are available, any detrimental impact of environmental factors is likely to be maximized (Hospitals & Health Services Commission Report 1976; Llorens 1971; 1976; Morris 1978; West 1973).

Diagnosing developmental delay

Court (1981) suggests that diagnostic evaluation should be directed toward answering four questions.

1. What are the concerns of parents, or the referring person?
2. Is there historical evidence that the child may be at risk for developmental disorders?
3. Objectively, is the child's development normal, delayed or uncertain?
4. Are there any abnormalities on general examination of the child?

Further examination of a child is indicated by a the presence of a large number of age-related factors, and also when parental or other adult concern is very high.

The process

While mothers are often vaguely concerned about their baby's behaviour in the first weeks of life, it is not uncommon for an adult outside the family circle to first draw attention to the child's suspected slowness. If, from the initial screening examination, it is thought appropriate to refer the child for further diagnosis, a specialist team will then take over. In centres where there is a developmental clinic, the team will usually follow a standard evaluation procedure. The procedure will usually comprise:

— A complete medical, including biochemical and neurological examination.
— The compilation of a developmental profile of the child by report of the mother, or other caregiver familiar with the child.
— A history of behaviour and events, from birth,

Age-related factors precipitating developmental delay

6 weeks
Abnormality in head circumference or general growth pattern
Restricted hip abduction
Assymetry of movements muscle tone reflex pattern
Developmental social delay
Visual or auditory delay
Any anxiety the mother may have

6 months
All of the above
Abnormal limb posture
Failure to turn to sounds
Poor response to people/objects
Inability to fixate visually
Failure to vocalize

1 year
Failure to bear weight on lower limbs and attempt to get upright
Retarded manipulative skill, and bimanual ataxia or tremor
Convulsions
Skin conditions
Failure to respond to sound
Limited or decreased vocalization
Inability to chew
Absence of smiling or laughing
Limited visual response

2 years
Clumsiness
Language — should be able to use 2–3 word sentences
Failure to comprehend
Defective vision
Poor co-ordination
Poor concentration, distractable or hyperactive
No observable imaginative play

---

which have caused the child's family to become concerned.
— A social history of the family — their ways of interacting, important events since the child's birth, attitudes to childrearing, and knowledge about child care.
— A standardized developmental assessment of the child.

From the data gathered it should be possible to define whether the factors which are giving rise to the behavioural picture of delayed development are primarily within the child, or arise from the environment.

Assessing and monitoring general developmental progress of children is a major professional activity for a paediatric occupational therapist. Judgements should never been made casually, or be based only on a therapist's unstructured observations. There are a number of excellent standardized assessment procedures available, which are used by all specialists who contribute to developmental assessment (see Lichtenstein &

Ireton 1984). A centre may have a policy about which procedures are to be used; and some are only available for accredited trained users. Because it is such an important area of occupational therapy practice, a detailed discussion is now provided about assessment of normal and delayed development.

Assessing developmental maturity

There are two types of procedures which will be employed routinely. The first procedure is called a screening test. The second procedure is called a developmental diagnostic assessment (Illingworth 1962; Knoblock & Pasamanick 1974; Sheridan 1975).

Some commonly used screening and diagnostic assessment instruments are listed in Table 12.1, and a more comprehensive annotated comparison of assessment tests and profiles is presented in Appendix VI.

Definitions
Screening is a cursory scan of a representative sample of some aspects of behaviour. Screening is the first step in diagnostic evaluation of developmental progress.
Developmental assessment is a comprehensive survey of detailed aspects of behaviour. The test verifies existence of delay and defines the problem area.

Screening development

Screening is the process of detecting an individual for some specific dysfunction or problem at a very early stage when the problem may not even be showing itself, or there are only vague worries on the part of the client or his family.

A screening test has the property that it will confirm either that (a) there is a high chance of a specific problem being found in a given individual screened. In this case further detailed evaluation must be undertaken; or (b) there is no problem — at least of the kind screened for. No further evaluation may be indicated, or a different focus for the investigation may be suggested.

Frankenburg & Dodds (1967) and Frankenburg et al (1976) provided useful criteria and justification for applying wide-spread screening to detect any condition, including developmental delay. The criteria are:

• Condition must be potentially treatable or controllable
• Early treatment must improve outcome
• The screening time must be adequate
• Firm diagnosis must be possible
• Condition must be relatively prevalent

Table. 12.1 Example of commonly used screening tests and assessments of a child's developmental maturity

Test	Purpose	Areas of assessment	Reliability	Age range
Denver Developmental Screening Test (1975)	Screening of development	Personal-social, fine motor adaptive language, gross motor	Good	1 month–6 years
Gesell Developmental Schedule (1975)	Developmental assessment	Motor adaptive, language, personal-social	Not reported	4 weeks–6 years
Griffiths Mental Developmental Scale (1954)	Developmental assessment	Locomotor, personal-social, hearing and speech performance	Good	1 month–8 years
Brazelton Neonatal Behavioural Scale (1975)	To index behaviour of neonate potentially relevant to social interactions	Behaviour and 20 neurological items	Good	first day–1 month
The Stycar test of Mary Sheridan (revised 1976)	Clinical testing procedure for paediatricians for diagnosis and management of developmental disorders	Stycar hearing test Stycar vision test Stycar developmental sequences Stycar language test	Good normative values from very large samples	6 months–7 years 6 months–7 years 1 month–7 years 1–7 years

- Condition must be serious to warrant the costs involved in screening large populations.

Other criteria should be applied when deciding whether a particular test will adequately provide answers. The criteria for evaluating screening procedures are:

- The test must be valid statistically
- Procedures must be simple
- Procedures must be accepted by those who use them, and those who are clients
- Follow-up services must be available
- Screening costs must be reasonable.

Perhaps the most widely used general developmental screening test is one developed by Frankenburg & Dodds (1967) — the Denver Development Screening Test (DDST). Not only does it admirably fulfil the criteria for a screening procedure, but it is very well supported by explicit easily understood self-training video and written instructions. The test is designed for children in the age span from birth to six years. Test items are arranged on the test form in four sectors:

1. Personal–social — that is, tasks which indicate the child's ability to get along with people and to take care of himself.

2. Fine motor-adaptive — that is, the child's ability to see and to use his hands to pick up objects and to draw.
3. Language — that is, the child's ability to hear, to understand, and to use language.
4. Gross motor — that is, the child's ability to sit, walk and jump.

The reader is referred to Frankenburg & Dodds (1967), Frankenburg et al (1971) and Frankenburg et al (1976) for instructions about administering the test, calculating the child's age, adjusting for prematurity and interpreting the results.

It is essential to remember two things about the DDST. The first is that the DDST is *not* an IQ test, but rather a screening test of development. The second is that the child *will not* be expected to do all that is asked of him. Should parents become anxious during the test, the tester should explain again that it is not expected that the child will pass all of the items. Screening procedures are further discussed Evans & Sparrow (1975) and Banus (1983).

Therapists could participate in routine developmental screening of infants and young children (Jaffe et al 1980). However, a child is usually only screened by an occupational therapist after being brought to attention for another reason, usually medical, such as the 'failure to thrive' syndrome.

Diagnostic developmental assessment

Diagnostic developmental assessment is a more detailed examination than screening. Developmental assessment is a diagnostic evaluation whilst screening indicates that further investigation appears warranted.

Purpose
1. To measure all facets of a child's development.
2. To promote health — physical, mental and social.
3. To diagnose — assess, treat and manage chronic physical and mental handicaps as early as possible.
4. To prevent any further handicaps from developing.
5. to obtain as complete a profile of child's abilities as well as disabilities as is possible.

Process.
Developmental maturity is assessed by the following:

- By observation of the child'd behaviour patterns
- By standardized testing
- By appraisal of the information gained (data) compared with normative data.

The areas of development that should be assessed are

Definition of the four areas of developmental assessment

Postural-motor development. All motor skills including gross bodily control and finer co-ordination, postural reactions, head balance, sitting, standing, crawling, walking, grasp and object manipulation.

Adaptive behaviour. Perceptual and conceptual abilities, ability to react to and/or use objects presented. Includes finer sensorimotor adjustments, co-ordination of eyes and hands in reaching and manipulation, and the ability to use equipment appropriately in solution of practical problems.

Speech, language (vocalization, comprehension). Language is used broadly to include all visible and audible forms of communication — facial expression, gesture, postural movements, vocalizations, words, phrases, sentences. Also includes mimicry and comprehension of communications of others.

Personal-social. Comprises the child's personal reactions to the social culture in which he lives. Includes play patterns, relationships with others, feeding and toileting. Here as elsewhere, the patterning of behaviour is fundamentally determined by intrinsic growth factors, e.g., bowel and bladder control and external factors such as cultural requirements, but the attainment depends primarily on neuro-motor maturity.

---

postural-motor, adaptive behaviour, speech and language, personal-social.

A complete assessment of development must also involve a general medical examination of the child. This may include taking measurements of height, weight, head circumference, examination of hips for subluxation, muscle tone and reflexes, examination of urine and blood for amino acids. As an outcome, genetic counselling can be given where indicated, and early detection and intervention can help to forestall secondary disorder.

Key ages. At certain ages individual skills which have been slowly emerging, and presumably refining through practice, appear as a constellation of integrated behaviour. To the observer, it is as if the child moved from one stage of maturity into a quite new stage. Distortions and abnormalities of development become particularly apparent at these 'key ages'. Assessment of developmental maturity assumes particular relevance and usefulness at these ages which are 6 weeks, 3 months, 6 months, 10 months, 18 months, 2 years, 3 years, $4\frac{1}{2}$ years.

Assessment instruments. Following on from the pioneering studies about infant development by Dr Arnold Gesell and his colleagues (Gesell et al 1940), various workers have produced standardized tests of developmental maturity.

Whereas the Gesell Developmental Appraisal (Knobloch & Pasamanick 1974) is perhaps the most widely known of all infant tests, it has poor normative data, lacks well-defined instructions and scoring systems. The most used standardized developmental maturity assessments were devised in the United States, for example the Bayley Scales of Infant Development, and the United Kingdom, for example, The Griffiths Test of Mental Abilities (Aldridge-Smith et al 1980; Griffiths 1954, 1970; Hanson 1982; Ramsay & Piper 1980; Stott & Ball 1965). Denton (1986) has presented a profile specifically for occupational therapists to use with infants who present with failure to thrive syndrome.

Presently available norms have application only to westernised, usually Caucasian children, i.e., the population from which the norms were derived. There are slight differences in the available norms which reflect cultural differences. For example, Australian children are very similar to both American and English children, though probably slightly closer to American children in terms of the timing of behavioural development. When used with children from very different cultural experience, e.g., Australian Aboriginal or American Indian, the scores achieved from standardized tests may be used as a guide only. The situation is like that in which an apple and a banana are measured (or compared) in order to make comments about the apple. Though both are classified as 'fruit' (children), the apple and banana cannot be meaningful compared.

The Griffiths Test is reliable in its results, simple to administer, and difficult to misinterpret. A therapist must undergo training in the use of the Scales, and become an accredited user. The Griffiths Test is one of choice when a clinician is new to the practice of developmental assessment (Aldridge-Smith et al 1980; see Frankenburg & Goldstein 1971). Later, either the Gesell Appraisal or the Bayley Scales may give more sophisticated results. However, both of these tests make strong demands on the competence and past experience of the tester.

In common with other developmental assessment tests, the Griffiths Test does not have predictive value for a child's general intellectual capacities. The value of developmental assessments is that the test provides a fairly accurate picture of the child's development and maturity, as compared with others of the same age at that point in time. The velocity of change over time is an important indicator of a child's capacities. For example, if a child gains eight months in mental age (MA) in a six-month period between tests, then that child is maturing rapidly and competently. If, on the other hand, a child only gains two months in the six-month period, then she/he is obviously falling behind

---

Advantages of developmental assessment

1. Comparison possible of the child's maturation in relation to peers.
2. Aids diagnosis of moderate and severe intellectual handicap.
3. Aids diagnosis of physical disorders, e.g., cerebral palsy.
4. Aids in the early diagnosis of hearing, visual defects.
5. Neurological defects can be diagnosed and treated in infancy.

Limitations of developmental assessment

1. There is no clear line between Normal/Abnormal. Diagnosis is based on the fact that the farther the child is from the norm in any aspect, the greater the likelihood of abnormality occurring.
2. Tests do not predict future performance ability, or IQ.
3. Mild cases of cerebral palsy or intellectual handicap are often missed in infancy. These can be very hard to establish by developmental assessment.
4. A normal result now does not preclude future mental deterioration, neurological or learning difficulties.

---

his peer group, and there is real cause for concern about the nature of the detected development delay.

Advantages and limitations. Thus in summary, there appear to be both advantages and limitations to the practice of assessing developmental maturity.

Testing the child

Make the child comfortable. Since the testing requires active co-operation of the child, every effort should be made to make him/her comfortable. A young child may be tested while sitting on the parent's lap. The child should be sitting high enough, and close enough to the table so that she/he can easily reach the test materials.

When testing, the tester should remove all test materials from the table except the one(s) being used, so that the child will concentrate on what is asked of him. The child should be praised or thanked for his efforts throughout the test regardless of passes or failures.

Arrange the environment. A quiet testing room, free from the sight and sound of other children, is recommended.

Motivate and attract the child. The principles of motivating and attracting the child to therapy should also be used to help gain the child's co-operation.

Give limited choices. With younger children it is suggested to begin assessment by saying, 'Do you want to sit on the blue chair or mum's knee?', rather than saying, 'Where do you want to sit?' or, 'Would you like to sit down?'

Testing order. The tester may begin the test by laying one or two of the test materials on the table in front of the child. While the child is playing with these materials, the parent is asked any relevant 'report' items. This gives the child a chance to become accustomed to the tester. A shy child will often withdraw if the tester commences the test by asking him/her questions. A shy child will also be more likely to do the Fine Motor-Adaptive items before the Language items because she/he can participate in what is being asked, and still not have to talk to you. It is best to give the Gross Motor items last since some children may be too shy at the beginning of the test. Other children may enjoy the hopping, jumping, throwing the ball, and other Gross Motor items so much that they will not want to sit down to do the items in other sectors.

Begin each sector by giving the child tasks which she/he can perform easily. This builds confidence to perform more difficult tasks, and reassures the parent.

Explaining the test. Using ordinary language, rather than technical terms, the therapist should explain the nature of the test to the child's parents. Mother and the child should be reassured that all items need not be passed. Some mothers may become anxious if the child appears to be having difficulties, or to be failing test items.

Interpreting the results. The tester should be particularly alert to the influence of the following factors on the test result:

1. The accuracy of reported history
2. Premature birth
3. Factors operating on the child at testing time, e.g., medication
4. Mother's presence throughout test
5. Infant's state, e.g., highly aroused, tired, crying, hungry
6. Infant's interest in environment other than the test task.

Results should be interpreted as a whole pattern, rather than in relation to each component section. Some aspects of development are more useful for purposes of assessment; the least important are the areas of gross motor, even though it is easiest to test; and sphincter control, which seems to be irrelevant. The most useful areas are fine motor manipulation, which provides a guide to general ability; speech, where early onset is a striking characteristic of generally gifted children though late onset does not necessarily suggest retardation. Comprehension of language rather than expression appears to be the crucial factor. There is some inconclusive evidence that difficulty or slowness in learning to chew is linked with general low intelligence level.

When a child is found to be delayed, either in one sector, or generally, then the tester must attempt to offer some possible explanations and recommendations for further action. Such action may be yet more detailed evaluation and/or therapy.

The diagnosis of developmental delay should never pre-empt other subsequent diagnostic findings, such as 'specific learning disability'. When a delayed child first presents for intervention the objective is to minimize or eliminate as many extrinsic factors as possible, in order to clarify which remaining intrinsic factors in the child then require special attention. From that point on, intervention should be targeted at the specific remaining dysfunction.

The case of Justin illustrates two important factors. Firstly, the contribution that an occupational therapist makes in the role of evaluation of intervention on a child's development picture. Secondly, the use of normal community resources to provide the direct service component of therapeutic intervention.

Aged three years five months at the time of initial referral, this little boy was referred to occupational therapy for developmental assessment of abilities, and therapeutic intervention, because of a medical diagnosis of intellectual retardation, thought to be of moderate to severe degree. Justin received 'early intervention' through attendance at the local kindergarten, complemented by a developmental play programme administered at home by his mother. No specialist assistance was available in their country town. However, the kindergarten programme met Lazar's criterion of 'bombardment' (Lazar et al 1982) as Justin attended five days weekly, 9.00 am to 2.00 pm.

Justin's experience is particularly interesting, as the diagnosis of 'intellectual handicap' was negated at age seven years. However, it also became clear that Justin had a moderately serious perceptual problem for which he received remedial teaching for development of reading skills, while remaining in a normal class situation in school. The final outcome could not have been predicted at age three, and Justin's case is one where, had therapy and specialist services been available, he would have received priority admission into a special therapeutic intervention programme. Here are excerpts from Justin's developmental assessment reports.

General summary and interpretation of results. The Griffiths Scales yield an estimate of general development maturity — not a score. The estimate is expressed as a 'general developmental quotient' (GQ) and an equivalent of mental age (MA).

Justin (Example 12.2) achieved a GQ of 85 when the mean for the population is 100. That is to say, Justin has an appreciable developmental delay. His mental age is calculated as 2 years 11 months when he is chronologically 3 years 5 months. Moreover, the delay appears more specifically related to the area of language — receptive and expressive. A profile summarising the test results is included below.

Example 12.2: Justin

Date of birth: 13.1.77 Age: 3 years 5 months 4 days
Date of assessment: 17.6.80 at the University Clinic

Justin attended the University Occupational Therapy Clinic with his mother, and the Griffiths Mental Development Scales, Extended Range, was administered. The duration of the test was about one hour and Justin remained apparently interested, alert and cooperative throughout. He was shy at the outset, but his mother was able to gain responses from him and Justin became more relaxed and interactive with the examiner as he found that he could successfully complete the test tasks. Mrs H commented that the test situation provided a very fair estimate of Justin's usual behaviour and performance.

Detailed results. The test examines six areas of maturity and development, and each will receive comment:

1. Locomotor scale: This is one of the more competent areas of Justin's skills, and no special comment is warranted.
2. Personal–social scale: Social experience is reflected on this scale. Mrs H remarked that Justin has made rapid progress in this area over the past six months. This is an important observation as it is the velocity of change over this time that indicates a child's ability to use therapy effectively.
3. Hearing and speech scale: Apparently there has been concern about Justin's hearing integrity, as his brother is hearing-impaired. In the test situation his behaviour did not suggest deafness. However, the delay is significantly more than in other areas, and full evaluation of his communication skills is indicated.
4. Eye-hand co-ordination scale: Justin does not show any evidence of a movement disorder as such. The fine manipulative skills tested in this scale were handled with ease and competence, where he was able to complete the task. On some items he failed because he was slow and could not meet the timing criterion, yet he was able to do the task.
5/6. Performance and Practical reasoning scales: These skills are linked and it is here that Justin's delay is very obvious. He clearly has difficulty understanding abstract concepts and perceptual relationships. It is in this area that intellectual deficit is likely to show increasingly.

Recommendations. They are as follows:

1. Top priority should be evaluation of all aspects of hearing and communication, specifically (a) receptive hearing testing through an audiology facility, and (b) evaluation of language reception with a diagnosis of aphasia in mind — by a speech therapist experienced with aphasic clients.
2. Continuation of present programme of developmental stimulation. Justin should be grouped with children of the developmental level of three years rather than the 3.5–4 years. Special focus should be on perceptual tasks and personal–social independence tasks.
3. Reassess in about six months or about November 1980, so that plans can be made for his therapy and schooling in 1981.

Re-test 1

Age: 3 years 10 months
Date of assessment: 12 November 1980 at the University Occupational Therapy Department Clinic

On the present retest, six months later, Justin achieved a general quotient of 103, when the mean for the population is 100. That is, Justin is now functioning within the normal developmental range for his age in all areas including language. He has gained 11 months of ability in six months. Such rapid change negates the possibility that Justin has any significant intellectual handicap. A profile is attached.

Detailed findings. By contrast with the initial test, in the re-test Justin performed the required tasks with ease and confidence. His speech, though intelligible, is difficult to understand. However, his receptive language skills appear to be developing rapidly and appropriately.

Justin has obviously had the benefit of consistent and carefully planned training, and he has been responsive to these efforts. This finding is an encouraging sign for continuing efforts. However, if the very significant gains are to be consolidated Justin's training must continue for the present time. It would be disappointing if he were to relapse or fail to progress in response to relaxed efforts.

However, this recent re-test has confirmed that he does still display specific delay in the area of performance, i.e., adaptive behaviour (Scale E).

This, finding strongly suggests that Justin is likely to find considerable difficulty with reading and numerical operations. Specifically, he appears to have difficulty recognizing abstract shapes in matching operations and with auditory sequencing of abstract symbols (numbers and letters). His performance suggests that the problems form both perceptual recognition skills and short-term memory skills.

It is very encouraging that he has continued to gain in achievements, and a tribute to those who have worked with him. My present view is that Justin should be regarded as a child of normal developmental ability who has a specific set of perceptual memory problems. He should respond to a remedial basic skills training programme, or preparation for reading and numbers work programme, which should run parallel to the normal first-grade class work. Thus, the following suggestions are offered:

Recommendations

1. Inclusion in a small class — the ideal upper number would be 20. Justin is a quiet, shy child who lacks confidence in his own abilities, and he is not likely to draw attention to himself or his needs. Thus, in a large class he could easily 'drift along', falling behind in his grasp of the formal material
2. Additional work in
   — visual perceptual shape recognition, matching and classifying of concepts;
   — development of sequencing skills, visually and auditorily;
   — practice in increasing his speed of response to solving problems. Some of his faliures in the current test came about because he failed to meet the timing criterion. His response was often correct but too slow. In a class situation slow responses could disadvantage him as he would not complete work in the time regarded as appropriate.

The readiness programmes could be given by a teacher with access to remedial programmes, an occupational therapist, or a psychologist specializing in the area of learning difficulties.

It may prove to be to Justin's advantage that he spend this year in Grade 1, developing confidence and basic skills, and a further year in Grade 1, consolidating his basic skills and developing more soundly the usual formal skills. However, that decision should depend on his performance.

It is of primary importance that the gains made over the past two years be supported. In my view, this will be best achieved if Justin is placed in a smaller class, with a kindly, supportive teacher who is prepared to allow some flexibility in his rate of responses to formal work.

Justin should take another re-test in six months.

SUMMARY

In conclusion, the term 'development delay' is a general one, to be applied whenever a child lags significantly behind his/her peer group in skill achievement, for whatever reason. The occupational therapist has an important contribution to make to the evaluation of a child's developmental abilities, to defining the aetiological factors leading to delay, and to designing and providing suitable therapeutic intervention.

In the next chapter, the discussion will focus on a group of developmentally delayed children who have been specifically singled out and classified by the designation 'developmentally disabled'.

REFERENCES

Aldridge-Smith J, Bidder R T, Gardner S M, Gray O P 1980 Griffiths scales of mental development and different users. Child: Care, Health and Development 6: 11

Banus B J 1983 The Miller assessment for preschoolers (MAP): an introduction and review. American Journal of Occupational Therapy 3: 333–411

Court J M 1981 Child development. Patient Management Nov: 21–29

Denton R 1986 An occupational therapy protocol for assessing infants and toddlers who fail to thrive. American Journal of Occupational Therapy 40: 352–358

Erickson M L 1976 Assessment and management of developmental changes in children. CV Mosby, St Louis

Evans R, Sparrow M 1975 Trends in the assessment of early childhood development. Child: Care, Health and Development 1: 127–141

Fraiberg S 1964 Studies of the ego development of the congenitally blind child. Psychoanalytic Study of the Child 21: 113–169

Frankenburg W K, Dodds J B 1967 The Denver developmental screening test. Journal of Pediatrics 71: 181–191

Frankenburg W K, Goldstein A D 1971 The revisited

Denver developmental screening test: its accuracy as a screening instrument. Journal of Pediatrics 79(6): 988–995

Frankenburg W K, Camp B W, Van Natta P A, Demersseman J A 1971 Reliability and stability of the Denver developmental screening test: Child Development 42: 1315

Frankenburg W K, Doonick W J, Liddell T N, Dick N 1976 The Denver pre-school development questionnaire. Journal of Pediatrics 57: 774–753

Gabel M D, Erickson M L 1980 Child development and developmental disabilities. Little Brown, New York

Gesell A, Halverson H M, Thompson H, Ilg F L, Castner B M, Ames L B, Amatruda C S 1940 The first five years of life. Harper & Brothers, New York

Goldberg S 1978 Prematurity: effects on parent-infant interaction. Journal of Pediatric Psychology 3: 137–144

Griffiths R 1954 The abilities of babies: a study in mental measurement. University of London Press, London

Griffiths R 1970 The abilities of young children: a comprehensive system of mental measurement for the first eight years of life. Child Development Centre, London

Hanson R 1982 Item reliability for the Griffith Scales of Mental Development. Child: Care, Health and Development 8: 151–161

Holt K S 1977 Developmental pediatrics. Butterworths, London

Hospitals and Health Services Commission 1976 Summary Report from 1976 Review of the Community Health Programme. Australian Government Printer, Canberra

Illingworth R S 1962 An introduction to developmental assessment in the first year. Medical Advisory Committee of the National Spastics Society, London

Jaffe M, Harel J, Goldberg A, Rudolph-Schnitzer M, Winter S T 1980 The use of the Denver developmental, screening test in infant welfare clinics. Developmental Medicine, Child Neurology 22: 55–60

Kennel J H, Klaus M H 1976 Maternal-infant bonding. CV Mosby, St Louis

Knobloch H, Pasamanick B (eds) 1974 Gesell and Amatruda's developmental diagnosis. Harper & Row, New York

Lazar I, Darlington R, Murray H, Royce J, Snipper A 1982 The lasting effects of early education: report from the consortium for longitudinal studies. Monograph of Society for Research in Child Development

Lichtenstein R, Ireton H 1984 Preschool screening. Grune & Stratton, New York

Llorens L 1971 Occupational Therapy in Community Child Health. American Journal of Occupational Therapy 25(7): 335–339

Morris A G 1978 Parent education in well baby care: a new role for the occupational therapist. American Journal of Occupational Therapy 32(2): 75–76

O'Neil S M, McLaughlin B N, Knapp M 1977 Behavioural Approaches to children with developmental delays. CV Mosby, St Louis

Parmelee A 1982 What are the functions of follow-up programmes for high risk infants? Paper presented at conference 'Environment intervention for infants at risk', Harvard Medical School Continuing Education Department, Boston

Ramsay M, Piper M 1980 Comparison of two developmental scales in evaluating infants with Down syndrome. Early Human Development, Elsevier/North Holland Biomedical Press, Utrecht

Sheridan M D 1975 The developmental progress of infants and young children. Reports on Public Health and Medical Subjects No 102, HMSO, London

Stott R S, Ball L H 1965 Infant and pre-school mental tests: review and evaluation. Monographs of the Society for Research in Child Development 101, Vol 30, No 3

West W L 1973 Professional responsibility in times of change. In: Llorens L A (ed) Consultation in the community. Kendall Hunt Dubuque, Iowa, pp 10–25

13. Applications for children with developmental disabilities

READERS' OBJECTIVES

After reading this chapter, you should be able to:
1. Name those medical conditions which are described as a developmental disability under the US Public Laws 1975.
2. Demonstrate knowledge of each condition, its incidence, aetiology, impact on development, and general approaches to intervention.
3. Describe the occupational therapy process with children affected by each of the defined developmental disabilities.
4. Present basic information about maturation of the motor behaviour system, with special reference to hand function.
5. Describe the role of an occupational therapist the practical management of activities of daily living.

The first part of this chapter presents a discussion of the concept of 'developmental disabilities', and the diagnostic conditions which are so classified. The second part focuses on motor behaviour dysfunction, a disability which affects very many developmentally disabled children.

THE CONCEPT OF DEVELOPMENTAL DISABILITIES

The term 'developmental disabilities' is a generic one covering medical conditions defined in United States Public Laws (1970, 1975). A developmental disability is defined as a condition that:

- Originates prior to the age of eighteen
- Has continued or is expected to continue indefinitely
- Constitutes a substantial handicap in the normal functioning of the individual in society.

Three conditions were named in the 1970 Bill, while two more were added, and the definition widened in the 1975 Bill. The discussion process in the 1960s and 1970s which led to formulation of the United States Bills attracted international interest, and the definition received worldwide acceptance. These Public Law definitions remain in use, and were recently re-affirmed as acceptable to the American occupational therapy profession in an official position paper (AOTA 1986).

The conditions which are designated as 'Developmental Disabilities' are:

1. Mental retardation, now referred to as intellectual handicap
2. Cerebral palsy
3. Epilepsy
4. Autism
5. Dyslexia of neurological origin and, 'any other condition . . . found to be closely related to mental retardation because such condition results in similar impairment of general intellectual functioning, or adaptive behaviour to that of mentally retarded persons, or requires treatment and services similar to those required for such persons' (United States Public Laws 94–103, 1975)

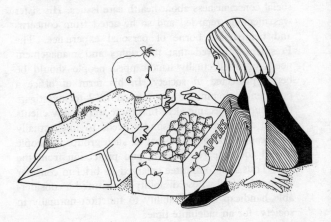

161

Developmentally disabled clients constitute a substantial proportion of the total occupational therapy population. Green & Souter (1977) reported the following international incidence figures per 1000 head of population.

- Intellectually handicapped 15
- Cerebral palsied 2.9
- Spina bifida 2.0
- Autism 0.45.

Factors which may be associated with a high risk of developing a handicapping disorder are as follows:

1. Family history
   a. Intellectually retarded parent or sibling
   b. Inheritable metabolic diseases
   c. Deafness
2. Pregnancy
   a. Rubella
   b. Syphilis
   c. Heavy alcohol intake
3. Perinatal period
   a. Small birthweight baby (<1500 g)
   b. Low APGAR scores (e.g., <5 at 5 minutes)
   c. Severe or prolonged jaundice (e.g., >300 mol/l)
   d. Convulsions
   e. Hypoglycaemia
   f. Cerebral haemorrhage
4. Early infancy
   a. Meningitis
   b. Convulsions
   c. Unexplained trauma, child abuse
   d. Failure to thrive
   e. Floppiness

History of policy changes

John F Kennedy, President of the United States from 1961 until his assassination in 1963, ushered in a new social consciousness about health care issues. His sister was mentally retarded and so he acted from concerns and compassion borne of personal experience. The President observed that the rights and management needs of intellectually handicapped people should be better protected in society. In his term of office a presidential committee was formed 1962 to investigate the issues. It became clear that there were many clients in the community with similar needs to intellectually handicapped people, and that all such groups of people lacked adequate recourse to, and protection from the law. Thus the Committee enlarged its brief to consider the needs of all whose disability constituted a considerable handicap to their ability to function normally in society, for an indefinite time.

It will be seen that the defined conditions all originate from factors within the child (intrinsic factors). The possible exception is autism (Kanner's syndrome), though most workers now agree that there is a high probability of some element of neurological disarray in the autistic child.

Implications

From the developmental disabilities legislation there flowed a general move to emphasize the functional needs of people (Hammer 1973). The United States Law specifically provided the following actions:

1. To eliminate inappropriate placement in institutions of persons with developmental disabilities.
2. To improve the quality of care and the state of surroundings of persons for whom institutional care is appropriate.
3. To provide for early screening, diagnosis, and evaluation of developmentally disabled infants and preschool children, particularly those with multiple handicaps.
4. To provide for counselling, programme co-ordination, follow along services, protective services, and personal advocacy on behalf of developmentally disabled adults.
5. To support the establishment of community programmes as alternatives to institutional living.

Perhaps the greatest advance from the introduction of the definition of 'developmental disabilities' is the removal of the arbitrary division of 'child' from 'adult' client. The 1975 Public Law initiated a new debate about society's role in providing care, services and resources for severely and multiply handicapped people. Many new directions have been suggested, however the exact form of service continues to be debated by specialists, government, and society alike — for all pay the bill. There is recognition that programmes begun in infancy should lead to others throughout the client's life. Concurrently, there has been official support for the development of care-giving centres and specialist resources to serve the client throughout his/her life. The modern emphasis is to encourage and support a family so that their child may grow and develop at home. However, there are still some children who, for various reasons, will live, grow and develop in institutional settings (Moersch 1978).

Impact on occupational therapy services

The impact of the Laws defining developmental disabilities on occupational therapy service may be summarized thus:

1. Where therapists traditionally worked with child clients 3–12 years of age, they now work with newborn infants, adolescents, and adults who are called developmentally disabled.
2. The professional boundaries between specialists has become less strict, and new agreements about roles and functions have become necessary. A discussion of team roles was presented in Chapter 11.
3. Occupational therapists now have the opportunity, and indeed, the responsibility to broaden their professional role of service to embrace community action, and legislative advocacy on behalf of clients (Moersch 1978). The American Journal of Occupational Therapy (1988) devoted a commemorative issue to examining the impact of the Public Laws on the practice of occupational therapy particularly in schools.

Diagnosis and intervention

Evaluation

Disability may be apparent at birth as in the case of a child with Down syndrome, spina bifida or even cerebral palsy. However, many children, such as those later designated as autistic, and/or intellectually handicapped, do not display obvious physical signs at birth. In some cases of intellectually handicapped children (approximately one-third), no conclusive diagnostic cause will ever be found. The diagnosis follows after parents become anxious because they think that their child's development is slower than normal. Indeed, there is often a long period of diagnostic uncertainty before specialists decide that a child is developmentally disabled, in the terms of the Public Law definition.

Regrettably, the range of specialist diagnostic and intervention services is usually limited because of service demands on specialists. Ideally, occupational therapists could assist in screening all infants in maternal and infant welfare clinics, child care centres and pre-school settings. As it is, developmental screening of infants and young children usually occurs only if doubts are raised about an individual child who attracts attention for another reason, usually medical.

Most mothers expect their child to be born normal and healthy, and to continue growing as such. Consequently, when the child is diagnosed as developmentally disabled, the parents are likely to respond with shock, bewilderment, and even disbelief. Thus, parents are often anxious and confused when first confronted with professionals (Cartwright 1981; Court 1981; Green & Souter 1977; Molony 1971; Smiley 1975; Tavormina et al 1981). This will affect the manner in which they perceive, understand, retain and recall information. Anxious people are less likely to perceive information correctly (Dick 1979).

An occupational therapist needs to approach the child's parents with sensitivity, and be prepared to allow them time to resolve their own conflicts and emotional responses to the diagnosis. It would be helpful to review Chapter 3, Foundations of therapy, and Chapter 9, Attracting the child and family to therapy.

The general principles of assessment and the process of diagnostic evaluation are the same as those already discussed for the developmentally delayed child. The occupational therapy evaluation report should provide other specialists with a global picture of the developmental competence, strengths and weaknesses.

Intervention

Early intervention is generally regarded as the most appropriate form of management for both developmentally delayed and developmentally disabled children. The reader is advised to review the general principles of, and procedures for, early intervention which are presented in detail in Chapter 11. Nurcombe (1972) suggests that the general aims of intervention should be to:

— Correct the effects of disability as soon and as far as possible.
— Educate the child to live with the disability.
— Provide general and special education (which may include special vocational training).
— Provide recreational and social opportunities.
— Provide parental guidance and/or counselling.

For many disabled children the process of therapy will continue for the greater part of their lives. For example, a cerebral palsied client may receive wide-ranging therapeutic services throughout his or her lifetime. On the other hand, occupational therapy services 'are discontinued when a child is functional in age-appropriate activities of daily living, has reached a maximum level of function or has derived maximum benefit from therapy' (AOTA 1986).

The five developmental disabilities are now described in terms of the clinical picture that each presents, as well as a general summary of the occupational therapy approaches.

INTELLECTUAL HANDICAP

Intellectual handicap has been recognized as a condition throughout recorded history. However criteria and definition have changed markedly over time. These persons have been labelled at differing times as idiots, imbeciles, mentally handicapped, mentally retarded, feeble minded, demented and simpletons (Clark & Clarke 1965, Clarke & Clark 1974, Gunzburg 1973).

The most accepted definition of intellectual handicap has been adopted from the American Association of Mental Deficiency (AAMD). The AAMD has defined mental retardation as 'significant sub-average intellectual functioning concurrent with deficits in adaptive behaviour manifested during the developmental period' (Ploy 1979). Such a definition implies satisfaction of three factors before a diagnosis of intellectual handicap may be used.

1. An individual's intellectual functioning must be below that considered 'normal' in the general population to which she/he belongs. 'Subaverage' generally means an intelligence quotient (IQ) on standardized psychometric assessments of more than 2 standard deviations below the population mean. In westernized cultures, the average intelligence quotient is considered to be 100; thus a person scoring below 70 on a standardized intelligence test would be considered as intellectually handicapped.

2. The individual must exhibit 'deficits in adaptive behaviour'. Broadly interpreted, this factor refers to an ability to cope adequately with the demands of the individual's society. Behaviour which is considered 'adequate' may vary widely from society to society and is often ambiguous. In addition, an inability to cope with societal demands may derive from factors which are not innate, e.g. an impoverished environment (Whelan & Speake 1979).

3. Intellectual handicap must originate in the developmental period, i.e. before the 18th birthday.

While neurological injuries beyond this age may be overtly manifested as intellectual handicap, they are referred to as brain injury or damage (Batshaw & Perret 1981).

Classification

Such a broad definition of the disabilities associated with intellectual handicap embraces a large group of individuals whose actual behavioural manifestations and capabilities are quite disparate. Hence intellectually handicapped individuals may be further classified in two ways.

Intellectual functioning. Classification is based on the individual's performance on standardized tests of intellectual functioning, e.g., Wechsler and Stanford-Binet. The degree of handicap is assessed in relation to standard deviations from the mean of 100, and the range is presented in Table 13.1

Table 13.1 Degree and incidence of disability in intellectually handicapped populations

Degree of IH	IQ test score range Stanford-Binet (SD = 16)	Percentage with disability
Borderline	68–85 ⎫	
Mild	52–67 ⎬	88
Moderate	36–51	7
Severe	20–35	4
Profound	<20	1

However, interpretation from IQ assessments is fraught with difficulty. Performance on these tests is not only a measure of innate ability, but also the result of experience with items similar to those in the test (Cronbach 1984). But there remains the problem that IQ may bear poor relationship to a person's ability to function in society with adequate training and support. This has

Table 13.2 Aetiologies for intellectual handicap

	Prenatal	Perinatal	Postnatal
Infections and intoxications	Syphilis, rubella, toxoplasmosis alcohol ingestion (fetal alcohol syndrome), maternal drug ingestion, radiation		Encephalitis, meningitis, drug ingestion, measles
Physical agents and trauma	Threatened abortion	Difficult or prolonged labour, anoxia	Child abuse motor vehicle accidents, falls, drowning
Disorders of metabolism, growth and nutrition	Maternal diabetes, toxaemia		PKU, galactosaemia, neonatal jaundice, malnutrition, hypothyroidism

---

Example 13.1: Medical conditions often associated with intellectual handicap

1. *Associated with gross brain disease*
   neoplasms
   tuberous sclerosis
   progressive encephalopathies

2. *Associated with diseases and conditions due to (unknown) prenatal influences*
   hydrocephalus
   craniostenosis, MR of unknown origin
   epilepsy, microcephaly, hypertelorism
   Von Recklinghausen's Disease
   Sturge-Weber Syndrome

3. *Chromosomal abnormalities*
   Down syndrome, Lejune syndrome, Cri du chat, Klinefelter's syndrome, Turner's syndrome
   Patau's syndrome, cretinism
   Edward's syndrome, Apert's syndrome, Crouzon's disease
   Lawrence Noon-Biedl syndrome, Lesch-Nyhan syndrome
   Chotzen's syndrome, Carpenter's syndrome, Pfeffer's syndrome

4. *Associated with prematurity*
   placental insufficiency, infections

5. *Following major psychiatric disorder*

6. *Psychosocial or environmental deprivation*

7. *Other and unspecified*

---

led to some classifications of disability according to functional ability.

According to aetiology Intellectual handicap may be classified due to its aetiological origins either biological or environmental or the time of onset, e.g., prenatal, perinatal or postnatal. Aetiological categories are presented in Table 13.2 and Example 13.1.

The more severe forms of intellectual handicap generally result from biological deficits and prenatal causes. The milder forms, in contrast tend to be multi-causal in origin, e.g., hereditary, environmental conditions and psychosocial deprivation.

Incidence

Only a few of the more severe forms of intellectual handicap can be recognized at birth. Milder forms may not be recognized until school age. Thus, it remains difficult to assess accurately the extent of the condition in the early years.

It is, however, generally accepted that 3.5% of the population may be affected, and it is the single largest handicapping condition affecting the Australian community.

Intervention

Normalization

Over the past twenty years, the principle of 'normalization' has had a profound influence on policy decisions and practical approaches to programme development and management with intellectually handicapped people. For example, The UN Declaration of the Rights of Mentally Retarded Persons is founded on the normalization principle. However, there has never been a satisfying consensus reached by workers on the

---

Definitions: The normalization principle
Normalization

- Making available patterns and conditions of everyday life as close as possible to the norms and patterns of the mainstream of society (Nirje 1969).
- Letting the mentally retarded person obtain an existence as close as possible to the normal (Bank-Mikkelsen 1969).
- Using culturally normal means to establish/maintain personal behaviour and characteristics like the normal (Wolfensberger 1972).

meaning of the word 'normality'. Briton (1979) observed perceptively that normalization has great intuitive appeal. Yet an objective assessment of the various interpretations of the concept suggest that normalization is a mirage — ethically and humanistically enticing, but nevertheless a mirage. Let us briefly examine the principle of normalization in the light of Briton's proposal.

A comparison of the two most influential interpretations of 'normalization' is summarized in the Example 13.2.

Example 13.2: Comparative views of 'normalization'

Nirje (1969)	Wolfensberger (1972)
Basic trust in normative environment	*Basic trust in normative behaviour*
Values self-image; self-confidence; sense of dignity;	Seeks to reduce visibility of intellectual handicap
Seeks an enlarged and more nearly normal behavioural repertoire — freedom of action	Eliminate those behaviours which mark retarded as deviant from others
Concerned with the range of behaviours	Concerned with the style rather than the range of behaviours
Assumes that: Enhanced life experience yields an enhanced self-experience; yields enhanced behaviour	*Assumes that:* Acceptable social behaviour yields enhanced social acceptance; yields enhanced self-experience and quality of life

---

Nirje emphasizes a *normative environment*, or *life conditions*. He divides this rather vague notion into two components, structural and social conditions.

Structural conditions are:

Normal standards of physical facilities
Temporal patterning — day work etc.
Developmental life cycle

Social conditions are:

Normal economic security
Normal sex
Normal respect from non-retarded.

This view inevitably leads Nirje to place high value on notions of *self-image, self-confidence, sense of dignity,* and *feelings of personal identity.* Nirje sees such perceptions as gained through therapy and training designed to develop a varied and as nearly normal as possible be-

havioural repertoire. The individual should enjoy normal freedom of action and response.

Nirje seems to suggest that there is a logical and predictable flow of benefits from his therapy proposal for the person. Furthermore, he claims that normalization (of the retarded individuals) will result in normalization of society's attitude.

Nirje's assertions remain untested, and therefore unsupported hypotheses for further study.

Wolfensberger (1972) has redefined the normalization principle to shift the therapeutic emphasis from concerns generally affecting the environment and thus behaviour, to concerns affecting the behaviour and presensation of the individual directly. Wolfensberger maintains that every effort should be made to increase the personal freedom of disabled people by establishing and/or maintaining 'personal behaviours and characteristics which are as culturally normative as possible' (Wolfensberger 1972, p. 28).

But it is abundantly clear that the degree of freedom will equal what specialists will allow or deem appropriate. The freedom of the intellectually handicapped individual to engage in sexual behaviour of his/her own choice provides a good example of the dilemma posed by Wolfensberger's proposition.

The difference between Wolfensberger's approach and that of Nirje is that Wolfensberger aims to reduce the visibility of the deviant individual in the community by eliminating marking out behaviours. He is concerned with *style* rather than variety/range of behaviours of the person.

Environmental planning for the care and training of intellectually handicapped people has undergone dramatic change (for example see Keane 1979). Wolfensberger and Dybward became strong and effective advocates of the dispersal and integration of intellectually handicapped persons into normal community living. (Kugel & Wolfensberger 1969; Wolfensberger 1972). The arguments used were:

— That dispersal reduces group visibility, hence is 'image normalizing'
— Dispersal of intellectually handicapped people in suburbs, houses, flats, apartments etc. maximizes exposure to normality and exposure of retarded to non-retarded, thus promoting acceptance.

Summary. Inherent in the normalization principle is a desire to offer opportunities to retarded people to live and behave as far as is possible like the rest of society.

Nirje focuses attention on making *adjustments to the environment* to accommodate the retarded individual. Wolfensberger focuses attention on making *adjustments* to the *individual*, to accommodate the retarded individual to society. The distinction is important for its influence on therapy design. The situation still remains that, while there is nothing wrong with intuitive ideas, there is a need for consensus on definition about 'normalization' to be reached, and an operational definition for the normalization principle. Assumptions need to be made explicit and examined.

Claims need to be made more circumspectly and backed by systematic study and research.

Occupational therapy

Intellectually handicapping conditions most often affect the global development of the child. Hence many specialists will be involved in the person's management throughout life. Treatment approaches must be co-ordinated, and there must be a consistent team approach.

Some problems that may be encountered in occupational therapy intervention include the varying degrees of cognitive, perceptual and sensory deficits clients may experience; behavioural difficulties, e.g., self-stimulatory behaviour, stereotypic behaviour; slow overall development; and lack of independence in the activities of daily living.

The general objective is to provide management that will facilitate the child's acquisition of skill in:

— caring for him/herself
— engaging in satisfying and appropriate social behaviour and interpersonal relationships
— performing activity that is expected and valued by the general community

The infant and young child

- Encourage parental bonding.
- Provide parents with practical and emotional support; give realistic and accurate information related to their child's needs about:
  — sensory stimulation and developmental facilitation through play;
  — behavioural management techniques.
- Instigate ongoing systematic evaluation procedures for developmental skills, perceptual/motor skills, general living skills, recreation and occupational skills.
- Provide parents with information on community resources, e.g. parental support groups, toy libraries, government, private and voluntary services for intellectually handicapped people and their families.

Later childhood

- Continue to assist parents to formulate realistic and constructive goals to achieve a lifestyle as close as possible to that of the average family.
- Provide specific remediation of cognitive and perceptual deficits.
- Assist other specialists in a team approach to behavioural management.
- Institute strategies to facilitate acquisition of age appropriate self help skills.
- Develop leisure and social skills.
- Train occupational and work skills and choices.
- Prepare for residential placement.

Specific aspects of programmes are discussed in Chapters 9, 10 and 14.

CEREBRAL PALSY

Incidence and aetiology

The term 'cerebral palsy' describes any disorder of movement and posture, resulting from non-progressive abnormality of the immature brain (Harryman 1981; Paine 1966). Because the term is a descriptive one, used broadly, it is difficult to gain an accurate estimate of affected individuals. However, Gordon (1976) estimated that there are probably about two to three infants in every 1000 live births who will be diagnostically classified as 'cerebral palsied'.

The clinical picture may result from many causes, and the precise cause will only be identifiable in about 60% of children diagnosed. The 'cerebral palsy' may originate from prenatal, perinatal or postnatal factors. These are presented in Table 13.3. The most frequently cited origin is complications occurring in the neonatal period.

Description and classification of the cerebral palsies

Clinical classification is determined according to the type of movement disorder which presents, and the degree of involvement of the body segments. Six types of movement disorder and levels of involvement have been described. They are as follows:

Classification by movement disorder

1. Spasticity in which there is damage, to the motor cortex or pyramidal tract. The 'spastic' individual presents with:

Table 13.3 Factors associated with motor abnormalities of the celebral palsies

Prenatal factors		Perinatal factors	Postnatal factors
1st trimester	Late pregnancy		
Congenital malformations	Threatened abortion	Toxaemia	Infection
Genetic	Maternal illness	Antepartum haemorrhage	Head injury
Threatened abortion	Toxaemia	Hypoxia	CVA
Radiation	Growth retardation	Ischaemia	Epilepsy
Infection		Birth trauma Infection Prematurity Hypoglycaemia Hyperbilirubinaemia Shock, e.g. due to haemorrhage Rh incompatability	

- Hypertonus with characteristic clasp knife quality. Flexor muscles are generally most affected, as are distal parts of the body.
- Hyperreflexia of deep tendon reflexes. Characteristically, there is a positive Babinski response. An increased resistance to passive movement can also be observed.
- Persistence of primitive reflexes, e.g., Asymmetrical Tonic Neck Reflex (ATNR), Moro.
- Difficulty in initiating voluntary movement.
- Increased tone, with resultant abnormal postures may result in permanent deformities.

2. *Athetosis*. Occurs when there is damage to the extrapyramidal pathways or basal ganglia, due primarily to perinatal insults (Davies et al 1979). The problem for the athetoid individual is not one of initiating movement, but of controlling movement and maintaining a normal background posture. There are two recognized types of athetosis:

a. Non tension athetosis characterized by:
- Variable or fluctuating tone.
- Purposeless writhing movements, especially of face and arms.
- Cog wheel rigidity.
- Less occurrence of deformities due to fluctuating tone.
- Facial involvement, causing swallowing and articulation difficulties.
b. Tension athetosis
- Generally increased tone.

However, the picture is distinguished from spasticity in that the rapid movements of tension athetosis lead to

decrease in tone.

3. *Rigidity*. Represents a severe presentation of spasticity in which there is:

- Extreme increase of muscle tone leading to a phenomenon called 'lead pipe rigidity'.
- Quadriplegic limb involvement.

4. *Ataxia*. Results from damage to or abnormality in the cerebellar region. Ataxia is characterized by:

- General hypotonia with resultant pendula deep tendon reflexes.
- Inco-ordination of movement and lack of trunk balance causing a 'rolling' gait.
- Intention tremor of the upper limbs and marked overshoot of hand and arm movement.
- Nystagmus, especially when the individual is resting.
- Normal reflex integration.
- Slow, slurred speech.

5. *Mixed movement disorder*. A clinical picture which includes elements of spasticity and athetosis. Usually, all four limbs are involved, suggestive of diffuse abnormalities in the brain.

6. *Atonia* (Flaccidity). Generally develops into one of the other types of cerebral palsy, as the child matures, and the clinical picture changes at about three years of age. It is characterized by:

- Hypotonia and hypermobility of joints.
- Absent or weak tendon reflexes.
- Absent or weak primitive reflexes.
- Hips are usually held in a 'frog-like' position,

abducted and externally rotated. Knees are held flexed.

- Absence of muscular contraction, which may lead to dislocation of shoulder and hips.

Classification by body segment involvement

1. *Monoplegia* — one limb involved
2. *Hemiplegia* — limbs affected unilaterally
3. *Paraplegia* — lower limb involvement
4. *Diplegia* — lower limb involvement greater than upper limb
5. *Triplegia* — three limbs involved
6. *Quadriplegia* — involvement of all limbs

Associated developmental deficits

Robinson (1973) plotted a pattern of incidence of other developmental deficits. The associated deficits which are most commonly seen in the clinical picture of cerebral palsy are:

Physical

1. Oral-dental: drooling, difficulty in swallowing and abnormalities of teeth.
2. Articulation: speech difficulties occur in 48–49% of affected children and may, for example, be dysarthria, dyspraxia.
3. Hearing loss: more commonly associated with athetosis.
4. Intellectual handicap.
5. Reading retardation.
6. Failure to establish lateral dominance.

Personality and behaviour

Emotional immaturity, dependence, lack of mature outlet for aggression, express other symptoms of central nervous dysfunction. The spastic child may be withdrawn, fearful, preferring to avoid overstimulation. The athetoid child is less fearful, more gregarious and affection seeking, with explosive temper and lack of insight into handicap. The ataxic child is similarly outgoing and affectionate, but readily frustrated.

Parents of the cerebral palsied child also seem especially vulnerable to react with guilt or shame. Parents may express their responses by setting unrealistic expectations and by clinging to the belief that training will lead the child to overcome the defect completely. They may become frustrated and disillusioned, and even reject the child especially as she/he approaches young adulthood. It would be helpful to review Chapter 3, the section on adverse effects of physical handicap, and Chapter 9.

Levitt (1977) provides a comprehensive, practical and well balanced description and discussion of the specifics of occupational therapy evaluation and intervention with cerebral palsied clients. As this area of work is quite specialized, the reader is referred to Levitt, and only the briefest summary is provided here.

Occupational therapy

Levitt cites the general aims of therapy as:

1. Developing forms of communication (speech, gesture, writing or sign language, typing).
2. Developing independence in the daily activities of feeding, dressing, washing and toileting.
3. Developing some form of locomotion.

The long-term objectives are those which apply for all developmentally disabled clients, such as a lifestyle which incorporates meaningful and remunerative work, satisfying recreation, and both within a social context of close interpersonal relationships.

If the cerebral palsied child also has intellectual, perceptual and sensory deficits, then the techniques to be used are those appropriate for all children with those deficits, and you should refer especially to those discussions in this book.

A helpful reference text is provided by Conner et al 1978.

EPILEPSY

Associated developmental deficits

There is a high incidence of psychological disorder in children with epilepsy because:

1. Cerebral dysfunction may have acute or chronic behavioural effects.
2. Emotional upset may accentuate epilepsy.
3. The disorder is psychologically traumatic.
4. The parents and social environment may react adversely.

Children with temporal lobe epilepsy seem to be more prone to behavioural disturbance, especially as time goes on. Behaviour disorder in epilepsy is of two types:

1. Secondary to cerebral dysfunction.
2. Secondary to the psychological effects of having a particular chronic illness.

Stevens et al (1968) claims that the fully developed picture of minimal cerebral dysfunction can be associated with epilepsy. The picture includes hyperkinesis, low frustration tolerance, impulsiveness, explosive rage, poor emotional control, perceptual and learning difficulties. In some cases overmedication (especially with barbiturates) may produce depression and poor concentration or accentuate hyperkinesis.

Intervention

Principles of management involve placing no more restrictions on the child than necessary. Physical injury is more likely to result from overprotectiveness than from an epileptic attack occurring while the child is engaged in sport, for example. Physical activity is generally beneficial, and precautions can be taken to protect the child during contact sport, climbing, swimming, bicycle riding.

Regrettably, the attitudes of the general community often reflect outdated notions of fear and repulsion — remainders from times when epilepsy was associated with 'demon possession'. Parents and teachers need to be reassured about the scope or limitations that should realistically be placed on an epileptic child, the importance of medication, the practical management of seizures, and the legal rights and limitations of an epileptic adult. There are special problems for the epileptic child who is also retarded and/or severely emotionally disturbed, and such children will require special educational and therapeutic facilities (Nurcombe 1972).

SPINA BIFIDA

Incidence

Spina bifida is the most common defect in the central nervous system in children. Its incidence tends to be extremely variable between areas and may vary from 0.1–4.13 per 1000 live births. On average the occurrence is thought to be 2–3 per 1000 live births (Bleck & Nagel 1975).

Description and classification

Spina bifida represents defective development of the spinal cord with accompanying defect in vertebrae. Several types are recognizable, and they occur most frequently in the lumbosacral region of the spine.

Meningocele. Is a lesion containing only the meninges and CSF. The spinal cord lies in the usual position and is normally formed; thus treatment is with corrective surgery. This condition is rarely associated with paralysis.

Myelomeningocele. Generally occurs in the lumbosacral region. In this case the spinal cord has failed to develop and protrudes into the lesion. Hence involvement of neural elements leads to paralysis and associated problems.

Encephalocele. Involves failure of fusion of the skull bones causing herniation of neural tissue through the skull. Surgical repair may indicate a favourable prognosis.

Spina bifida occulta. Failure of formation of the posterior vertebral arches with outpouching of neural and subcutaneous elements. To superficial examination the defect may not be obvious, but there may be pigmentation of the skin or tuft of hair over the area.

Associated developmental deficits

— Sensory impairment of the segments below the lesion.
— Lower motor neurone (flaccid) paralysis of the muscles below the level of the lesion.
— Bladder paralysis (neurogenic bladder). The child is unable to control the emptying and retention of urine. This inability causes overdistension of the bladder with subsequent overflow and incontinence. If urine is allowed to back up into the ureters, urinary tract infection (UTI) becomes a recurrent problem.
— Paralysis of bowel, anal sphincter and rectum. Inability to voluntarily empty the bowel may lead to chronic constipation and soiling.
— Bony deformities occur as a result of muscle paralysis and imbalance. Deformities of the spine may include lordosis, kyphosis and scoliosis. Characteristic deformities of the feet may occur including club foot (equinovarus), rocker bottom feet (calcaneal valgus) and dislocation of the hip (Bleck & Nagel 1975).
— Hydrocephalus occurs simultaneously in 90–95% of spina bifida children. A defect of the brain prevents the circulation of CSF leading to increased intracranial pressure, compression of brain structures and an abnormal increase in skull size.
— Mental retardation may occur if the hydrocephalus is not surgically corrected, and subsequent damage to the brain occurs.

Intervention

Medical

The complex medical and functional problems of the

child with spina bifida necessitate the intervention of a multitude of medical and therapy, educational and psychological specialities. Medical and surgical measures include:

— Surgical repair of lesion
— Ventricoperitoneal shunt to minimize hydrocephalus
— Orthopaedic correction of hip and lower limb deformities
— Provision of orthotic device, e.g., braces, parapodium or crutches
— Frequent urinalysis to detect UTI
— Catheterization
— Ileal diversion and stoma therapy
— Bowel management, e.g., suppositories

Physiotherapy

— Strengthening weak muscles
— Enhancing mobility and motor functions
— Preventing deformity

Occupational therapy

The range of associated problems to which an occupational therapist usually pays attention is:

— Limited mobility
— Postural insecurity
— Motor planning problem
— Bowel and bladder incontinence
— Diminished sensation
— Absence of proprioceptive input
— Clumsy fine finger movements

Here is a summary of the general programme of occupational therapy; the details are naturally designed for each client:

1. To determine factors which have an impact on the child's developmental progress and to predict what the impact is likely to be; and
2. To provide management techniques to facilitate competence in:
   — caring for him/herself;
   — interacting socially with others; and
   — performing satisfying activity.

The therapeutic process

Short term goals

1. At birth provide constructive and realistic goals and information for parents.

2. Encourage attachment and bonding between parent and child.
3. Instruct parents in handling and positioning techniques appropriate for their child's needs.
4. Begin developmental evaluation and planning long-term goals.

Long-term goals

1. Develop the child's fine motor skills and hand skills.
2. Assess and develop the child's ADL skills, e.g., bowel and bladder management, dressing, independent mobility. Assess the need for adaptive equipment and clothing.
3. Assess and provide therapy in specific areas, e.g., directed at problems associated with perception, body image.
4. Develop basic work related skills leading to employment preparation.

AUTISM — KANNER'S SYNDROME

Autism has been described as a pervasive developmental disorder which is manifest during the infancy period (birth to 30 months) (Rutter 1985). Kanner's evidence for his original description of 'early infantile autism' (Kanner 1943) rested on observations of eleven children only, eight boys and three girls. These children, who varied in age up to twelve years, had shown a striking failure to make affective contact with other human beings from very early in life. Kanner spoke of this as 'extreme aloneness' and postulated an innate inability on the part of the children to form affective relationships with other people. Other symptoms included an anxious obsessive desire for the maintenance of 'sameness' in the environment, and a range of language and speech disorders ranging from mutism to failure to use language as appropriate communication.

Kanner implicated a particular parental type associated with the behavioural disorder in the children: notably, the parents were 'for the most part strongly preoccupied with abstractions of a scientific, literary or artistic nature, and showed limited genuine interest in people'. Most of the eleven families were previously known to Kanner and he argued that the parental traits were in evidence before the child's birth. By arguing thus, he rejected the notion that the parents' aloof mechanized, interpersonal responses were a direct response to exposure over time to an abnormal condition in their child. This finding is supported generally and there has been considerable research into the family characteristics, prenatal and postnatal factors, genetics, anatomy and neurology of autistic children and their families. Many of the studies are inconclusive and do not readily explain the behavioural and intellectual deficits of these normal looking children (Cantwell et al 1978; Clancy & McBride 1975; DeMyer et al 1972; Ney & Mulvihill 1985)

The original descriptive criteria represented several dimensions of organization, for example, a structural dimension, e.g., the upper age for the appearance of the symptoms; a functional dimension, e.g. language involvement; and an operational dimension — the interpretation of observed behaviour, e.g., 'desire for the maintenance of sameness'.

These criteria subsequently generated many varying deductions about the nature of the condition, and a few examples follow: O'Gorman (1967) considered that infantile autism could be considered within the general framework of schizophrenia. Van Krevelin (1952) and Rutter (1965), however, regarded infantile autism as separate from schizophrenia, and thought that it resulted from unknown organic changes in the central nervous system. Rimland (1964) considered it to be a specific dysfunction of the reticular system. Hutt et al (1964) also implicated the reticular system but, in contrast to Rimland's suggestion of under-arousal, they hypothesized a chronically high state of arousal in autistic children. Others (e.g., Creak 1964; Menolascino 1965) have suggested that infantile autism is a variant of mental retardation. Yet others regarded the condition as a severe response to stress (Bettelheim 1967). Clancy & McBride (1975) suggested that autism is a developmental process, operating within a social system, the family. While they considered the possibility of a predisposing condition, they saw the primary developmental condition as the failure to develop a bond with the mother, and consequently with the others in the family. The child does not develop the stranger response because all are strangers. She/he develops a standard pattern of responses to all, family and outsiders alike. Members of the family have interactions with him/her, but none find these reinforcing or affiliative, so all relationships develop abnormally. The child is tolerated with as much affection as it is possible to engender in a one-sided relationship. Thus they saw the disorder as one of relationship processes, and its treatment involving therapy aimed at the relationships, not the child.

Modern thinking is that autism is distinct from the psychoses of childhood such as schizophrenia, and that it does represent a serious abnormality in the developmental processes (Clancy & McBride 1969; Eisenberg 1972; Newsom 1980; Robinson 1986; Rutter 1970, 1985). All of the findings indicate important genetic influences at work. The findings also suggest that probably the child inherits some broader predisposition to language and cognitive abnormalities (Rutter 1985).

Incidence

Kanner's observation that males appeared more commonly affected than females has been confirmed and generally accepted (ratios of 2 : 1 to 4.25 : 1 were suggested by Rutter & Lockyer 1967, and Treffert 1970). Figures resulting from the few epidemiological studies relating to childhood psychoses including infantile autism suggest that the latter is a rare syndrome (2 per 10 000 to 4.5 per 10 000) (Gillberg & Schaumann 1982; Wing & Gould 1979).

Rutter (1985) notes that if severe mental retardation with some autistic features is included, the rate rises to 20 per 10 000. Clancy & McBride (1975) considered that this latter group should not be considered as autistic — they proposed a separate clinical entity, the isolation syndrome, as providing a more appropriate clinical definition of such children.

There have been some attempts to establish generally acceptable diagnostic classificatory systems for children older than three years (Clancy et al 1969; Creak 1961; Polan & Spencer 1959; Rimland 1964) and while all are in use, no one has become predominant. Furthermore, diagnostic criteria for use in the earliest years of life are not generally used.

Behaviour

Definition Autism is defined by reference to the following criteria (Rutter 1978, 1985; Rutter & Garmezy 1983):

1. Onset before 30 months
2. Deviant social development
3. Deviant language development
4. Stereotyped behaviours and routines
5. The absence of delusions, hallucinations and schizophrenia-type thought disorders

The characteristic behavioural picture is described below.

Birth to 30 months. Mothers have consistently reported:

— Lazy sucking associated with long and tiresome feeding periods. Weaning difficulties are common, particularly refusal of all solids.
— Absence of smiling response. When a smile was remembered it was dated towards the end of the first year.

— Quiet undemanding behaviour when left alone but irritation when disturbed. Baby often wriggled and squirmed when held but was pacified by putting alone in cot.
— Unresponsive to human voice, but selectively responsive to other sounds.

These behaviours were all described retrospectively and therefore not observed; they are also not specific to autism. Schaffer & Emerson (1964) found lazy sucking and non-cuddliness in normal children. Autistic children seem different in that parents report a range of these behaviours, and it seems that these behaviours potentially function to express and shape an abnormal mother–child bond. It further suggests that the autistic process can be established very early, perhaps even before the smiling response is normally acquired (Clancy & McBride 1975).

30 months onward. Language is absent or markedly abnormal. The child may echo, reverse pronouns (you for I), or use stereotyped language. The overriding principles are:

— The child fails to use language appropriately to communicate in a reciprocal manner with others. Language, if used is devoid of symbolic thought representations, imaginative content, or ability to talk about future or past. Approximately 50% of autistic children never gain language.
— Social behaviour is developmentally inappropriate. The child actively avoids interaction with others and expresses this by failing to make eye contact, by maintaining physical distance from others, and engaging in excessive 'tantrum' behaviour, such as screaming if his/her rituals are interrupted. It appears that the child organizes the social world to make isolation, and resists intrusion from others.

An autistic child does not play in the normal sense of the word. She/he manipulates objects, often with great skill, but in a repetitive unimaginative manner. The child may collect curious objects and become intensely attached to these objects, or be preoccupied with one activity to the exclusion of other activities, and engage in stereotyped, repetitive movements (especially hand and finger movements). Other behaviour may include extreme food fads; over activity (often develops into underactivity in adolescents); short attention span; and extreme fears, which may be expressed through aggressive behaviour and tantrums.

Intervention

The most common intervention approaches to autism include psychotherapeutic, behavioural and special education. Newsom (1980) states that in light of current research, behavioural approaches appear 'demonstrably superior'. Pharmacotherapy may be used as an adjunct, aimed towards making older children more receptive to behavioural and educational intervention (Campbell 1978).

Occupational therapy

There is no clearly defined and generally accepted profile for occupational therapy with the autistic child. In Chapter 14, there is an account of an integrated treatment regime with severely ill autistic children living in an institution. However, Clancy & McBride (1969) suggest that the ideal situation is for the child to remain within the family. Because they see this serious disability as a disorder of social processes, they argue that it is fruitless to target therapy at the child. Intervention must be targeted at the social system of the family relationships.

These authors see the clinical picture as one where predisposing factors act with initiating situations to establish a self-perpetuating autistic process. The first object of therapy is to achieve primary socialization, that is, to develop affiliations or bonds between the child and the family. The second stage of the treatment aims to foster the acquisition of behaviours normally developed in the socialization process, especially language. A simple approach is used throughout. The therapist leads in every step, and when successful, hands over to the appropriate member of the family. Naturally most attention is given to promoting the mother—infant bond.

The first step is to intrude on the child. The most successful method has been to correct the feeding problem. The treatment has been described previously (Clancy et al 1969; Clancy 1970).

Mother and child are hospitalized together because the programme is directed at strengthening the bond between them. The programme consists of the therapist offering the child new food, camouflaged by the preferred food, at each successive mealtime. Soon hunger becomes the prime motivation for the child to extend his/her food range. When eating begins, usually within a week, the programme becomes the mother's responsibility under the continuing guidance of the therapist. The feeding time becomes a play time, so that strong social reinforcement is added to food.

During the period of starvation, a programme is developed for the mother and child. Young autistic children do have favoured activities, such as rough and tumble, water and bubble play. These are used throughout the day to provide a context for pleasant interaction between child and mother. Social facilitation is used to initiate each activity. For example the mother starts to blow bubbles to attract the child's attention so that she/he begins to join in her activity. At first the child's response is only to the medium, in this instance the bubbles, and the mother is simply the means by which the bubbles are provided. The child uses her as she/he would an object to meet his/her demand for the activity. However, this manipulation is not allowed to continue. Demands are made on him/her before his/her need is met. For example eye contact is required, then sounds are demanded, so that the therapist's or the mother's intrusion is maintained throughout. The child's demands are *never* met until she/he meets the requests of the therapist or mother. The child becomes more amenable to physical contact throughout this stressful period, and the mother is encouraged to give long sessions of cuddling and physical comfort.

The therapy developed strong bonds between the mother and child in about a month. These bonds are manifested in a strong preference for the mother (previously absent), the appearance of the stranger response, a marked change in the quality of emotions, and the *spontaneous* appearance of babbling in previously silent children. Each child progressed from babbling to speech, though it is stressed that the pattern was almost always abnormal in the manner described by Rutter (1965). It is always necessary to give special attention to language defects.

While in hospital, the only bond developed is with the mother, so that a programme is used to integrate the child into the family when, she/he returns home.

Basically all of the activities used to foster affiliations are common sense. Any normal activity enjoyed by the child can be used as a reinforcer for social contact, as long as the unit of therapy is the social relationship rather than the child (Clancy & McBride 1969).

MOTOR DISABILITY AND DEVELOPMENTAL COMPETENCE

Disordered motor function is a major component of the clinical picture for many developmentally disabled clients. Occupational therapy intervention deals with the practical consequences. For example, a child with cerebral palsy may require special support in order to sit unaided, so that she/he can eat, play, and participate in schooling. Thus it is relevant to examine the general principles of therapy for children with motor function disorder, in the context of this discussion about the full range of developmental disabilities.

The knowledge base needed, and some therapeutic techniques for dealing with disturbances of motor function will be examined.

The word 'motor' refers to muscular movements. Motor function represents the ability of a person to perform a sequence of voluntary, co-ordinated motor movements leading to a *functional* end point, for example walking along a footpath, cleaning teeth, threading a needle. Holle (1976) reminds us that good co-ordination is not inborn, but develops in conjunction with maturation of the nervous system, aided by the kinesthetic, touch and sight senses, as well as by experience. All systems are interdependent. Table 13.4 shows the usual pattern of development of the motor system, compared with the sensory-perceptual systems.

Table 13.4 Usual pattern of development of the motor system compared with the sensory-perceptual system after birth

Motor system	Sensory-perceptual system
Relatively undifferentiated response	Tactile, vestibular, proprioceptive, olfactory, gustatory, auditory, response. Visual senses are mature at birth
Partial patterns arise More specific local movement Reflexes interact, more patterns evolve	Sides of body integrate e.g. can cross midline — bilateral activity Depends on maturing proprioceptive system Primitive reflexes integrate, body image, body scheme mature
Equilibrium sense gained Moves from static postures Freer movements in environment	Gross motor planning skill develops (engages in non-habitual movements) Depends on intact tactile and proprioceptive systems Visual-space perception Fine motor planning
Maturity: Maturation of higher nervous centres, assimilation and inhibition of reflexes e.g. rides bicycle	*Maturity*: Ability to conceptualize e.g. reads, does math

Motor abilities also have far-reaching consequences on the social relationships that the infant makes with others. For example, the 'windy' smiles of the newborn infant encourage the mother to pick up her infant, hold him upright, look at him, and smile and coo. Maternal handling is one of the strongest influences on a child's motor experience, for it involves inhibitory sensory input, deep tactile input, vestibular system stimulation, balance practice, visual location and exploration (Korner 1971, Lee & Aronson 1974). Later, the child starts to push on the hands, providing himself with deep proprioceptive and tactile input. This experience heralds

the beginnings of co-contraction of the muscles and head rotation, which in time stimulate the semi-circular canals and the vestibular system. All of these experiences are necessary precursors for fine manipulative skills to emerge and mature.

In the first year of life, maturational forces are the chief ones determining the rate, the level of readiness, and the pattern of an infant's early motor responses. Figure 13.1 illustrates the maturation of motor skills from prone lying to independent walking.

Progress is influenced by a number of factors, for example:

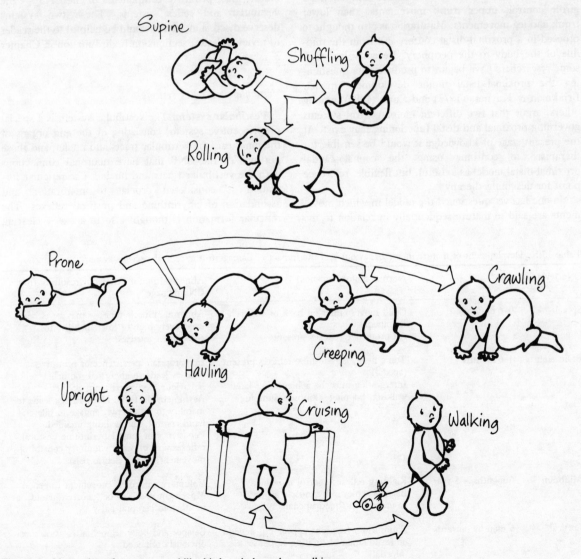

Fig. 13.1 Maturation of gross motor skills, birth to independent walking

- opportunity to practise the motor skill
- the child's attitude to learning the skill
- physiological inhibitions to learning (presence of a meningoecele)
- psychological (i.e., environmental) inhibitions to learning (for example an impoverished care giving environment).

Principles

It has been widely accepted that maturation occurs from the head to feet direction, i.e., in a cephalo-caudal direction. The significance of this is that a child gains head control integrated with shoulder and shoulder girdle control, upper trunk movements, then lower trunk and leg movements. Maturation is also thought to proceed in a proximal-distal course, and from the midline of the body to the periphery. Recently however, some researchers have begun to produce data questioning the proximal-distal motor development model. Brinkman & Kuypers (1973) and Loria (1980), among others, argue that two different motor control systems governing proximal and distal functioning may exist. At the present stage of knowledge it would be sensible for therapists to continue using the cephalo-caudal proximal-distal model as a useful, but flexible, reference point for designing therapy.

No one has yet questioned the model in which movements are said to mature sequentially in relation to the planes and axes of the body. Thus flexion is held to precede extension patterns, adduction precede abduction patterns, and ulnar proceed radial patterns. Gross movements precede fine movements, and rotation completes the process as the most complex movement in relation to body axis. The development of mature motor behaviour, and the impact on it of damage to the central nervous system is presented in Table 13.5.

Muscle function also follows a developmental sequence, commencing with automatic reflex contraction present at birth, and maturing into voluntary controlled contraction. In fact the ability to move about in the environment is most significantly influenced by two of the oldest, most primitive components of the CNS — the vestibular and reflex systems. These two systems deserve discussion, and it would be helpful to the reader to review relevant sections on brain function in Chapter 3.

Vestibular and reflex systems

Vestibular system. The vestibular system is a special proprioceptive system, consisting of the end organs of the inner ear, the vestibular tracts and nuclei, and those portions of the CNS that have neuronal connections with the vestibular tracts and nuclei. The reticular formation is considered crucial to maturation and assimilation of labyrinthine and postural reflexes. The reticular formation is thought also to act as a clearing

Table 13.5   Development of mature motor behaviour and the impact of damage to the central nervous system

CNS level	Age	Normal motor behaviour	Abnormal motor behaviour resulting from CNS damage
Spinal	0–6 months	Child moves either on back or stomach i.e. apedal All protective reflexes present	Abnormal muscle tone — may be either excessively high or low. Inability to co-contract muscles.
Brain stem	4–6 months	Tonic neck, labyrinthine reflexes present (apedal) Intergration must be achieved for later walking, hopping, skipping, jumping	Inappropriate persistence of primitive reflexes leads to abnormal motor behaviour. e.g. persistence of the Asymmetrical Tonic Neck Reflex leads to inability to roll, crawl, engage in bilateral hand control, and walking unaided Persistence of tonic labyrinthine postural reflexes also impedes voluntary control of movement, as in celebral palsy.
Midbrain	6 months – 5 years	Righting reflexes control movement Balance achieved by muscle group co-ordination (quadrupedal)	Voluntary control of movement impeded Movement is sail to be 'choreoathetoid', as in athetoid cerebral palsy
Cortical	6 months onwards	Equilibrium reactions appear but depend on assimilation of righting responses (bipedal)	Balance and body segmental rotation most obviously impeded

house for the cerebellum, and to be influenced by the vestibular system.

Functionally, the vestibular system operates to enable a person to detect motion, both acceleration and deceleration. Other functions include maintenance of equilibrium, and the monitoring of the relationships between body motion and the visual field. The functions of the vestibular system are mediated primarily at the brain stem level, to influence reflex behaviour. Thus, it is not possible to discuss motor function development without considering reflex and vestibular activity as intimately connected. Weeks (1979) provides a useful discussion of the vestibular system.

Reflex system. Reflex activity is that which occurs independently of the individual's will, as an involuntary and predictable response to nervous stimulation. The mechanism is a stimulus–response one. Reflex responses appear to perform the following functions:

• Those concerned with facilitating vital survival functions e.g. sucking and swallowing reflexes necessary for feeding. The reflexes concerned are mediated through the spinal cord and brain stem and are present at birth.
• Those concerned with achieving mobility and stability. Reflexes act to range muscles and joints through different patterns of movement — these are called phasic reflexes. Others called tonic reflexes give stability to different groups of muscles. (Barnes et al 1978; Hopkins & Smith 1978)

Some reflexes are present at birth, while others appear later on. Individual reflexes may be affected so that an individual who has movement dysfunction may exhibit a 'patchy' overall picture of maturing reflex behaviour. A useful analogy might be drawn between an orchestra performing a symphonic movement, and the human reflex system emerging and integrating. In the orchestra, one set of musicians will take up a theme and extend it, while other musicians will weave into that theme and extend it further. The orchestra combines to produce a complex, and fully integrated performance. In much the same way, different reflexes weave and flow into each other giving rise to smooth and integrated motor performance. Non co-operation or distortion leads to disharmony and awkward performances — both in the orchestra, and the human reflex system.

Within the classification of specific response patterns, there are motor behaviours which are primarily concerned with the organization and orientation of bodily movement in space. These are called *general static reactions*, which further subdivide into two categories:

1. Those concerned with movement itself — *equilibrium reactions*
2. Those concerned with resulting body position — *righting reactions*

The general pattern of appearance and assimilation (i.e., integration) of reflexes and the general static reactions are presented in Table 13.6.

Table 13.6 Pattern of development of reflexes and general static reactions

Reflex	Normally present	Assimilated
Flexor withdrawal	Birth	8 weeks
Extensor thrust	Birth	8 weeks
Crossed extension	Birth	8 weeks
Rooting, sucking, swallowing	Before birth	10 months
Moro (vestibular)	Before birth	12 weeks
Startle (sound response)	Before birth	12 weeks
Grasp	2 weeks	8 weeks
Placing, walking	Birth	3–4 weeks
Asymmetrical tonic neck (ATNR)	Birth	12 weeks
Symmetrical tonic neck (STNR)	Birth	20 weeks
Tonic labyrinthine	4 weeks	16 weeks
Positive supporting reactions	Birth	16 weeks
Negative supporting reactions	Birth	16 weeks

General static reaction		
Righting reaction	Birth–6 months	3 months (strong)
Neck righting	3 months (strong)	6 months
Body righting	6–7 months	6–7 months
Labyrinthine righting acting on head	2 months	10 months (strong)
Optical righting acting on head	4–8 weeks	4–8 weeks
Equilibrium reactions	6 months	6 months
Prone/supine lying	6 months	6 months
4 point kneeling	8 months	8 months
Sitting	10–12 months	10–12 months
Standing — hopping, dorsiflexion, see-saw	15–18 months	15–18 months

Movement disorders

Movement disorders present themselves in a wider range of clinical pictures. Though this chapter is concerned with the five identified developmental disabilities, we believe it is important to present a general classification of movement disorders.

One of the major and complex sets of motor tasks is hand function, which must be learned in early childhood, if the child is to become competent in daily living tasks.

Classification of movement disorders

1. Those resulting from damage directly to the central nervous system.
2. Those resulting from damage to anatomical structures and associated soft tissues.
3. Those resulting from damage directly to musculature.

Resulting from direct CNS damage

— congenital, e.g., spina bifida; arthrogryphosis; failure of limb development (due to, e.g., thalidomide)
— traumatic injury before/during birth, e.g., cerebral palsy
  traumatic injury after birth, e.g., car accident — non-specific, brain damage paraplegia/quadriplegia
— disease process — meningitis, encephalitis, polio/guillain-barré syndrome
— familial inheritance — Down syndrome, Friedrich's ataxia

Resulting from damage direct to anatomical structures

— e.g., juvenile rheumatoid arthritis — a condition which also has direct general systemic effects on the individual.
  Osteogenesis Imperfecta.

Resulting from damage to musculature

There is thought to be a genetic factor involved in some forms of damage to musculature, so this could also be classified as 'congenital'.

— by trauma, e.g., amputation
— by infection/disease process, e.g., musculature dystrophy
— dermatomyositis
— polymyositis
— spinal muscular atrophy

HAND FUNCTION

Hand use is a central focus of human activity, and thus, of occupational therapy practice. The meaningful use of a variety of tools is a distinguishing characteristic of man, and of some other primates (Connolly 1973). By approximately 15 months of age a child has normally acquired the patterns which will persist throughout life, in refined forms. The acquisition of mature hand function is dependent on CNS integrity, and opportunity for practising the manipulation and use of objects.

Maturational

Four components, each with its own predictable pattern of development, lead toward increasing hand use competence. The components are:

1. Vision: its role in directing hands to objects
2. Posture: its role in promoting effective object use
3. Grasp: its role in securing objects
4. Manipulation: its role in achieving the goal of object use.

Programme to develop reach, grasp and release skills

1. *Clients*: Moderately and profoundly retarded children
2. *Age*: 5–9 years
3. *Developmental level*: Variable, but at least 16 months, with reach and grasp skills potentially available
4. *Objectives*:
   • To train functional reaching and grasp skills.
   • To train the child to use his reaching skills in daily activities, e.g. feeding and play
5. *Training materials*:
   Jolly Wobbler
   Dandy Dangler
   Roly Poly
   Feeding materials
   Sandwiches and other finger foods
   Spoon
   Cup
   Positioning Chair
   Water Play Materials
   3 inflatable swim pools
   1 inflatable mattress
   1 inflatable ball
   1 blue plastic sieve
   3 kiddicraft mumbo jumbo
   6 black/white ping-pong balls
   6 plastic bubble pipes
   5 wooden bubble pipes
   9 assorted small plastic floating fish
   1 large yellow plastic duck
   2 plastic sponges
6. *Training programme*:
   a. Position child in selected aid and leave 10 minutes to habituate to position.
   b. Present novel object. Observer mark on a checklist any intentional reaching movement.
   c. Contingent on step b. administer the previously selected reward (reinforcer).
   d If no intentional movement noted in 5 minutes after presentation, discontinue task.
   e. Represent second novel object. The reinforcement schedule will move from reward to any response to fixed interval to random schedule (variable interval).
   Total training session should last 15 minutes and be repeated three times in one $\frac{1}{2}$ day session, i.e. each child will be trained 3 times × 7 sessions = $10\frac{1}{2}$ hours over entire programme.
7. *Data collection record*:
   (Figure 13.2 gives an example of the record form used.)

Appendix VIII provides an overview of the emerging developmental patterns.

Voluntary reaching behaviour requires more than just the flexion and extension of the fingers, supination or pronation of the forearm, and integration of reflex patterns. The infant must be able to formulate a movement plan and must have developed visual regard (see Appendix VIII. Wolff (1965) reported that the visual pursuit and fixation behaviour of a four-month-old is similar to that of an adult. By seven months, the baby is visually monitoring the entire movement while reaching and grasping the object (Halverson 1931). By this stage, the infant also holds and inspects objects. Thus it appears, that from five months onward, the infant is able to formulate the necessary action plan to enable him or her to co-ordinate movement and visual information, sufficiently to occasionally reach and grasp an object in the environment, though still in a very immature manner.

The reflex grasp present at birth is different from the voluntary grasp of later life, in that it is a digital rather than a palmar grasp. That is to say, the thumb is not used to oppose the forefinger, but rather, is placed in the palm of the hand, under the object. Twitchel (1970) asserts that thumb and finger opposition is not possible until there is a disintegration of the grasp reflex somewhere between eight and ten months of age. At five months there is still no true grasp, the child corrals the object with the hand, pressing the object to his body. Over the first year, the progression in developing a true grasp release pattern is from whole hand closure, to scis-

---

Department of Occupational Therapy
MULTIPLE HANDICAPPED CHILDREN'S UNIT
SAMPLE: DATA COLLECTION RECORD — REACHING SKILLS TRAINING PROGRAMME

INSTRUCTOR .... DATE ....

CHILD'S NAME .... WARD ....

TIMES   Commence... Finish ....

Session No...

OBJECT	TIME INTERVALS 1 Minute					REMARKS
1. Roly Poly						
2. Jolly Wobbler						
3. Dingle Dangle						

CODE O — no movement
      X — slight movement towards object
      Y — definite reaching movement
      Z — reach and grasp

Signed...

Fig. 13.2   The record form used in a programme to develop reach, grasp and release skills.

sor type closure, to pincer prehension. That means that by one year of age, a child can hold a crayon and scribble, but without control, whereas by two and a half years she/he will copy vertical and horizontal lines.

Exploration and practice

There is evidence that practice of basic manipulative skills in infancy, will lead to higher levels of proficiency in 'tool use' at an earlier age. Kopp (1974) demonstrated this to be so in two groups of infants aged between 32 and 36 weeks, both having normal grasp patterns for their age, but one group having an enriched experience of handling a variety of objects. The 'enriched', children had significantly better controlled co-ordination at eight months of age. Saida & Miyashita (1979) demonstrated a similar finding when they compared young Japanese children, brought up to use chopsticks, with same aged British children. The element of practice is an important one to be built into therapeutic intervention programmes designed to facilitate hand skills and use of 'tools'.

The infant begins to explore and practise hand skills by 'mouthing' objects, she/he then progresses to finding out what the object will 'do', for example by hitting and banging things. Eventually the maturing child becomes socially organized, and includes other children in his/her play, handing play objects around, and so on. In the most sophisticated form, hand skills are used to hold implements for writing and other fine creative work. A discussion of the skills reflected in such fine motor activity is beyond this presentation, and the interested reader should refer to specialised literature.

Summary

The goal of this section has been to provide essential information about the normal development of motor skills, with specific attention to hand skills. Fiorentino (1981) has summarized the acquisition of motor skill into four basic components, providing a fitting conclusion to this discussion. The four components of motor skills are:

1. Head control — influential in the development of tonal distribution and much of motor movement.
2. Increasing generalized extensor tone — necessary to establish and maintain positions against gravity.
3. Rotation with the body axis — necessary for the development of righting reactions and higher levels of sensorimotor development.
4. Equilibrium reactions — necessary for maintaining balance in sitting, standing and walking.

There are a number of intervention approaches which propose that unwanted abnormal muscle and motor movement can be inhibited by reference to the general principles governing motor behaviour. The reader is referred to Chapter 15 for a review of these approaches.

Hand skills — reaching, grasping, manipulating and releasing objects — are essential for meaningful 'tool' use and independent performance of normal everyday activities. For these reasons the facilitation of hand skills and tool use is fundamental to all occupational therapy practice.

We will now consider practical application of the basic knowledge of maturation of motor behaviour to therapy programmes designed to develop a child's competence in everyday living skills.

PRACTICAL MANAGEMENT OF DAILY LIVING ACTIVITIES

Principle and applications

The objective of all therapeutic and educative procedures in activities of daily living skills is to encourage a disabled child to become as efficient and/or independent in self-care as the disability allows. The following factors will have to be considered:

1. Appropriate physical positioning — to prepare the child for activity, in the most facilitating manner.
2. The task itself must be organized in terms of (a) materials and equipment suitable for the particular child; (b) the sequence of therapy task steps, organized to lead from dependence on another to self-reliant performance.
3. Physical aids/assistive devices must be prescribed, fitted and incorporated into task performance.

Occupational therapy procedures are directed at achieving movement patterns and behaviour which facilitate functional activity by the child: feeding, dressing, toileting, play and school. All therapy should be related to the normal daily routine as far as possible. For example, feeding training should take place at normal meal times; dressing training should occur for the older child in the morning and again at night. The concept of special therapy sessions of half-an-hour duration three times a week, to fit department schedules, is particularly inappropriate training in activities of daily living. Similarly, therapists should not be overly enthusiastic in devising elaborate training programmes for the child's mother or primary caregiver to implement. The tasks of caring for a disabled and handicapped child are onerous enough. Johnson & Deitz (1985) investigated the amount of time taken in the everyday tasks of caring for their children by the mothers of physically handicapped preschool children, compared with a matched group of mothers of normally developing children. These authors found that the mothers of handicapped preschoolers spend more time in physical child care than the control mothers. In fact, Joosten (1979) found that mothers of young spina bifida children spend twice as much time in normal daily care tasks associated with the child, than do mothers of normally developing, similarly aged children.

Positioning

Before beginning any fine motor activity it is necessary to have a child positioned in an optimum position. Finnie (1978) identified key points of body control which provide useful positioning guides. The child must be well supported with his/her trunk stable, and hands free to grasp and manipulate. Generally, there are several principles which apply.

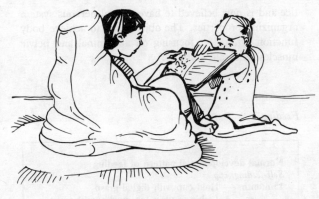

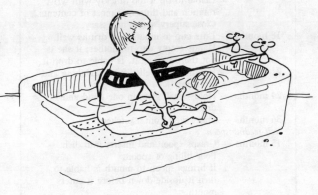

Key points of control

- The head is held steady in the midline to enable the child to see what she/he is doing with the hands, to approach grasp and release objects
- The body is held steady in the midline body posture to provide stability to carry out an activity
- The hips are positioned well back in the chair
- The knees are flexed
- The work surface should be at the appropriate height to enable freedom of hand and arm movement.

With experience, a therapist develops sensitivity in his/her own touch, and this becomes an important skill which allows him/her:

- To monitor varying change of muscle tone.
- To estimate/detect difference between stiff rigid limb resistant to movement, and light, flexible or overly flexible limb.

Fig. 13.3 Examples of aids and positions which facilitate more normal movement and activity by a spastic child (top), and a 'floppy' child (bottom).

While general principles are applicable to all clients, they should be interpreted differently for children with different conditions. For example, the spastic child should be moved and positioned to achieve inhibition of unwanted movements and patterns. Bringing the child into a flexion posture enables him/her to reach out and grasp at objects, to visually explore, and to experience bodily and visual symmetry. A 'trough pillow' tilts the head forward, and thus helps to inhibit excessive extension of the neck, which leads to a tonic thrust mouth/tongue pattern, and inhibited sucking and swallowing. It is important to keep the stimulus toy or food below eye level for a child, whether she/he is in both the flexion posture, and in sidelying.

On the other hand, the athetoid or 'floppy' child requires positioning and movement experience which achieves stability and proprioceptive input, through firm physical pressure on muscles (see Fig 13.3).

Stability of the pelvis is essential to upper limb functioning. The infant with motor dysfunction will stay in the 'frog-leg' position longer than the normally developing infant. The outcome is pelvic femoral tightness, leading to adducted, internally rotated femoral joints and scissor gait by age 6–7 years. Williamson (1982) counsels that it is not necessarily the achievement of motor milestones that is the important assessment guide, because the accentuation of the extensor pattern can make milestones seem precocious. Rather, it is the *quality* of movement that offers the key. For the child who is hemiplegic, Williamson (1982) advises swaddling, that is wrapping the limbs and body very firmly like an Egyptian mummy. Swaddling is an ancient practice and is now believed to have central nervous system organizing properties. The objective is to achieve body function symmetry, focusing on abdominal and pelvic muscles, and thus stability.

Feeding

Normal developmental pattern of feeding
Self-feeding: cup
15 months — Hold cup with digital grasp
Liable to tip it too quickly with wrist rotation and thus spill most of contents.
Close supervision is necessary.
18 months — Lifts cup to mouth and drinks well.
Hands empty cup to mother; if she is not there to take it, is liable to drop it.
21 months — Handles cup well; lifting, drinking and replacing.
24 months — Holds small glass in one hand and drinks.
36 months — Pours well from a pitcher.
Self-feeding:spoon
15 months — Grasps spoon and inserts into dish.
Poor filling of spoon.
If brings spoon to mouth is liable to turn it upside down before it enters mouth.
18 months — Fills spoon.
Difficulty in inserting spoon in mouth; liable to turn it in mouth.
Considerable spilling.
24 months — Inserts spoon in mouth without turning.
Moderate spilling.
36 months — Girls may have supinate grasp of spoon.
Little spilling.
Social behaviour at meals
15 months — Exhibits grasping of dish.
Interested in participating in eating.
18 months — Hands empty dishes to mother.
24 months — Continues to need help in feeding.
Is apt to dawdle and play with food, especially stirring it.
Refuses foods.
Very little conversation with meals.
36 months — Rarely needs assistance to complete a meal.
Interest in setting the table.
Either talks or eats.
Frequent getting up from the table.
48 months — Sets the table well.
Desires to choose menus.
Combines talking and eating well.
Rarely gets up from the table.
Likes to serve self.
60 months — Eats rapidly.
Very social and talkative during meal.

Assessing feeding problems. Feeding problems are jointly assessed by speech therapists, physiotherapists and occupational therapist, though each has a slightly different focus.

The starting point is to assemble a history from the child's mother or caregiver about:

— the child's food preferences and dislikes including textures
— a description of the mealtime situation
— method of feeding and time taken to feed
— position of child during feeding
— the child's response to foods
— implements used to assist feeding
— if the feeding experience is positively rewarding for the child/mother.

Erickson (1976) also offers suggestions for useful questions. As well as a thorough history, the therapist needs to assess the child's developmental maturity in skills needed for independent feeding. Skills to be formally assessed include:

— primitive postural reflexes
— orofacial reflexes: swallowing, biting, coughing
— muscle tone and jaw stability
— oral and tactile sensitivity
— tongue movements
— general bodily posture, but with emphasis on upper limb and head control.

On the basis of the data gained, the therapist devises a feeding-training programme.

Devising a feeding programme. A training programme will need to pay attention to the following areas.

1. Designing positioning for the child and caregiver, in preparation for the child's mealtime.
2. Prescribing the range of foods and fluids to be offered to the child.
3. Identifying the sequence of steps that the child needs to master in order to achieve competent feeding behaviour.
4. Prescribing appropriate assistive devices, either for positioning of the child, or the presentation of the food.

Positioning the child for meals. The underlying principles are that:

1. The chosen position allows adequate control of the child's body by the caregiver.
2. The position must allow the child a clear view of the food, and eye contact with the mother or caregiver.

Diet. With developmentally disabled children, pureed food will usually be offered for a longer period of time than for a normally developing child. Care must be taken to introduce a range of taste and flavours and to maintain a balanced nutritional diet. Gradually the puree can be made thicker and lumpier until the child graduates to soft food such as biscuits and finally to solids (Holle 1976).

While even normally developing children can have narrow food preferences, some developmentally disabled children, for example autistic children, have quite bizarre food preferences. Such children commonly only eat one or two foods and then only when presented under quite peculiar circumstances. For example one autistic child would only eat orange peel and salted crackers, at particular times of the day and in particular parts of the family garden. This situation presents a challenge to the occupational therapist, and Clancy et al (1969) have devised a successful programme for correcting such feeding abnormalities.

Training independent eating skills. The following steps are essential to independent self-feeding:

— Orienting to food by looking at it
— Looking at the spoon
— Reaching for the spoon
— Touching the spoon
— Grasping the spoon
— Lifting the spoon
— Delivering the spoon to the bowl
— Lowering the spoon into the food
— Scooping the food onto the spoon
— Lifting the spoon
— Delivering the spoon to the mouth
— Opening the mouth
— Moving the tongue and mouth to receive food
— Closing the lips
— Swallowing the food
— Returning the spoon to the bowl

If any steps are missing, helping the child master them must become a part of the feeding programme (Erickson 1976).

These steps represent all that an occupational therapist could design into a child's programme. Children will be different, and programmes must be related to the individual child's needs. Some precautions apply if feeding techniques are allied to facilitation procedures such as brushing, stroking, and using ice, to reduce hypersensitivity in and around the mouth. The precautions are:

1. A child should be assessed by a therapist before any form of oromuscular facilitation, e.g., ice,

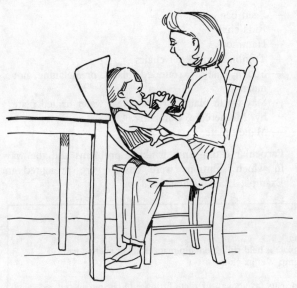

Fig. 13.4 Positioning the infant child with little or no sitting balance. The child is semi or fully upright, right angled at the hips. Her/his legs are parted with the adult's knees between them. The child's head/shoulders are brought forward from the shoulders, and the adult maintains the position by placing the flat of her/his hand or forearm on the child's lower chest.

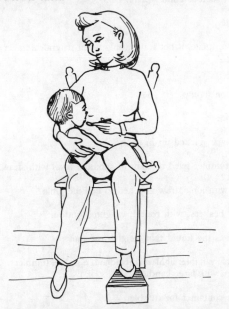

Fig. 13.5 Positioning the infant/child with some sitting balance. The child is seated on the adult's lap — the child's hips are flexed and legs abducted. One of the adult's legs is placed under the child's knee; the other leg is lower, under the child's buttocks to inhibit extensor pattern movement. The child should be positioned in an aid of some kind, a chair preferably, as soon as balance control has been achieved.

brushing, vibration is implemented.

2. Facilitation techniques can be dangerous for children with heart conditions or epilepsy.

3. Children should only be fed by nasogastric tube when supervised by trained staff. (Poulsen & Rodger 1981 Personal communication)

Prescribing assistive devices. Here are some examples of useful assistive devices for developmentally disabled children.

— Firm foam wedges
— Firm commercial 'bouncinette' with adjustable back angle *or* other modified seat

— Bean bag chair
— Rida chair
— Hammock
— Tumbleform feeder chairs
— Spoon, shallow, rounded, plastic or melanine, not metal
— Stay warm plate, for example a water heated plate by 'Mothercare' Company, UK
— Manoy plate

Particular eating and drinking problems and the way in which solutions were devised are presented in Example 13.3 (Nichols 1978).

Example 13.3 Solving eating and drinking problems

Eating problem	Problem solving
Plate moving on a table	Important that plate is held still. Non-slip mats. Rubber suction pads ('Octopus'). Damp Wettex cloth.
Inco-ordination and tremor	Heavy plate, on mats (as above), or plate fitting into cut-out in tray or table, or suction pads fitted to base of bowl.
Inability to 'catch' food on plate	Ideally, plate with low rim at point of entry of spoon, and high rim on opposite side to push against, as Manoy Melaware. Clip-on plate buffer guard.
	Plate with deep rim, such as child's plate.
Slowness in eating or swallowing	Specially heated plate.
	Plate placed over soup plate of hot water (only when parent/caretaker feeds child).
Inability to lift: From table	Use straws, clipped on to cup.
	Tipping-cup on stand.
	Plastic mug, softer type, picked up in teeth.
In wheelchair	Drop in holder for tumbler fixed to chair at shoulder level with straw.
In bed	Cycle-bottle carrier with long straw attached to bedside table.
Difficulty in lifting without spilling	Children's 'training' beakers, with round, weighted bottom.
Weakness in grasp and lifting	Only half-fill cup, it is the liquid that weights the most.
	Choice of implements available: lightweight ridged, e.g. Bex tumblers and mugs. Select cups with large handles.
	Two-handled plastic container for tumbler.
Slowness — need to keep drink warm	Insulated plastic picnic mugs
Lack of sensation and risk of burning, e.g., quadriplegics who tend to balance cup on wrist or forearm, or hold between palmar surface of both wrists.	Insulated plastic mugs. Plastic containers.

Toileting

Normal developmental sequences leading to independent toileting

15 months — Co-operative toilet response especially for bowel movement. Indicates wet pants or puddles, usually by pointing. May awake dry from nap.

18 months — Toilet regulated for both bowel and bladder control. May awaken at night and cry to be changed.

21 months — Beginning to tell of toilet needs and usually uses same word for both functions. Increased frequency of

24 months — Verbally differentiates bowel and bladder functions but is not dependable.
Has to be taken to toilet at special times.
Rarely has bowel movement accident. Dry at night if taken up.

30 months — Longer periods between eliminations. May show resistance to toilet if taken too frequently.

36 months — Responds to routine times and usually does not have to go to the toilet between these.
Takes responsibility for toileting, but always tells that, she/he is going.
Is liable to hold off too long, dances up and down, and just begins to wet pants before reaching toilet.
Is able to go by self, but needs help on back buttons.

Attempts to wipe self but is not very successful.
Verbalizes difference between boys and girls; girls sit down, and boys stand up to go to the toilet.
Girls may attempt to urinate standing up in imitation of boys (42 months).
Is dry at night without being taken up (42 months).

48 months — Goes by self and can manage clothes without difficulty.
May still tell before she/he goes, but insists upon going by self and often prefers to have the bathroom door shut. Likes to go in bathroom when others are there.
Marked interest in bathrooms in other people's houses.
Shows excessive interest in bowel movements and asks many questions about humans and animals in relation to this function.

60 months — Takes complete charge of self, including wiping.
Does not mention to adult that she/he is going to the toilet.
Boys and girls are usually separated for toileting at kindergarten.
Becoming self-conscious about exposing self.
Beginning to be reticent about going to the toilet.

Assessment. A child requires a number of skills in order to achieve the self-care task of toileting (Lansky 1984). In essence, the child needs to be physiologically ready, i.e., have sphincter control; have the required motor and physical skills, i.e., standing, balance and co-ordination; and also have had a comfortable and trusting relationship with a caretaker. Several researchers have asserted that a child is not normally ready to achieve independent control of bowel and bladder functions before the age of 20 months (Brazelton 1962; Sears et al 1957). Many developmentally disabled children will never attain this level of maturity, and one of the tasks for the occupational therapist will be to design compensatory procedures in order to ease the stresses for both the child and the caretaker.

In the course of taking a toileting history from the child's main caretaker, Erickson (1976) suggests some questions, and presents a scholarly and practical discussion of managing a toileting programme. The reader is referred to this discussion for the principles on which successful toilet training for any child are achieved.

It is wise to keep a formal assessment of a child's level of competence, and the reader is referred to Coley's Time Oriented Record, Activities of Daily Living Assessment (Coley 1978). An example of the time oriented is included in Figure 13.6.

Devising a toileting programme. A toileting training programme will need to pay attention to:

1. Positioning the child on the toilet or the pot.
2. Designing the reinforcements to be used to facilitate the child's mastery of bowel and bladder control.
3. Identifying the sequence of steps that the child needs to master in order to achieve competent toileting behaviour.
4. Prescribing appropriate assistive devices and clothing modifications.

Positioning the child for toileting

● The pot must have a wide firm base and preferably be of clear plastic to allow the mother or caregiver

| | | CHILDREN'S HOSPITAL OCCUPATIONAL THERAPY

TIME-ORIENTED RECORD

ACTIVITIES OF DAILY LIVING ASSESSMENT |

Key to scoring: 4 ... Independent
3 ... Independent with equipment and/or adaptive technique
2 ... Completes but cannot accomplish in practical time
1 ... Attempts but requires assistance or supervision to complete
0 ... Dependent—cannot attempt activity
— ... Nonapplicable

The **Year-Month** vertical column represents the Order of development sequence or approximate age when the child accomplishes the activity; the horizontal column represents the chronological age of the child being assessed.

Visit number		1		2		3		4		5		6		7		8	
	Yr. Mo. Order of dev. seq.	R.	L.	R.	L.	R.	L.	R.	L.	R.	L.	R.	L.	R.	L.	R.	L.
FEEDING—cont'd Utensils																	
21 Bottle	0.10																
22 Spoon	3.0																
23 Cup	1.6																
24 Glass	2.0																
25 Fork	3.0																
26 Knife	6.0–7.0																
TOILETING																	
27 Bowel control	1.6																
28 Bladder control	2.0																
29 Sit on toilet	2.9																
30 Arrange clothing	4.0																
31 Cleanse self	5.0																
32 Flush toilet	3.3–5.0																
HYGIENE																	
33 Turn faucets on/off	3.0																
34 Wash/dry hands/face	4.9																
35 Wash ears	8.0																
36 Bathing	8.0																
37 Deodorant	12.0-																
38 Care for teeth	4.9																
39 Care for nose	6.0																

Fig. 13.6 A time-oriented record of activities of daily living competence (Coley 1978).

ACTIVITIES OF DAILY LIVING

to see if the child is finished, without altering the child's position

- The child's hips must be flexed and abducted
- The child's back and head must be supported.

One of the greatest difficulties for the child with a disturbance of motor function, for example cerebral palsy, is the child's inability to sit and relax in a position that allows him or her to press down, and empty the bowel or bladder.

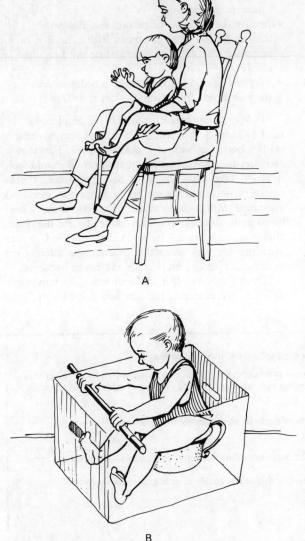

A

B

Fig. 13.7 Two ways of creating a comfortable and functional toileting situation. Note the caretaker flexing and abducting the child's legs.

Figure 13.7 illustrates helpful positioning techniques for promoting independent toileting in children with different levels of motor maturity.

Reinforcement. The primary goal of toilet training is to help the child experience success (Erickson 1976). Reinforcement of successful toileting and co-operative behaviour is one means of achieving this. Erickson offers useful advice for facilitating toilet training:

— The parent or caregiver should have a relaxed attitude.
— The goals of the programme should be reasonable and realistic. Directions should be simple.
— The child should be placed or led to the pot regularly, timing should be associated with daily routines, for example, first thing in the morning, before and after snacks and meals and before bedtime.
— Help the child only if necessary, that is to say, promote independent behaviour.
— Show approval for co-operative behaviour, for example, helping to undress, signalling desire to eliminate and trying hard to eliminate.
— Reward immediately after co-operative and or successful toileting occurs. For example, 'Good boy, you've done a wee in the toilet'. Ignore mishaps. Refrain from anger, scolding and threatening.

The occupational therapist should advise parents and caregivers not to use suppositories, enemas and other invasive techniques unless directed to do so by a medical specialist.

Prescribing assistive devices. There are many simple but effective manufactured and homemade training 'potties'. The reader should refer to available distributors' catalogues for descriptions and prices of potties and other toileting devices.

Dressing

The normally developing child is about one year old before she/he begins to co-operate with dressing, and five years before reaching independence. Do not set unrealistic expectations of the disabled child, but rather check his or her developmental, not chronological, level.

Assessment. The reader is once again referred to The Time Oriented Record, Activities of Daily Living Assessment for a formal assessment of a child's competence in dressing and undressing (see Fig. 13.3). O'Neil and colleagues (1977) consider it useful to make a video-tape of the child in the assessment. This provides realistic feedback to the child and family later on during the training programme.

Normal developmental sequence leading to independent dressing

15 months — Co-operates in dressing by extending arm or leg.

18 months — Can take off mittens, hat and socks.
Can undo zippers.
Tries to put on shoes.

24 months — Can remove shoes if laces are untied.
Helps in getting dressed — finds large armholes and thrusts arms into them.
Helps pull up or push down panties.
Washes hands and dries them, but does neither very well.

36 months — Greater interest and ability in undressing. May need some assistance with shirts and sweaters.
Is able to unbutton all front and side buttons by pushing buttons through buttonholes.
In dressing does not know back from front. Apt to put pants on backwards, has difficulty in turning socks to get heels on behind. Puts shoes on but may put them on wrong feet.
Intent on lacing shoes, but usually laces them incorrectly.
Washes and dries hands.
Brushes teeth with supervision.

48 months — Is able to undress and dress herself/himself with little assistance.
Distinguishes between front and back of clothes and puts them on correctly.
Washes and dries hands and face.
Brushes teeth.

60 months — Undresses and dresses with care.
May be able to tie shoe laces (usually at 6 years).

Devising a dressing program. A dressing training programme will need to pay attention to:

1. Positioning the child for dressing.
2. Training the child in the steps needed to master dressing.
3. Prescribing appropriate clothing modifications and assistive devices.

Positioning the child for dressing

- The dressing position should inhibit extensor patterns or habits.
- Have the clothes in easy view and reach prior to commencing dressing.
- Involve the child in the procedures. Begin the activity for the child but try to let him/her complete the task, give time and do not hurry the child.
- Vary the positions for dressing in order to discover the easiest one for the child. (Levitt 1977)

Modifying clothing. Finnie (1978) emphasises the need to keep clothes within reach, and suggests that a clothes horse or back of a chair be used. Finnie also discusses how important it is that the child should look nice and take pride in his or her appearance. Fortunately modern technology has reduced the workload associated with soiled clothes. Synthetic fibres, combined with natural fibres, are comfortable for the child, attractive, and easy to care for. Velcro and zip fasteners often provide very acceptable fastenings as alternatives to difficult buttons, press studs and hooks and eyes.

For infants and older children who find movement difficult, for example, the cerebral palsied child, the

---

Example 13.4: A dressing program for a child with cerebral palsy, ataxia, inco-ordination

Complete dressing independence may be attained with repeated practice and persistence in a calm atmosphere. Where the child has unwanted movements which interfere with the dressing process, the following clothing choices are suggested.

Choice of clothing
Loose fitting clothes of stretch materials which can be put on over the head are preferable to jacket style
Raglan sleeves are preferable to inset sleeves
Fastenings should be avoided
Zips are difficult to manage and Velcro may not stand up to the continuous pull of athetoid movements — buttons on strong elastic or tape shanks are preferable
Firm, lace-up shoes with toe reinforcement – children with severe ataxia will probably need help in tying shoelaces.

Method
Must be individually arranged

Adaptations
Openings should be reinforced with tape or extra machine stitching
The tongue of the shoe must be sewn firmly to the upper at one side to keep it in place while foot is pushed into shoe.

modern stretch fabrics ease the dressing operation, and are comfortable to wear. Finnie also noted that many parents have found thermo-insulated clothing to be very useful. (See Finnie 1978) Cauenbach (1978) also provides excellent practical advice and patterns of clothing for developmentally disabled children.

SUMMARY

Introduction of the generic classification of 'developmental disabilities' has had a major impact on health policy planning, and on the delivery of therapy and other specialist services to clients. The notable positive impacts appear to be:

- A previously dominant medical model of 'illness' has been replaced by a model centred on adaptive functioning of the affected individual.
- There has been a recognition that developmentally disabled clients require facilities, programmes, and services throughout their life. The objective of all programmes is to achieve a lifestyle for the child and family that is personally satisfying for all, ensures personal dignity and legal protection for the affected person, in environments that are integrated with the non-disabled community.
- General principles of assessment and intervention have replaced action 'recipes' for specific conditions. Thus, assessment procedures seek to establish a profile of the infant, later child, and

then adult's developmental competence and delayed or dysfunctional area. The preferred intervention approach is early intervention, and strategies are related to identified competence and dysfunction.

This chapter has provided a general discussion of the concept of developmental disabilities, and the history of the policy change which gave rise to the generic classification. The five medical diagnostic conditions have been described, and a summary provided of occupational therapy assessment and intervention procedures and objectives.

The development of motor skill competence is an important component of occupational therapy intervention with most, if not all, developmentally disabled children. For this reason, a discussion of the developmental emergence of gross and fine motor skills is provided. The knowledge base is then related to clinical applications for promoting competence in activities of daily living.

Several underlying themes have emerged from the practical occupational therapy procedures discussed in this chapter. Firstly, the occupational therapy procedures are directed at achieving movement patterns and behaviours which can facilitate functional activity by the child, in this case, feeding, toileting and dressing. Secondly, the child should be positively reinforced for effort. Thirdly, the therapy should be embedded in social relationships, the most usual being the mother–child relationship. Finally, therapy should be related to normal daily living.

REFERENCES

American Occupational Therapy Association 1986 Roles and functions of occupational therapy in early childhood intervention. American Journal of Occupational Therapy 40(12): 835–838

American Journal of Occupational Therapy 1988 42(11): 701–731

Bank-Mikkelsen N E 1969 A metropolitan area in Denmark: Copenhagen. Part iv: Model of service models. In: Kugel R B, Wolfensberger W (eds) Changing patterns in residential services for the mentally retarded. President's Committee on Mental Retardation. US Government Printing Office, Washington

Barnes M R, Crutchfield C A, Heriza C B 1978 The neurophysiological basis of patient treatment. Stokesville Publishing, Atlanta

Batshaw M L, Perret Y M 1981 Children with handicaps: a medical primer. Brookes, Baltimore

Bettelheim B 1967 The empty fortress Free Press, New York

Bleck E E, Nagel D A 1975 Physically handicapped children: a medical atlas for teachers. Grune & Stratton, New York

Brazelton T B 1962 A child-oriented approach to toilet training. Pediatrics 29: 121–128

Brinkman J, Kuypers H C H M 1973 Cerebral control of contralateral and ipsilateral arm, hand and finger movements in the split brain rhesus monkey. Brain 96: 653–674

Briton J 1979 'Normalization' what and what for? Australian Journal of Mental Retardation 5: 6 224–229

Campbell M 1978 Pharmacotherapy. In: Rutter M, Schopler E (eds) Autism: a reappraisal of concepts and treatment. Plenum, New York

Cantwell D, Rutter M, Baker L. 1978 Family factors. In: Rutter M, Schopler E (eds) Autism: a reappraisal of concepts and treatment. Plenum, New York

Cartwright S 1981 Why my child? Rigby, Adelaide

Cauenbach 1978 Pas mode aan; Kleding tips voor handicaps.

Clancy H G 1970 A group family holiday: an innovation in the therapeutic management of the autistic child. The Slow Learning Child 17(3): 149–162

Clancy H, Entsch M, Rendle-Short J 1969 Infantile autism: the correction of feeding abnormalities. Developmental and Child Neurology 11: 569–578

Clancy H G, Dugdale A, Rendle-Short T J 1969 Diagnosis of infantile autism. Developmental Medicine and Child Neurology 11(5): 569–578

Clancy H G, McBride G 1969 The autistic process and its treatment. Journal of Child Psychology and Psychiatry 10: 233–244

Clancy H G, McBride G 1975 The isolation syndrome. Developmental Medicine and Child Neurology 17: 198–219

Clark A M, Clarke A D B 1965 Mental deficiency: the changing outlook. Methuen, London

Clarke A D B, Clark A M 1974 Recent advances in the study of subnormality. National Association of Mental Health, Bethesda

Coley I A 1978 Paediatric assessment of self-care activities. CV Mosby, St Louis

Connolly K V 1973 Factors influencing the manual skills of young children. In: Hinde R A, Stevenson-Hinde J (eds) Constraints on learning: limitations and predispositions. Academic Press, London

Connor F P, Williamson G B, Siepp J 1978 Program guide for infants and toddlers with neuromotor and other developmental disabilities. Teachers College Press, New York

Court J M 1981 Child development. Symposium. Patient Management November: 21–29

Creak M 1964 Schizophrenic syndrome in childhood: Further progress report of a working party. Developmental Medicine and Child Neurology 4: 530–535

Cronbach L J 1984 Essentials of psychological testing, 4th edn. Harper, New York

Davies P A, Drillien C M, Foley J et al 1979 Cerebral palsy. In: Drillien C H, Drummond M B (eds) Neurodevelopmental problems in early childhood. Blackwell Scientific Publications, Oxford

DeMyer M K, Pontius W, Norton J A, Barton S, Allen J, Steele R 1972 Parental practices and innate activity in normal autistic and brain-damaged infants. Journal of Autism and Childhood Schizophrenia 2: 49

Dick R 1979 Communication skills — non-defensive communication for improving relationships and problem solving. Organisation Study Units, Department of Management and Psycholgy, University of Queensland, St Lucia

Eisenberg L 1972 The classification of childhood psychosis reconsidered. Journal of Autism and Childhood Schizophrenia 2: 338–342

Erickson M L 1976 Assessment and management of developmental changes in children. CV Mosby, St Louis

Finnie N R 1978 Handling the young cerebral palsy child at home. William Heinemann Medical Books, London

Fiorentino M R 1981 A basis for sensorimotor development — normal and abnormal. Charles C Thomas, Springfield

Giampa F L 1982 A curriculum guide to the training of mentally retarded people. Northland Residential Training Centre, California

Gillberg C, Schaumann H 1982 Social class and autism: total population aspects. Journal of Autism and Developmental Disorders 12: 223–228

Gordon N 1976 Paediatric neurology for the clinician. Heinemann Medical Books, London

Green A C H, Souter G B 1977 The family and the young handicapped child: the importance of the right start. Medical Journal Australia 1: 254–57

Grosman H J (ed) 1973 Manual on terminology and classification in mental retardation. Garamond/Pridemark Baltimore

Gunzburg H C 1973 Advances in the care of the mentally handicapped. Bailliere Tindall, London

Halversen H M 1931 An experimental study of prehension in infants by means of systematic cinema records. Genetic Psychological Mongraphs 10: 107–285

Hammer P B 1973 Community attitudes towards the developmentally disabled in the coming years. In: Manpower projections for the developmental disabilities centre. Temple University, New York

Harryman S 1981 Cerebral palsy. In: Batshaw M L, Perret Y M (eds) Children with handicap: a medical primer. Brookes, Baltimore

Holle B 1976 Motor development in children. Blackwell Scientific Publications, Oxford

Hopkins H L, Smith H D 1978 Willard and Spackman's occupational therapy. Lippincott, Philadelphia

Hutt S J, Hutt C, Lee D, Ounsted C 1964 Arousal and childhood austism. Nature 204: 908–909

Johnson C B, Deitz J C 1985 Time use of mothers with preschool children: a pilot study. American Journal of Occupational Therapy 39(9): 578–583

Joosten J 1979 Accounting for changes in family life of families with spina bifida children. In: Johnson C B, Deitz J C (eds) Time use of mothers with preschool children: a pilot study. American Journal of Occupational Therapy 39(9): 578–583

Kanner L 1943 Autistic disturbances of affective contact. Nervous Child 2: 217–250

Keane D 1979 L'Arche — Australia. Australian Journal of Mental Retardation 5(6): 209–211

Kopp C B 1974 Fine motor abilities of infants. Developmental Medicine and Child Neurology 16: 629–636

Korner A F 1971 Individual differences at birth: implications for early experience and later development. American Journal of Orthopsychiatry, 41: 608

Kugel R B, Wolfensberger W (eds) 1969 Changing patterns in residential services for the mentally retarded. President's Committee on Mental Retardation. US Government Printing Office, Washington

Lansky V 1984 Toilet training. Bantam, New York

Lee D N, Aronson E 1974 Visual proprioceptive control of standing in human infants. Perception and Psychophysiology 15: 529–532

Levitt S 1977 Treatment of cerebral palsy and motor delay. Blackwell Scientific Publications, Oxford

Loria C 1980 Relationship of proximal and distal function in motor development. Physical Therapy 60: 167–172

Menolascino F 1965 Psychiatric aspects of mental retardation in children under eight. American Journal of Orthopsychiatry 35: 852–861

Moersch M 1978 Developmental disabilities. American Journal of Occupational Therapy 32: 93–99

Molony H 1971 Parental reactions to mental retardation. Medical Journal of Australia 1: 914–917

Newsom C D 1980 Childhood psychoses. In: Gabel S, Erickson M T (eds) Child development and developmental disabilities. Little Brown' Boston

Ney P G, Mulvihill D L 1985 Child psychiatric treatment: a practical guide. Croom Helm, London

Nichols P J R 1978 Training the retarded child. Butterworths, London

Nirje B. 1970 The normalization principle. British Journal of Mental Subnormality 16: 62–70

Nurcombe B 1972 An outline of child psychiatry, New South Wales University Press, Sydney

O'Gorman G 1967 The nature of childhood autism. Butterworths, London

O'Neil S M, McLaughlin B N, Knapp M B 1977 Behavioural approaches to children with developmental delays. CV Mosby, St Louis

Paine R S 1966 Cerebral palsy: symptoms and signs of diagnostic and prognostic significance. Current Practice in Orthopedic Surgery 3: 39–58

Ploy S C 1979 The Year 2000 and mental retardation. Plenum Press, New York

Polan C G, Spencer B L 1959 A check list of symptoms of autism of early life. West Virginia Medical Journal 55: 198–204

Poulsen A, Rodger S 1981 Personal communication

Rimland B 1964 Infantile autism — the syndrome and its implications for a neural theory of behavior. Appleton-Century-Crofts, New York

Robinson M (ed) 1986 Practical paediatrics. Churchill Livingstone, Melbourne

Robinson R O 1973 The frequency of other handicaps in children with cerebral palsy. Developmental Medicine and Child Neurology 15: 305

Rutter M 1965 The influence of organic and emotional factors on the origins, nature and outcome of childhood psychosis. Developmental Medicine and Child Neurology 7: 518–528

Rutter M, 1978 Diagnosis and definitions. In: Rutter M, Schopler E (eds) Autism: a reappraisal of concepts and treatment. Plenum, New York

Rutter M 1985 Infantile autism and other pervasive developmental disorders. In: Rutter M, Hersov L, (eds) Child and adolescent psychiatry: modern approaches. Blackwell Scientific Publications, Oxford

Rutter M, Garmezy N 1983 Socialization, personality and social development. Vol 4, Handbook of child psychology. 4th edn. Wiley, New York

Rutter M, Lockyer L 1967 A 5–15 year follow up study of infantile psychoses. 1: Description of the sample. British Journal of Psychiatry 113: 1169–1182

Saida Y, Miyashita M 1979 Development of fine motor skill in children: manipulation of a pencil in young children aged 2 to 6 years. Journal of Human Movement Studies 5: 104–113

Schaffer H R, Emerson P E 1964 The development of social attachment in infancy. Monographs of the Society for Reseach in Child Development 29(94)

Sears R R, Macoboy E E, Levine H 1957 Patterns of child rearing. Row Petterson, New York

Smiley C W 1975 Feelings and reactions of parents to their retarded child. British Journal of Occupational Therapy 38: 29–31

Stevens J R, Sachdev K, Milstein V 1968 Behaviour disorders of childhood and the electroencephalogram. Archives of Neurology 18: 160–177

Tavormina J B, Ball T J, Dunn N J, Luscomb R L, Taylor J R 1981 Psychosocial effects on parents raising a physically handicapped child. Journal of Child Psychology 9: 121–131

Treffert O 1970 Epidemiology of infantile autism. Archives of General Psychiatry 22: 431–438

Twitchell T E 1970 Reflex mechanisms and the development of prehension. In Connolly K (ed) Mechanisms of motor skill development. Academic Press, London

Uzgiris I C, Hunt J McV 1971 Ordinal scales of psychological development in infancy. In: Haywood H C (ed) Social-cultural aspects of mental retardation. G Peabody-NIMH Conf, Appleton-Century Crofts, New York

van Krevelin A 1971 On the necessity for limiting the concept of autism. Proceedings of the 13th International Pediatric-Neuro-Psychiatry Conference, Wien

Weeks Z R 1979 Effects of the vestibular system on human development. Part 1, Overview of functions and effects of stimulation. American Journal Occupational Therapy 33(6): 376–81

Whelan E, Speake B 1979 Learning to cope. Souvenir, London

Williamson J G 1982 Therapeutic intervention for infants with sensorimotor dysfunction. In Brazelton T B, Newberger E (eds) Environmental intervention for infants at risk. Symposium of Harvard Medical School held at Dedham

Wing L, Gould J 1979 Severe impairments of social interaction and associated abnormalities in children: epidemiology and classification. Journal of Autism and Developmental disorders 9: 11–30

Wolfensberger W 1972 The principle of normalization in human services.

Wolfensberger W National Institute on Mental Retardation, Toronto

Wolff P H 1965 Visual pursuit and attention in young infants. Journal of the American Academy of Child Psychiatry 4: 473

14. Minimizing the effects of impoverished environments

READERS' OBJECTIVES

After reading this chapter, you should be able to:

1. Name and discuss the three stages of children's response to hospitalization, as presented by Bowlby (1952) and Robertson (1958).
2. Discuss parental responses to their child in hospital.
3. Discuss occupational therapy intervention with hospitalized children.
4. State indicators of physical, emotional, and sexual child abuse.
5. Describe intervention approaches with an abused child and the family.
6. Discuss ways in which design of the physical environment can influence behaviour.

In Chapter 4 we defined 'environment' as 'those parts of the surroundings (i.e., space and everything in it around an individual or group) to which the person pays attention'. We discussed the interrelation between context, surroundings and environment, and the special relationships which an individual develops with people, and with the spatial and object environment. In this chapter we examine particular ways in which a child's environment may be impoverished, and as such may impede healthy growth, development and maturation. We discuss the approaches that an occupational therapist may use to minimize the detrimental effects of an impoverished environment on a child.

The conditions and situations to be discussed are representative of environments which are considered impoverished, because close attachment relationships between child and family are either absent, interrupted, inappropriate or pathological, and/or the physical environment is deficient in providing sensory stimulation, opportunities for exploration and for mastery of motor and other skills.

The following conditions and situations will be discussed:

1. Young children in hospital
2. Children living with their parents, but exposed to abuse — physical, emotional and/or sexual
3. Children living in institutions

The unifying feature is that there is a distortion in the normal primary attachment relationship between the child and mother. In the hospitalized child, the distortion is imposed temporarily, on a presumably appropriate relationship. At the opposite extreme end of a normality/abnormality continuum, the child who lives in an institution lacks an appropriate attachment relationship.

The normal process by which attachment develops, and socialization proceeds, was discussed in Chapter 3. In summary, the critical elements are that an infant develops within the context of the family, and learns the skills of communication through a process of reciprocal interaction and response. A mother's social stimulation

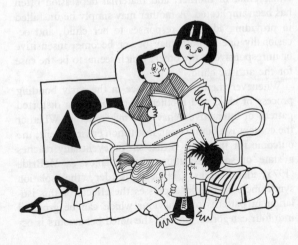

193

(by touch, speech or visual stimuli) is an effective reinforcement of her baby's behaviour. The baby in turn responds with behaviour (e.g., smiling, cooing, attendtion) which reinforces the mother's stimulation and overtures (Clancy & McBride 1975). For a child and his mother or caregiver to develop a mutually rewarding relationship, both must display sensitivity, perceptiveness and responsiveness to each other. The available data suggest that an optimal situation for growth and development exists when caregiving is restricted to a very few people interacting *consistently* and *predictably* with the infant, at least in the first two years of life (Lutkenhaus et al 1985; Maine et al 1985; Singer et al 1985; Sroufe 1983).

The isolation syndrome

Anything which lowers mutual responsiveness between a young child and significant adult must affect the quality of the emerging relationship. It is only when the behavioural adaptations of the child are outside the fairly wide range considered as 'normal' that they attract sufficient attention to be investigated and diagnosed. If the child lives in a family, the mother's adaption to the child attracts little attention because she is seen in other normal relationships. A child may rock, for example, in order to satisfy a need for stimulation which is not available in the social world. Yet it is no more abnormal for the child to sit and rock all day, than it is for the mother to ignore such behaviour. In cases like this example, the abnormal behaviours often represent attempts by both mother and child to adapt to each other's inadequate communication.

A breakdown in mutual responsiveness may have its origins in many situations. There may be illness in either child or mother, and maternal depression often has been implicated. A mother may simply be unskilled in providing adequate responses to her child, and occasionally one or both may be, or become, insensitive or unresponsive to the other, which seems to be the case for the autistic child.

Whenever there is interference in the early bonding process of child and mother (or caregiver), a distorted pattern of interactive behaviours may emerge. Whether the context is a family or an institution environment, the outcome for the child is that she/he eventually reaches a state of social isolation which Clancy & McBride (1975) identified as a clinical disorder, 'the isolation syndrome'. The child expresses the effects of this isolation in patterns of behaviour which can be grouped into four categories. Each of the noted behaviours is oc-

casionally observed in normally developing children. However the characteristic constellations of abnormalities have been described in children with a primary disorder, or in some situation which has hindered the development of a communicative bond with their mothers or caregivers.

The four behavioural categories are:

Defective social interaction and communication

Many of the normal affiliative or affective behaviours associated with the maternal bond are absent. These behaviours include attending (to the mother), eye contact, social responses such as smiling, and cuddling. Isolated children develop attachment bonds which are at the extreme ends of the scale of (parent) dependence/independence.

Disorders of perceptual function and motor skills

The child fails to make the appropriate visual responses (by becoming alert and orienting) to sources of stimulation — tactile, visual, auditory or olfactory. In particular, the child fails to respond normally when addressed vocally, and appears to be deaf. She/he may eat substances which are considered by adults to be unpleasant and she/he may fail to communicate with cries when in pain. These abnormal responses probably arise partly from perceptual dysfunction and partly from inadequate socialization.

Excessive self-stimulation (stereotypes)

Self-stimulation is common among isolated people and animals. It seems that, when inadequately stimulated, an individual will provide the missing stimulation, and by so doing reinforce his/her own behaviour. Children may spend considerable time in hand-regard or in rocking or bumping themselves or, when older, in masturbation.

General developmental retardation

This is seen especially in language. In many primary disorders of young children (e.g., blindness, deafness or mental retardation) the disorder is associated with developmental retardation. There appears to be a direct effect of the particular deficit on the normal developmental processes, but there is also an indirect effect in that the child fails to develop efficient means of communication with his mother or caregiver, who is then unable to provide the stimulus for effective socialization.

These four behaviour patterns develop because the child's attention is not directed in the normal manner towards the mother or primary caretaker. Instead the child develops an attitude of self-attention and self-stimulation which is more typical of very much younger children.

Isolation effects seem to be rare among infants in low-technology societies. Two possible reasons are that children who are vulnerable at birth, because of some physical abnormality, may not survive the neonatal period; again, child-rearing practices usually provide much continuous bodily contact with the mother or caretaker and thus provide consistent social and sensory intrusion, stimulation and interaction.

The three conditions and situations which are representative of impoverishing environments will be examined in some depth.

THE YOUNG CHILD IN HOSPITAL

A stay in hospital is a common experience in childhood. The experience provides an important example of the way in which an environment which is designed with the child's best interests at heart — his or her restored health — can at the same time be impoverishing.

Wooton (1979) observed that children's hospital conditions in the 1930s were such that practices, 'successfully sterilized the surroundings of the child from germs, and also (sterilized) his psyche!' The hospital became an impoverishing environment for the child because it deprived him/her of the security of the close attachment to mother and family.

All visiting was greatly restricted, often to only one hour per day. The hospital environment was also one of considerable austerity — toys were regarded as carriers of disease. Thus, the availability of sensory stimulation that promotes healthy development was improverished. Further, during a highly stressful time, the strange environment imposed an additional demand on the child. Namely, that he or she be highly attentive in order to try to make some sense of the unfamiliar routines and procedures of the hospital environment, and of the very many strange people who attended to him or she every day. These environmental effects were compounded by the necessary infliction on the child of frightening, painful and physically restrictive medical practices.

It was the trail blazing theoretical work of the British psychiatrist John Bowlby (1952) that first aroused interest in studying and changing hospital environments for children, though others had already drawn attention to detrimental effects on children as a result of hospitalization (see Bakwin 1942; Heinecke 1956; Schaffer & Callender 1959; Spitz 1945).

We owe our understanding of the characteristic response process of young children largely to researchers such as Bowlby (1952; 1973), Robertson & Robertson (1958), and others (Geist 1965; Mason 1965; Prugh 1965). These researchers have increased our understanding of both the detrimental effects, and also those factors and intervention approaches which minimize such effects, and protect the child against long-term psychological damage.

Parents now visit frequently, for example, ward routines are much less strict, and children may bring some of their own personal belongings to hospital with them, for example, the battered and questionably clean teddy bear. Newer policies encourage open visiting, and most children's hospitals make facilities for mothers to 'room in', particularly in the case of breastfeeding mothers and mothers from rural or distant locations. Parents are seen as 'partners' (Hart 1979), who can help with personal care of their child, as well as providing for the child's psychosocial needs. There is acceptance of residential admission of parent(s), not only assisting in nursing and medical treatment where appropriate, but also having a part in the decision making process of their own child. Parents can also influence ward policies.

Nevertheless there still remains the danger of staff forgetting that adequate care of the sick child must also involve consideration of the psychological aspects of illness. The most painstaking efforts in physical treatment cannot compensate for neglect of the child's emotional needs.

The importance of communicating effectively with hospitalized children has been recognized and accepted (Duberly 1974, Heagarty et al 1973, Klitzing et al 1977, Plank 1971, Puchinger et al 1975). Attempts have been made to describe or assess such communicative interactions, but we still do not understand what factors influence the occurrence of these interactions. Several authors have noted certain factors which appear to have some influence.

Bergmann (1965) noted that the quality and quantity of a hospitalized child's relationship with staff may depend, in part, on the child's personality. Others, such as Bryne et al (1968) have suggested that physical attractiveness predisposes individuals to improved interpersonal relationships. These workers also found that the unattractiveness of a sick child had a negative effect on caretakers. The severity of the illness appears to have an impact on interactions between the child and hospital personnel. When a child is seriously ill, workers appear to give less supportive attention to that child. Such behaviour must compound the stress of hospitalization and separation from the family for the child.

Perhaps one explanation is that personal interactions may be difficult for the first few days of hospitalization especially with the unhappy, negativistic or seriously ill child. A situation exists in which complete devotion to a helpless patient is demanded of the nurse, while the child regards him/her with hostility and rejects efforts at giving comfort (Bergmann 1965). Often the quiet or unhappy child has the greatest need for attention, but is neglected (Dimock 1960). Further investigation is needed to synthesize information, and determine more clearly which factors influence the attention a child receives in hospital.

Children's responses

The child who has developed predictable and consistent trusting relationships within a family is more likely to react to separation with extremely vigorous, noisy, angry, prolonged protest. This response is often misinterpreted by nursing staff. The same child is likely to accommodate the separation experience with fewer ill effects, given that subsequent parent—child relationship continues to be consistent.

Factors influencing children's response to hospitalization

- personality traits
- previous developmental experience
- previous separation from parents
- nature and severity of the illness
- duration of separation
- time spent by parent(s) with the child
- the attitudes of nurses, doctors and others
- amount of anxiety communicated to the child by others
- number of children in the ward and number of staff available to meet the child's needs
- culture, socioeconomic class, religion

Geist (1965) feels that children who cope with hospitalization best, are those who have an interest in other children, who before hospitalization were interested in games and toys, and who can express themselves indirectly by crying, anger and naughtiness, with only moderate limitation of self-control.

Some of the more common responses include anxiety, regression, overdependence, attention seeking behaviour and/or depression.

and/or depression.

— Anxiety may produce restlessness, tension and negative attitudes toward the staff, making treatment difficult.
— Regression is almost universal. The child reverts to infantile behaviour, becoming clinging and difficult. Well established habits may break down, for example, toilet training. Auto-erotic behaviour may appear, for example, rocking and excessive thumb-sucking.
— Overdependence on parents or staff may become manifest.
— Attention-seeking behaviour is common. In an effort to boost sagging confidence, the child tries to manipulate the staff with noisy behaviour or whining. She or he may terrify younger children with stories of hospital — what goes on in the operating theatre is a common theme of the hospital veteran.
— Depression may result from the illness itself (for example, viral hepatitis) or from the stress of hospitalization. The depressed child then becomes apathetic and withdrawn, refuses food and loses interest in books and toys. Adolescents are naturally prone to wide mood variations and may occasionally become severely depressed.

Bowlby (1952) and Robertson & Robertson (1958) described the characteristic responses observed in children as falling into a three phase process of protest, despair and detachment.

The first four years

Detrimental effects accrue with increasing age, with the most vulnerable period being from about seven months – the time of primary bonding with the mother – to four years. In the first four years, the child suffers chiefly from separation from his family, especially his mother. The three phases are:

— *Protest*. The child is grief stricken by separation, in particular, the loss of mother. She or he cries loudly and thrashes about the cot, pushing away hospital staff if they try to offer comfort. This phase may last a few hours or a few days.
— *Despair*. This stage is characterized by apathy and behaviour suggesting a feeling of hopelessness. The young child has a poorly developed sense of time and cannot comprehend that mother will return. The child cannot conjure up the mother's image mentally either — when she leaves, she goes forever. The child cries softly and monotonously. Because he/she is quieter staff often assume she/he is 'setting-in', and mistake this withdrawal for improved emotional adjustment.

— **Detachment**. This stage emerges if the child's stay is prolonged and staff changes do not allow consistent care by one person. The child cuts off from relationships with others. She/he has been so badly hurt by what she/he feels to be desertion by the mother that she/he will not risk further hurt by forming a loving, trusting relationship again. She/he shows more interest in the surroundings, and is sociable, but this is superficial. She/he then becomes quite gregarious, going to anyone in a manner quite atypical for his or her age. She or he develops on excessive interest in material things.

Middle childhood

Anxieties relate to anaesthetics, operations and the meaning of illness. Parents sometimes threaten hospitalization as a punishment; for example, a child who sucks his/her thumb is warned, that unless she/he stops 'doctor will cut if off'. The child may be puzzled, wondering what she/he has done to deserve admission to hospital, or feel guilty because she/he has been bad enough to be punished this way. Certain organs such as heart and genitals have a primitive significance, and a child may be very threatened by pathology in relation to these. Misinterpretations of the actions of staff are common; the hypodermic needle is perceived as a dangerous weapon. It is not so much the prick which the child fears but what might happen afterwards. Fantasies relate to the needle remaining embedded permanently, letting out vital elements, and causing changes in feeling and behaviour. Sibling rivalry may also be aggravated. The child in hospital may feel rejected by the parents in favour of brothers and sisters at home. Older children may worry about the financial aspects of their stay in hospital.

Around the age of eight or nine, there is a growing awareness of the meaning of death. Before this the child regards it as a going away process which is reversible. Now she/he grasps the concept of its finality. An illness or stay in hospital at this stage may precipitate a great deal of anxiety as the child faces this basic issue.

Adolescence

With the onset of puberty the child becomes sensitive about his or her physical growth changes. As the criterion for admission to a children's hospital usually depends upon chronological age and not physical development, children who are well developed for their age find themselves with little privacy among children who lag far behind them in the development of secondary sexual characteristics. The adolescent who is in the process of establishing an identity may also be devastated if their physical appearance is altered by disease, disfigurement and/or loss of function. There are several factors which influence how a child responds to separation.

After hospitalization

Geist (1965) reports that severe reactions after hospitalization can be twice as high in the two-to five-year age group as in the six-to twelve-year age group, and children under four years of age show persistent signs of emotional disturbance three months after hospitalization.

Young children may show the following behaviour manifestations on going home after a period of hospitalization:

— Anxiety over being separated from mother, even for a short time.
— Outbursts of screaming, crying, or panic etc., when approached by an adult.
— Specific fears, e.g., strangers, the dark, needles.
— Disturbances in feeding and sleeping, e.g., nightmares.
— Regressions to earlier levels of development, e.g., loss of control over bowel and bladder functions where the child may previously have been toilet trained.
— Psychological symptoms such as rocking and thumb sucking.
— Children who experienced long-term hospitalization may develop severe behaviour problems, and become hyperactive, destructive and affectionless on return home.

The growing child cannot afford to interrupt the cycle of daily living and growth as can the adult.

Parents' response

Many parents become guilty when their child is sick; they feel as if they have failed in some way by allowing this to happen. For example, they may wonder if they sought treatment early enough, or they may blame themselves for accidental injury. Some may be acutely anxious; young children regard their parents as being omnipotent and it is very frightening to them to see a parent becoming emotionally disturbed. Richmond & Weinburger (1970) have described parental reactions as occurring in three stages.

1. Initial denial and disbelief — 'my child can't be ill'.

2. Fear, frustration and guilt, when they blame themselves for the child's illness.
3. Intelligent enquiry and planning, when they face the situation with courage and attempt to make the best of it.

Unfortunately many do not achieve the third stage. If hospitalization is a necessary interruption, the child and parents should be helped by the treatment team, to cope with the stress of separation, consequent lags in development, and proper management of the child on return home (Bell 1969; James & Wheeler 1969; Mason 1965; Prugh 1965; Rousseau 1967; Shope 1970).

Parents should demonstrate their confidence in the hospital staff, offer a simple explanation for any operative procedures to be performed, and give the child a chance to express anxieties about the coming event. Parents are helped greatly by practical advice about how to cope with their child's difficult behaviour in the hospital and when she/he returns home. Otherwise, they may blame themselves for what has happened, and mother's self-esteem may be diminished if the child is more difficult to manage than before she/he went to hospital.

The child's symptoms must be evaluated in the context of the parent–child relationships. Unsatisfactory relationships may produce distortion of symptoms; some unhealthy relationships may be encouraged because they fulfil a parent's needs. On occasions a child is punished because the parents cannot tolerate the child's symptoms.

Other problems which parents can face include:

— Chronic tiredness through meeting the needs of the child as well as the siblings and spouse at home. Lack of sleep through anxiety, and long hours spent at the hospital as well as meeting the needs of the family at home.
— Feelings of helplessness and frustration and loss of control.
— Difficulty in dealing with child's aggression, negativism and distress.
— Difficulty in coping with anger. At times parents may feel angry with the child and towards hospital staff.
— Separation from spouse, family and home.

Intervention

Children's hospitals need not represent an impoverished environment, and the effects of a hospital stay need not be detrimental to a child or young person. There is a body of research and clinical experience accumulating which offers directions for intervention. Three approaches are suggested.

1. Preparation of the child for admission to hospital, and support programmes for adults.
2. Planned and therapeutic play for the child while hospitalized.
3. Design of the physical hospital environment to minimize detrimental psychological and emotional effects.

Preparing the child, supporting the parents

Where the hospital stay is elective, the child should be prepared well ahead of time. There are many excellent commercial publications available about going to hospital, and these are designed for children of varying ages.

The child should be told of the impending admission to hospital with an explanation suited to developmental level. She/he should be allowed to pack belongings, go on a preliminary visit to the ward to meet nursing and other staff. The occupational therapist is a logical specialist to organize such visits, and to plan activities which do inform the child about what to expect. For example, children can be taken to visit the radiology department, or the operating theatre. In these situations the child should be allowed to work some machinery, e.g., turn on the lights over the operating table, or raise the hydraulic table. She/he should also have the opportunity to get dressed in the strange clothing. The object of such visits is to familiarize the child with the hospital, the places, the routines and the equipment.

Planned and therapeutic play

The benefits of planned and therapeutic play for hospitalized children have been well recognized, and recommended readings are provided at the end of the chapter. The distinction between 'planned' and 'therapeutic' play, arose because a new group of professional people has emerged, 'play leaders' (Hart 1976). Their role is to provide planned play experiences to promote healthy ongoing development for hospitalized children. The role of the occupational therapist, on the other hand, is to provide play experiences by prescription, to meet specific identified needs of a child, as well as defined intervention objectives. She/he should be willing to act as consultant and co-ordinator of a planned play programme involving play leaders or volunteers. Consultative team interaction increases the effectiveness of all programmes designed to minimize the detrimental effects of hospitalization on young children.

As early as 1953 Prugh and colleagues were able to demonstrate positive effects of therapeutic play programmes on young hospitalized children. These effects were evident during hospitalization, and in the longer term after discharge. It was noted that the children who received therapeutic play were less depressed, showed only half the amount of thumb sucking, rocking, overtly aggressive behaviour. On return home sleep disturbances were markedly less in the experimental group children. Kielhofner et al (1983) have noted similar positive effects in young children hospitalized for extended periods for problems associated with tracheostomy.

The play experience should provide a haven in which a child can express and resolve fears, guilt and anger. Preparation for special procedures, such as surgery, can also be accomplished through role playing. The important general principle is that the child has one context in which she/he exerts control over the environment. The form of play is limited only by the imagination of the therapist. For example, a fish bowl or small acquarium placed within sight of a bed-bound child will provide endless variation of activity, and absorb the child's curiosity and interest for long periods of time. Occupational therapists have always recognized the value of pets for sick children, and carefully chosen and cared for pets present no particular problems in a hospital ward. There is now a branch of the psychology profession which is concerned with amassing research data about the therapeutic use of pets. Audio tapes of stories and music can also be useful for the child who is immobilized, or in an isolation ward.

Guidelines which will be helpful to interacting with the child have been presented in the box.

The premature or low birthweight infant is particularly vulnerable to the effects of separation from mother in hospital. Much research has accrued since Kennell et al (1974) first described detrimental effects of long hospitalization on prematurely born infants (Brachfield et al 1980; Crawford 1982; Crnic et al 1983).

In Chapter 4 an example set of equipment is provided for 'infant exploration kits'. These kits were devised in response to a perceived need to provide sensory stimulation to hospitalised infants, birth to one year. The kits comprise play materials which will attract the infant to explore them without the need for an adult to be present. The kits comprise an overhead frame which is easily clamped to the back of the infant's cot, and which swivels 180 degrees thus allowing the arm to be swung aside for caregiving and medical attention to the child. Different items are attached to the overhead arm, and also to the side bars of the cot. The selected play materials are appropriate for the skills of a particular developmental period. Thus, for example, kits are prepared for infants birth to 6 weeks, 6 to 12 weeks, 3 to 5 months, 6 to 9 months, 9 to 12 months.

Finally, the potentially impoverishing effects of a hospital environment can also be minimized by careful design of the physical environment.

Guidelines for interacting with hospitalized children

She/he should be approached with quiet confidence.

Questions should be answered truthfully and at a level which the child can comprehend. If treatment is going to hurt, the child should be warned, it is breaking trust not to do so. The child should not be expected to be stoical beyond his years, otherwise she/he will suffer not only the pain but also from the feeling she/he has let his attendant down.

All medical and other specialists should avoid talking about the child and his/her condition and progress in the child's presence. Children comprehend far more than adults realize, and may become very frightened by talk that they do not understand fully.

Encourage the child to be independent, and not to develop an attitude of 'invalidism'. Some children find it helpful to develop a special relationship with a staff member, with whom to share anxieties and the feeling of being 'special'. The occupational therapist has a particular role here because she/he is less readily associated with the painful and frightening aspects of hospital, and yet she/he is an authority figure who can be trusted.

Designing the physical environment

Environmental design features are particularly important as variables which may influence the type of interactions between sick children and their caretakers. For example, Hoyle-Parent (1978) noted that hospital intensive care units or immobilization of a child by any means, e.g., plaster cast or bandages replicate the low stimulus environments of the classic sensory deprivation studies of the 1940–60s. Lindheim et al (1972) produced a challenging analysis of the physical environment of children's hospitals. Others have also studied specific aspects of the interaction between behaviour and physical environment of children's hospitals. For example, Jacob (1953) studied the number and type of interactions between staff and children and concluded that contacts were fleeting, focused on practical tasks such as toileting, or medical procedures. Only 1.1% of contacts over a 10 hour period were in anticipation of the children's needs. The children consistently met too many different adults. The implication of this finding is

---

Example 14.1 Hospital environments for toddlers (1–3 years) and preschoolers (3–6 years)

Does the environment allow direct visual supervision of young children at all times?
— unobstructed visual field from nurses station to all indoor and outdoor patient areas within the nursing unit
— glazed partitions
— other techniques for visual supervison

Is the environment safe for young children?
— single, well-controlled entrance to unit
— low beds or cribs
— no oxygen outlets, electrical outlets, hot or sharp objects, or other potentially dangerous objects below fifty-five inches
— all glazed areas made of tempered glass or unbreakable plastic
— glazed doors
— medication preparation area well-equipped, quiet, and lockable
— other safety features

Can the young child keep in touch with his family?
— available telephones
— windows overlooking streets and parking area used by visiting parents and linking the child with the outside
— facilities for parent to live in and stay overnight
— other ways to maintain contact

Is the scale of the environment appropriate for both young children and adults?
— small groupings of a social scale comprehensible to young children
— raised facilities for eating, playing, and bathing so that an adult can help a child without bending
— variations in ceiling heights and changes in levels to allow a child to feel big and adult to look small by contrast.

Reprinted by permission from Lindheim et al 1972 Changing hospital environments for children, Havard University Press. © 1972 by the President and Fellows of Harvard College.

---

that a child could not develop a close relationship with staff who rarely got to know the child. Other studies have revealed that seriously ill children attract less, rather than more attention from nursing staff.

Lindheim et al (1972) have examined ways in which the physical environment should be arranged to promote optimal physical and psychological care for a hospitalized child. An example of guidelines which these authors have developed for the differing developmental groupings of child from birth to adolescents, is shown in Example 14.1.

The specialist knowledge that a paediatric occupational therapist has about growth, development, play and effects of hospital equips him/her to contribute to new planning of hospitals for children or modification of existing facilities.

Summary

It is generally acknowledged that there are detrimental effects associated with hospitalization, for children who are separated from their family for treatment. The younger the child, the more serious and long lasting are the effects on the child's developmental progress. However, we also know that it is possible to minimize the negative effects, if there is no alternative to admitting a young child to hospital without his/her mother. Effective intervention is through careful preparation of the child and family, in anticipation of the hospital experience; provision of continuing empathetic support to parents, especially the child's mother before, during, and after hospitalization; provision of planned and therapeutic play in co-operation with colleague play leaders; and systematic design of the physical hospital environment to promote optimal caring interactions between caregivers and the sick child.

The discussion now moves to consider an extreme example of an ordinary family home environment which should be considered as impoverishing for the child who resides in it. The decision to include a discussion about abused children in this chapter was taken after much debate. We recognise that some readers would believe that the subject is more appropriately placed with discussion of child psychiatric issues. However, our reasoning was that abuse can only occur where a range of complex factors combine to produce a context and environment which allows abuse — in any form — to happen and be maintained. The child who is exposed to abuse, lives in an environment which stultifies healthy growth, development and maturation. Such an environment impoverishes his/her developmental experience. The implications for intervention from this view are that approaches must be targeted at changing the whole environment, and not focused on the child as the unit of treatment.

THE FAMILY-LIVING ABUSED CHILD

Contributed by Frances Forbes B Occ Thy(Qld)

To some degree, child abuse has been culturally endorsed in human society for decades (Soukup et al 1984; Committee for Children 1984a, b; Parton 1985). Yet the practices of abuse still continue, even though children are no longer regarded as 'property', but as 'people' with rights (Adams et al 1971).

Definitions of 'child abuse' are not consistent (Adler 1986; Dates 1985), and Helfer's (1978) has been chosen as a focus for the present discussion.

Definition

Abuse is 'any interaction or lack of interaction which results in non-accidental harm to a child's physical, emotional, psychological or developmental state'.

In fact, whatever definition is applied, the descriptive label of 'child abuse' represents a generic classification for specifically harmful behaviour inflicted on a child, usually, but not exclusively, by parents. The harmful behaviours are:

- Physical abuse
- Neglect
- Emotional abuse
- Sexual abuse or exploitation.

The categories are not mutually exclusive, and often the abused child has suffered more than one form of abuse (Adler 1986; Kashani et al 1987; Oates 1985). For example, it has been suggested that emotional abuse is always a component of the other forms. A child who is being hurt physically or sexually is receiving the emotionally destructive message that she/he is worthless and deserving of such treatment (Garrison 1987, Hart & Brassard 1987).

Societal contribution

Reimer (1984) and Parton (1985) have stated that child abuse must be viewed in the social context of each culture. Beliefs regarding harsh discipline and child rearing may contribute to an acceptance of violence toward children. Several studies of childrearing attitudes have shown that a disturbing number of parents still believe that violent acts are acceptable methods of discipline.

A generation ago, people married relatively young, brought up their children close to their extended family and were involved in community groups, such as church and service groups. A mother with young children obtained assistance or babysitting from her informal social network. However, the increasing trend toward geographical mobility, two income families and later childbirth has meant that parents have access to fewer of these informal community support networks to assist them in reducing the stresses of parenthood.

Incidence

Physical and emotional abuse. Estimates vary from 0.01% to 1% of children, per annum (Gil 1970; Helfer 1978; Light 1973). Surveys conducted in South Australia and New Zealand reported an incidence of 3 per 1000 children (Ferguson et al 1972; Oates 1984). Springthorpe et al (1977) estimated 40% of children under five years admitted to the casualty department of a general children's hospital had injuries suggestive of abuse.

While accurate statistics are difficult to obtain, it is certain that most countries have experienced a substantial increase in child protection notifications in the past decade. The reasons for this increase are unclear, but may result from increased community awareness of the problem and procedures for reporting suspected cases.

Sexual abuse. As in other forms of abuse, incidence is difficult to establish as official statistics reflect underreporting. However, several studies have given remarkably consistent results. It is estimated that 1 in every 4 girls and 1 in every 8 to 10 boys will be sexually assaulted before they reach 18 years (Morgan 1985). Many authors feel that sexual abuse of males is seriously underreported as boys are reluctant to admit victimization which is opposed to the expectations of masculinity (Finkelhor 1986). In addition, it is speculated that the homosexual nature of most abuse of boys may label them as homosexuals. Children are sexually abused in all age groups from birth onwards. Although the median age of the victim is 11 years, this reflects the age at which it is reported rather than when the abuse commenced. About 85–90% of the victims are female, but increasingly, boys are also victims.

It has become clear that child abuse only flourishes in

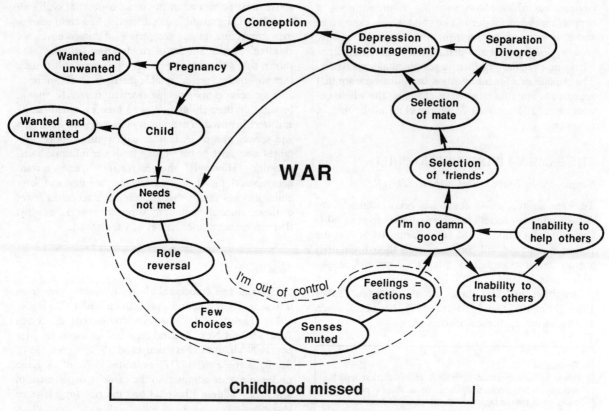

Fig. 14.1 Helfer's World of Abnormal Rearing (WAR). From Kempe C H, Helfer R E (eds) 1980 The battered child. University of Chicago Press, Chicago © The University of Chicago. Reproduced with the publisher's permission.

an environment where a number of complex conditions interact (Steele 1980). Helfer (1980) has provided a conceptual model which he has described as the world of abnormal rearing (WAR). This model depicts the multi-causal aetiological complexity of the child abuse syndrome, and is presented in Figure 14.1.

Descriptions

Physical abuse

> **Terminology**
> *Physical abuse* includes severe beatings, shaking, burns, human bite marks, grab marks, strangulation which may result in unexplained bruises or welts, lacerations or abrasions, fractures or dislocations, severe head or internal injuries, or death.

The Committee for Children (1984) has characterized the differences between abuse and safe effective dis-

cipline as one of a difference of parental intent. Discipline is designed 'to help children control and change their behaviour' (Committee for Children 1984). On the contrary, abuse is characterized by its 'orientation toward satisfying needs or expressing the negative feelings of parents'. While abuse may temporarily change children's behaviour, it has a tendency to build resentment, hatred and hostility in children. Eventually to avoid further abuse, children may lie, run away or avoid the abusive parent. Abuse has a tendency to damage all parties' self-esteem and does little to teach children more appropriate behaviours. Physical abuse most often results from normal parental anger that is inappropriately expressed by a parent that has few coping skills (Oates 1985).

Detection of physical abuse is generally based on the presence of repeated physical injuries. The child may also display a concomitant range of behavioural indicators that may serve to underscore concerns. Furthermore, the parental reaction to and interaction with the child may characterize an abusive family.

Neglect

> **Terminology**
> *Neglect* is the failure to provide a child with the basic necessities of life, e.g., food, clothing, shelter, emotional security, medical and dental care and adequate supervision needed for the child's optimal growth and development (Queensland Centre for Prevention of Child Abuse 1986).

While other forms of abuse and their associated injuries are generally episodic, neglect tends to be a chronic condition. It has been estimated that the incidence of neglect may be as much as three to five times greater than other forms of abuse (Polansky 1985; Reimer 1984; Young 1981). Evidence also suggests that chronic severe neglect may be more resistant to intervention than other forms of abuse.

In general, neglect is more obvious amongst poor families faced with a complex combination of social, economic and emotional problems. Such families may be characterized by chaos, disorganization and an absence of routine (Young 1986). Frequently, neglectful parents suffered a childhood history of abuse and neglect and display emotionally immature personalities (Polansky et al 1981; Steele 1976; Young 1986).

Emotional abuse

> **Terminology**
> *Emotional abuse* involves excessive or unreasonable parental demands that place expectations on a child beyond his/her capabilities.

Examples of emotional abuse include constant criticism, belittling, terrorizing, rejecting, ignoring, corrupting and isolating (Garbarino & Gabarino 1980, Queensland Centre for Prevention of Child Abuse 1986). The problem for the specialist is that the less overt damage of emotional abuse may be overlooked. (Garbarino & Vondra 1987). Navarre (1987) considered that emotional abuse was conveyed through physical, verbal and interactional actions that assaulted the individual's perception of the self as valuable and competent.

Child sexual abuse

Child sexual abuse shares some common features with other forms of abuse, though the precipitating dynamics and intervention are quite distinct.

> **Terminology**
> *Sexual abuse* is the exploitation of a child for the gratification of an adult or older person. Child sexual abuse involves a continuum of behaviour from non-touching sexual behaviour, e.g., exhibitionism, provision of pornographic material, verbal suggestion, to touching behaviour, e.g., fondling, sexual intercourse, masturbation and sodomy.

Dynamics

Sexually abusive behaviour is sometimes mistakenly viewed as a problem of sexual behaviour deviance. Often, the abusive behaviour is a response to non-sexual but personal emotional needs. Groth & Burgess (1977) report that sexually abusing adults attempt to meet deep seated needs for self-worth, recognition, for power, domination and nurturance. Abusing adults are unable to make and sustain mature adult relationships, and turn to children who are less powerful and less demanding (Sgroi 1984). However, recognition of these dynamics does not lessen the reality that an adult is always responsible for his/her actions and the child is always more vulnerable to physical and psychological harm.

Responsibility. A disturbing trend has been to blame the child victim for seductiveness, or inviting abuse. This justification ignores that:

- The adult perpetrator chose to interpret the child's behaviour as seductive
- The child may have learnt from adults that seductive behaviour gains adult affection and attention
- It is the adult's responsibility to set limits on inappropriate behaviour.

Abusers. Most often the perpetrator is a male, who takes advantage of his position of trust and the child's innocence and desire for affection. Offenders may be of any age, ethnic or socioeconomic background (May 1978). In at least 85% of sexual abuse cases the offender is someone known and trusted by the child. Thus, for the child victim there exist powerful reasons for not disclosing abuse when the offender may be a family member, relative, babysitter or family friend. Sgroi (1984), Reimer (1984) and Finkelhor (1986) have developed a profile of the sexual offender.

Contexts. Finkelhor (1986) considered that preconditions are necessary for sexual abuse to occur: access and attraction to a child; lack of internal and external controls.

As well as having the motivation to sexually abuse the

child, a perpetrator must overcome internal inhibitors that sex with children is illegal, inappropriate and taboo. Such values are often overcome by rationalizations such as, 'I'm teaching her about sex in a loving way' or, 'She asked for it'. The abuser must also overcome external inhibitors such as detection. The last obstacle requires strategies to overcome a child's resistance.

High-risk children and families. The following factors have been cited as indicative of high risk children, and Sgroi (1982) and Reimer (1984) have identified the following characteristics which differentiate high risk families.

- Preadolescent (8–12 years) female
- Social isolation
- Parental absence, particularly mother, and/or unavailability
- Conflict between parents
- Poor parent-child relationship
- Step or blended families
- Low self-esteem
- Parental history of abuse
- Poorly defined role boundaries between family members
- Ambiguous family communication patterns.

The sexually abused child who has few avenues for adult affection and regard may well enjoy the attention lavished upon him or her under the guise of sexual abuse (Sgroi 1984). Problems may arise for the child to whom sexual abuse has not been unpleasant. This is particularly so upon disclosure when those around him or her express shock, horror and disgust. Such a child, faced with these attitudes, may experience much guilt that she/he derived only pleasure from the abuse.

Disclosing abuse. Surveys of adults have made it clear that many children never tell of abuse. Such a phenomenon is hardly surprising when it is considered that most children are abused by an adult they know and trust. Fear of reprisals and not being believed and feelings of guilt and shame are some of the reasons why children do not disclose about abuse.

Sexually abused children more commonly deny or minimize abuse, but rarely do young children lie about abuse. Considering how difficult it is for a child to reveal the secret of sexual abuse, it is clear that there are many easier ways to seek attention. When false allegations do occur as in custody matters, such allegations are generally made by the adult.

Some common themes have also been distinguished in the child's reactions immediately after disclosure. These themes include, anger, hostility, psychiatric disturbance, guilt, anxiety and revenge (Finkelhor 1986).

Many children express anxiety that they are permanently physically harmed. Abused adolescent girls may worry about future relationships and their ability to have a family subsequently. In such cases children may require sensitive assurances from an experienced medical practitioner. Older children may need accurate sex information. Surprisingly, many victims are extremely misinformed on sexual matters.

Society's response to the child's victimization can contribute to the 'damaged goods' syndrome (Sgroi 1984). A child who has been sexually abused may evoke pity, disgust, intense curiosity, hostility for the 'trouble' she/he has caused. Parents need guidance about how to respond to the child appropriately, and not as different.

Indicators of abuse

Physical

- Unexplained
  bruises and welts
  burns
  fractures
  lacerations and abrasions
  abdominal injuries
  human bite marks
  bald spots and scalp bruises
- Failure to thrive
- General developmental delay
- Hunger, poor hygiene, inappropriate clothing
- Lack of supervision in dangerous situations
- Excessive fatigue or listlessness
- Unattended medical conditions

Behavioural (Child)

- Wariness of physical contact with adults
- Displays extremes of behaviour
- Fears parents
- Fears going home
- Is overly compliant
- Is frequently late or absent from school, or consistently arrives early or leaves late
- Rare attendance at school
- Inappropriately seeks affection
- Exhibits habit disorders and neurotic traits
- Begging or stealing food
- Constantly falling asleep in class
- Addiction to alcohol or other drugs
- Delinquency
- Low self-esteem
- Speech disorders
- Sleep disorders

As well as the above indicators, children who have been sexually abused may show the following sexual behaviour indicators.

- Unusual interest in and/or knowledge of sexual acts and language inappropriate to the child's age
- Seductive behaviour

- Abnormal awareness of touch, or related behaviour and/or reluctance to undress
- Abrupt change in behaviour, personality or school performance
- Extreme avoidance of, or over-attention to adults of a particular sex
- Suicidal threats, gestures; causing deliberate harm to self

Parental

- Uses harsh discipline
- Complains that the child cries too much or causes trouble
- Has unrealistic expectations of child
- Is angry, defensive or uninterested about child's problems
- Offers unconvincing explanations for child's injury
- Misuses drugs
- Home life appears disorganised
- Family is socially isolated
- Parent(s) in ill health
- Uneducated about child rearing
- Predominantly negative verbal and non-verbal interaction with the child
- Expresses belief that child seeks to hurt or annoy
- Expresses belief that child is physically 'deformed', 'bad' or 'different'

Sequelae

Attempts to study long-term effects of abuse on children have been fraught with methodological problems. Most studies are retrospective, lacking in control comparison with non-abused children, and anecdotal in nature. Observations of sequelae which have been reported suggest that physical and emotional abuse may be associated with the full gamut of disturbances and distortions of normal behavioural development, ranging from 'failure to thrive' as an infant, (Bullard et al 1967; Evans et al 1972; Leonard et al 1966) to repeating the pattern of abusive behaviour in the next generation (Anthony & Cohler 1987; Blager & Martin 1976; Egeland & Srouffe 1981; Elmer & Gregg 1967; Garbarino & Vondra 1982; Kaufman & Zigler 1987; Oates 1985; Sandgrund et al 1974; Steele 1986; Toro 1982).

Evaluation

A child may be referred for assessment of developmental maturity, because some form of abuse is suspected, but not substantiated. In this instance the therapist's responsibility is to provide a detailed assessment of all aspects of the child's developmental competence. There should be special attention given to examining the content of the child's symbolic play, particularly the verbal content if she/he is old enough. Symbolic play may give an indication of the nature and quality of family and other close child/adult relationships.

On the other hand, abuse may be substantiated, and then the purpose of evaluation is more specifically to determine the extent of any effects on the child's development and maturation. The reader is referred to Sgroi (1984), Oates (1985) and Jones & McQuiston (1986) for detailed guidance.

Assessment of the abused child may include the following:

— Full developmental assessment
— Play assessment
— Assessment of self concept
— Observations — behavioural interactions, specifically that of mother-child interactions
— Perceptual and sensory assessment
— Interviews with child and with parents
— Emotional and psychological assessment
— Consultation with other agencies such as schools, child care centres, etc.

Intervention

The family of an abused child is truly the unit of treatment, whatever intervention approach is chosen. It was policy in most societies to remove the abused child from his/her family — presumably to safeguard the child. Specialists now take the view that the family unit should be maintained intact and supported while special therapy proceeds with parents and children. Unfortunately, there are no reliable statistics which allow decisions to be made about which of the available approaches are more effective in re-orienting dysfunctional family interactions. The United States national survey of child abuse demonstration projects reported that only 42% of parents who received intervention did not abuse their children again (Cohn 1979).

Occupational therapy

No single form of treatment will be successful in all child abuse cases because the abuse is symptomatic of many individual and family problems. Intervention must be specifically targeted, and thus a detailed diagnositc evaluation is critical to effective intervention planning. The differing aspects that might be targeted for intervention have been discussed widely throughout this book, and will not be addressed any further.

The child

Intervention with abused children requires a combination of many of the approaches employed with children with other problems (Salter et al 1985). However, while there are some overriding intervention processes, there are also factors which relate particularly to the abused child and family. For example, the parents of an abused and developmentally delayed child may not be supportive. Thus the therapist may have to enlist the support of other people in the child's environment, e.g., teacher, foster parent or others. The Committee for Children (1984a, b) has proposed some general intervention guidelines which apply specifically to children who have been abused.

Guidelines for intervention with abused children

- Recognize the child's need for authority. Offer choices and tasks at which she/he can succeed. Break these tasks down into their simplest elements and repeat often, building up towards total accomplishment.
- Watch for signs of recurring abuse. Let the child know that you are available to talk. However, do not dwell on the issue or allow it to become a means of gaining attention.
- If the abuse is discussed in a group, deal with it then, matter-of-factly and briefly. Try to talk to the child alone later. Offer reassurance and continue to support and care for him/her.
- Teach and model appropriate behaviour. Do not allow the child to climb all over you.
- Refrain from touching a child who has been sexually abused. For these children, all touch may mean sexual touch. A non-intrusive touch, such as an arm around the shoulder, should be given only with caution and the child's permission.
- Do not tolerate inappropriate behaviour. If a child is sexually acting out with other children, respond to the behaviour as you would with any inappropriate behaviour.
- Be aware and respectful of the family. Following disclosure of abuse, the family may feel shame, fear and isolation. Respect their feelings and privacy. Do not discuss the abuse with those not involved.
- Be prepared for depression weeks or months after disclosure of abuse. Withdrawal and acting out may recur.
- Maintain contact with the caseworker or therapist and the non-offending parent when sexual abuse has occurred.
- Be aware of your own reactions and get support and help for your own feelings of pain, fear, anger and powerlessness. If you made the notification remind yourself that it was right to notify. Remember the alternative to not notifying — further abuse of the child.

Approaches

Play and arts therapies. Play and art therapy techniques have been frequently used with abused children to facilitate the child's disclosure of abuse, to aid in evidence gathering and to assist the abused child to express and deal with his or her experience. For the abused child, play may be a vehicle for the safe expression of painful experiences and emotions. Furthermore, through play the victim has the opportunity to master situations in which she/he has been helpless, thus mitigating the effect of traumatic events (Petrillo & Sanger 1972). The self-expression gained through play may help the child cope with his or her conflicting environment and thus move toward emotional maturity.

This technique may be particularly useful for younger or less verbal children who may not possess the language or verbal skills to tell accurately of their experiences. Furthermore, the use of this media may be less threatening to a child who has experienced the trauma of legal intervention, disclosure, and perhaps temporary foster placement. In such cases, play or art may be a comfortable method to establish trust and a therapeutic relationship.

One special application of play techniques has been the use of anatomically correct dolls. Through the use of these dolls clinicians have been able to elicit information from abused children that is clear and accurate. This method is more common in the treatment of sexually abused children but may be useful in other forms of abuse (see Axline 1989; Jones & McQuiston 1986; Sgroi 1984; Chapter 16).

Behaviour management. Teachers, parents and other staff may ask the occupational therapist to provide strategies for effective management of problem behaviours. Principles of behaviour management are discussed in Chapters 9, 10 and 16.

Group therapy. There is much benefit from group therapy for abused children. Adolescents particularly may benefit from peer support. Further benefits may be increased social skills and peer acceptance. The use of groups can provide a secure setting where a child can test out new behaviour. Through finding more appropriate patterns of behaviour and interaction patterns, abused children can eliminate some of the behaviours that may have labelled him or her as a problem (Cooke 1982) in both the family and in school.

In the group, abused children can benefit from some limits on group rules, e.g., confidentiality within the group, compulsory attendance, unacceptability of antisocial or destructive behaviours. Activities for the group allow for both self-expression and individual success, e.g., cooking, arts and crafts, sand and water play, dramatic arts.

Inclusion of parents into groups with their children is another form of group therapy.

The parents

Parents have been the primary focus for intervention from the earliest intervention efforts. The establishment of a trusting and respectful relationship with abusing parents may be difficult to effect, but once gained may provide a powerful vehicle for prevention of further abuse.

Helfer's (1980) conceptual model of the WAR cycle points to abuse being the result of a disorder of parenting which includes the parent's own unmet needs, limited knowledge of child development, discipline difficulties and limited coping skills, and a limited support network.

The therapist's personal attitudes toward the abusive parent are vital in determining the outcome for both parent and child. Barnes (1988) has suggested that professionals should reject a superior and punitive attitude, in favour of 'being alongside' the parent. The therapist works from the client's level, recognizing that the parent's perceived needs and priorities may be divergent from that of the therapist's. Most parents presenting for treatment for child abuse differ from other parents in that they are often involuntary clients. Thus in initial sessions these clients may be resistant and unmotivated. However, Sgroi (1984) notes that a hostile facade generally conceals a desperately needy person who is eager for someone to show a caring and supportive approach to them. Thus, an initial task for the therapist may be to allow the parent to diffuse anxiety and acknowledge that parenting can be stressful and difficult.

Timeout. As many cases of abuse present as the culmination of a crisis, it may be useful to eliminate some of the immediate stress for the parent by providing respite care for the child. Generally placement of the child will be handled by child protection authorities and may include temporary foster care with relatives or foster families, family day care, child minding, etc.

Parent education. The family must be assisted to treat the child in a manner appropriate to his/her developmental age in order that the child may complete missed developmental tasks. Therefore, parents may be included in structured parent education programmes.

These programmes offer many benefits including the opportunity to provide role models, supportive environments and practical instruction about child rearing and development. One problem about parent education with abusive parents is that formal parent education may not meet parental needs. Many programmes focus upon the children's needs. Many abusive parents are so absorbed with their own needs that they may have difficulty recognizing their children's needs. Hence serious consideration should be given to personal development programmes for parents. One such easily implemented programme is the Parent Burnout Kit (see Batdorf & Krebill 1983); and in Chapter 10 there is an extended discussion of parent education.

Helpers. A study by Cohn (1979) has suggested that while experienced professional workers are necessary to conduct initial diagnosis and case management the use of 'natural helpers' or lay counsellors are more likely to improve outcomes. These natural helpers can include supportive relatives, friends of the family or trained volunteers such as parent aides and homemakers. These workers are able to work more intensively in the family's home and may be seen as less threatening than professionals. Ballew (1985) stated that too often professionals undervalue the role of natural helpers who may be an invaluable resource. In a survey of natural helpers Ballew found that 85% of such interventions were seen by both professionals and client families as effective. These workers were able to provide long-term, intense and effective therapy. The benefit of such workers is often that they can obtain a more accurate picture of the family in their environment as well as providing practical assistance. Using natural helpers can allow more intensive treatment with the professional acting as a consultant or resource.

Self help groups. Cohn (1979) also commented on the success of self help groups for abusive and 'at risk' parents. Sgroi (1984) also proposed that self help groups are powerful tools that can provide a safe and supportive environment for participants to discuss their fears and problems openly. This author suggests that guidance by a therapist is effective as a resource, to answer questions, maintain group direction and model appropriate behaviours. Groups such as Parents Anonymous may also provide an ongoing support long after therapy has ceased. Such groups vary considerably in terms of duration, content and structure. They may either be time limited or open ended, closed or open groups. Opportunities also exist for these parents to experience helping and supporting others.

Prophylaxis. From a young age children learn rules about water, fire, traffic, bicycle and poison safety. Personal body safety should be added to that list. Prevention education programmes therefore should also include personal safety rules about okay and not okay touching to prevent children from being exploited or harmed. The concept of personal safety training for children is believed to be useful in preventing sexual abuse. Ideally such education should be given to all children before victimization occurs. However, personal safety information may be particularly pertinent to abused children to prevent recurrence of abuse.

The principles of sexual abuse prevention and safety training are that children can make judgements, speak up for themselves and play an important role in looking after their own well being. Three basic elements of a personal safety programme are:

1. building self-esteem
2. training for assertiveness
3. teaching self-protective skills and behaviours.

Summary

Society has had a long history of mistreating children. Unfortunately, families are not always the loving and happy units which we would like to think they are. Child abuse, be it physical, emotional, sexual or by neglect, is a very real problem and one which is, sadly, emerging as a major area of contemporary occupational therapy practice.

Children receiving treatment for other stated reasons (e.g., developmental delay, behaviour disorder) may disclose or show behaviours or signs indicative that abuse may be taking place. While there has been considerable research into the characteristics of abusers, there is clearly more research needed into various treatment regimes. The role of prevention and education may prove to be effective (Boss & Goddard 1986). Child abuse is a multifaceted problem where social, environmental and individual factors interact. Intervention should be holistic, and it provides a prime, if sobering, example of occupational therapy intervention with the family as a unit of treatment.

CHILDREN LIVING IN INSTITUTIONS

The institutional effect

Behavioural scientists have become increasingly interested in the relationship between behaviour and the environment — not only in the laboratory, but also in naturalistic settings. Studies of human behaviour interacting with the physical environment are relevant to the design of a variety of therapeutic regimes. For example, studies of the play behaviour of children in hospitals and nursery settings (Hutt & McGrew 1967; McGrew 1972), 'open plan' designs in hospitals (Canter 1975),

'therapeutic institutions' (Brown 1966; Clancy 1976; Richer & Hutchings 1973) and low stimulus environments (Schultz 1965, Zubek 1969) have practical and theoretical implications for occupational therapy. There is now quite a body of research data that examines the natural environments of institutions, for example, long-stay psychiatric treatment institutions, and the effectiveness of changing behaviour through systematic study and modification of the physical environment (e.g., Esser 1971; Newman 1972; Richer & Nicholl 1971; Sommer 1973).

Working with children and adults who live in residential institutions presents caregivers with a very special dilemma. Usually, staffing is inadequate, attention to individual residents is necessarily low, and the process of institutionalization is added to the primary developmental disability (see Clancy 1976; Lieberman 1977; Lutkenhaus 1985; McBridge & Clancy 1973; Main & Weston 1981; Oswin 1973; Provence & Lipton 1967; Rutter 1973; Thompson & Lamb 1983). The spatial environment is characteristically barren, to minimize destruction of property, and facilitate the tasks of domestic and caregiving staff.

Dunning (1972) said that though the physical environment is one component of the total environment 'whatever component is extracted, it is clearly evident that it not only acts upon other components and thereby changes them, but in so doing it changes the "total" environment and thereby induces changes in itself'. Therapy has many components. 'patients' — the children — interact with each other and with doctors, nurses, therapists and those concerned with the delivery of ordinary services such as food, linen and housekeeping. There are also the specific tasks associated with the treatment or therapy. These tasks are directly related to servicing some aspect of the 'patient, and may include personal care and development of a range of physical, social and intellectual skills of normal development and living. In all activities there will be a multitude of small daily interactions between the 'patient' and his or her social and physical environment which appear to have little or no relevance to the therapeutic process. However, we postulate that by designing the physical environment to harness the potential usefulness of these seemingly irrelevant interaction, the therapeutic process may be positively influenced. For example, environment design may foster skill development in the following ways:

— Sensory awareness and skill may be fostered
  through design of spaces which differ in
  (a) texture and shape (tactual and visual senses)
  and (b) colour (visual sense).

— Environmental mastery and personal confidence may be fostered through responsive environments which, for example, respond to physical approach or touch with sound or a visual display.
— Social skills may be promoted by designing environment features which foster interaction between people, and/or bring them into a face-to-face relationship, in a rewarding manner.
— Personal identity may be fostered by the design of space which is identified with an individual. For example, photographs of the person can be displayed beside a mirror in which the person can identify him/herself. Belongings also confer personal identity, such as clothing, though this variable is very difficult to monitor in an institution.
— Task skill development can be facilitated by environmental design. Motor and perceptual skills can be designed into ordinary daily tasks, e.g., feeding, dressing, bathing. In this way, the opportunity for practice and increased proficiency is facilitated.

Thus the spatial environment is viewed as an interactive and communicative channel. The objective is not to replace therapists and caregivers, but to maximize their efforts where they are in short supply, and the demands on their skills are heavy. Design of the physical environment may also complement therapeutic efforts in the long hours outside of the specific therapy session (Stout 1988). Too often in institutions the skills fostered by one set of specialists are ignored by others, so that skills become situation specific. By attending to the design of the spatial environment it is postulated that there can be generalizing effects from the specific therapy interventions.

Evaluating physical environments

Dunning (1972) provides some practical guidelines for examining the environment. She does this by means of an 'environmental grid' which analyses the component parts of the environment — space, people and the task. While 'environment grid' is exploratory in nature and applied to an adult psychiatric population, the basic principles nonetheless have properties which can be generalized to other client populations and which can assist the therapist in assessing environments.

Space. Can the furniture be arranged to promote social interaction? Does the grouping of objects provide cues to their use? Can space be used to increase or decrease the feeling of privacy or crowding? Is the furniture a fixed feature or a semi-fixed feature?

People. Can the distance between the individual and those with whom she/he wishes to communicate be narrowed? Can the environments be selected to increase the likelihood for social stimulation and interaction?

Task. Do the presence, availability, desirability and feasibility of the objects and space in the environment have potential for use?

This discussion concludes with an example of how the environmental design component was integrated with other components of therapy in one institution.

Intervention

Integrating the environment in therapy

An experimental programme was implemented in an institution for 24 severely disturbed autistic children under the age of 12 years. The prime focus of the programme was the structuring of people's attention — transferring the child's attention from self-involved trivial activities, to the physical and social environment, while affiliative relationships were fostered between the child and others. The living environment was modified to be interactive, and to redirect the attention structure of staff and children alike. A complete description of the project is available elsewhere (Clancy 1976).

The features of the programme were:

1. Master planning of the children's waking time, in terms of skills required by a child in the open social and educational community.
2. Facilitation of the master programme by a division of specialist staff labour based on individual skill related to programme requirements.

Such a division recognized that professional education usually prepares a specialist to work in special skill areas, but it avoids the problems of allowing children to be packaged according to traditional concepts of specialist 'territory'. The approach is problem oriented, and leads to the integrated treatment programme. Treatment priority is shifted from individual child training to whole group training, recognizing that some children also have a need for specialist individual attention.

Data collection. This step occupied one week and was followed by implementation of the experimental therapeutic regime with the following objectives:

Terminal objectives:

— To facilitate primary socialization, that is, the development of affiliations or bonds between a child and important adults, and
— To foster the acquisition of behaviours normally developed in the socialization process.

Enabling Objectives:

— To establish a total daily programme so that the children's waking time would be occupied in a manner contributing to therapy, i.e., demanding attention of them.
— To integrate the therapeutic team by co-ordinating skills to provide minimum overlap and expenditure of effort, with maximum effectiveness.
— To develop an interactive spatial environment in the living area of each apartment.

The procedure chosen because of the institutional context was to link each child to a restricted number of adults so that she/he gained effective security, with 'insurance' against withdrawal of one caretaker.

Roles and function. The paradigm for all child training was behaviour modification, aimed at relationships in naturalistic settings, rather than at individuals, insofar as this is possible in an institution. Reinforcements were generally social, though occasionally supplemented by other rewards. Handling techniques were, allowing for the human factor, consistent between all workers. Emphasis was always on eliciting and consolidating non-verbal and verbal communicative skills, with all other training embedded in the resulting social relationship. Particular emphasis was paid to the following ranked behaviours:

— Non-verbal social communicative skills, e.g., eye-contact.
— Pre-verbal visual perceptual skills, e.g., concept and vocabulary development leading to shaped verbal language skills.
— Gross and fine motor skills, and training in self-care independence.

The school was to provide the future context for further formal education, and the shaping of increasingly complex social skills.

Total daily programming was conceived as a relatively inflexible 'architectural structure.' Five out of seven days were so planned and the plan is presented in Figure 14.2. The remaining two days were organized by the cottage parents.

The roles and functions of all workers were redefined in relation to the daily programme. The cottage parents continued as caretakers, but they also became students, involved with the children from their unit in each component of the day's programme. The assumption here was that the cottage parents should become conversant with the functions of the other team members as well as with special techniques of handling. the children. All meals were treated as opportunities for extending the children's eating skills and social behaviour. A midday rest period remained temporarily in the programme in order to give staff an opportunity to meet daily for dis-

Period	Group activity	Apartment 1	Apartment 2	Apartment 3	Apartment 4
am 8–9	Breakfast Kitchen activities				
9–10		OT	Language	Social skills	School
10–11		School	Social skills	OT	Language
11–12		Social skills	School	Language	OT
pm 12	Lunch Rest time				
1–2	Team meets				
2–3		Language	OT	School	Social skills
3–4	Play				
4–5	Story time — TV 'Sesame Street'				
5–6	Dinner				
6–8	Structured indoor play Bath				
8.00	Bed time				

Fig. 14.2 A fully integrated daily intervention plan for children 4–12-years-old living in an institution in apartment groups of 8–10 children and 2 adults. From Clancy H G 1976 Integrating the environment in therapy. Man-Environment Systems 6: 305–12. Reproduced with permission of the publisher.

cussion and teaching. Volunteers were brought in to supervise the rest period, but it was generally agreed that most of the children required increased activity rather than sleep periods.

The occupational therapist was assigned two new functions, the first being to teach cottage parents how to train children in feeding, dressing and toileting independence. To this end, the occupational therapist designed a weekly activities programme for each apartment. She then spent one morning in each apartment helping the cottage parents improve their skills in implementing the activities.

For example, there were practical demonstrations in teaching non-cooperative, poorly skilled children to dress, and ways of encouraging feeding independence in children. After breakfast, activities were located in the kitchen, because it had been noted that cottage parents were regularly engaged in kitchen duties at that time. Activities with the children included washing breakfast dishes, tidying the kitchen as a group, followed by small tasks, for example, simple cooking, or preparing the day's finger-paint or dough, or sorting the cutlery drawers.

The second function of the occupational therapist was to implement social skills training of the children. All children required specific guidance in learning how to handle interpersonal skills and appropriate feelings, such as anger, warmth, sharing property and affection, with others. This function could well have been assumed by a different specialist but in the experimental institution the most efficient division of labour was for the occupational therapist to do this job. Such training occupied the time designated 'occupational therapy' in the daily programme structure. Sometimes the context was a conventional play therapy setting, centred on group participation in co-operative activities such as finger painting and imaginative games using farm and doll's house equipment. On other selected days the setting was an apartment, and the activities provided gross motor skill and body image development.

The school room was always the context for special education activity. The teacher was assigned formal responsibility for training the children in cognitive pre-formal and formal educational skills. Again, this represented a sensible division of labour in this institution, as other specialists are often equally skilled in the area of cognitive, perceptual pre-formal skill training. In addition to their role as monitors of the children's medical care, the registered nurses in the institution assumed responsibility for social skills training away from the institution. This became loosely referred

to as 'the socialization programme'. The group, comprising the children, cottage parents and one or two nurses, would leave the unit and on one day would practise crossing the street at pedestrian lights. On another day, the group might travel to and from the shopping area by public transport, the children paying their own fares. Five distinct areas of public behaviour would be practised in one week. This programme was expanded in a most imaginative and exciting way. For example, children were taken to visits in the houses of friends, and to eat in public restaurants.

The speech therapist was responsible for all language programming, in groups and for individuals. She designed and implemented programmes in each apartment. Her purpose was to teach the cottage parents how to establish a language environment, translate it into activities, and how to elicit verbal and vocal exchanges with the children. A formal story time provided another medium for language programming. The aims were to further language stimulation, and teach the cottage parents the skills of telling stories to isolated inattentive children, so that this activity could be incorporated into the repertoire of the cottage parents' skills.

There was a gradual process of handing over the story time to the cottage parents and the final step was that they should plan the day's stories and implement the activity, in consultation with the speech therapist.

An unstructured 'free' time was allowed for both children and staff to 'let off steam'. The way in which the children used this time also provided a valuable informal guide to the effectiveness of the integrated treatment programme.

Programming for the time between dinner and children's bedtime presented more difficulties than for the remainder of the day. There appeared to be several problems. The time was approximately two hours at the end of a hectic day, the children were tired and thus more prone to isolating behaviour. A staff of volunteers who were not engaged in other aspects of the programme assisted the cottage parents and nurses during this time. As well, the daily clothes washing and the children's bath time were incorporated into the evening therapy sessions.

Television, such as the programme *Sesame Street*, was included in this evening session. Whenever the television was used, the cottage parents watched with the children, thus directing their attention to it. Neither the radio nor the television was used to provide a general noise background, or just to keep the children quiet.

There were not enough machines to allow each apartment group to participate in daily washing, so a roster was organized. The dry washing was kept over, and at bath time one cottage parent directed a folding and sorting operation with the group, while the other cottage parent engaged one or two children in bathing. Cottage parents were again shown how to extend the value of the bath time to promote social and play interactions between children. Again, the children could also practise dressing and self-care skills. In institutions there is a danger that children will fail to develop the normal sense of identity and ownership of property. A special effort was made to allot each child his or her own clothing and personal items, and mirrors were to be installed in the living area, where the evening activities normally took place.

The social worker maintained the role of providing the link between families and the institution, with the focus on providing supportive therapy with the parents — a conventional and important role. The psychiatrist, by general agreement, was to direct the integrated treatment programme after the experimental period.

The physical environment

Situation to be modified. The living room of one apartment housing six children and two caretakers (see Fig. 14.3).

Why modify? The children spent at least an equal amount of time in the apartment to that spent in 'therapy'. Thus it was assumed that the apartment experience either reinforced and facilitated other treatment strategies, or negated them.

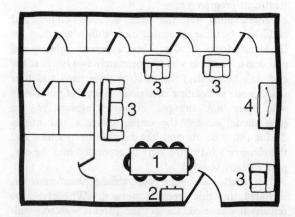

Key
1—Dining table and chairs
2—Buffet
3—Couch and lounge chairs
4—TV

Fig. 14.3 Experimental apartment before modification.

Observed behaviour. The children habitually ignored all others, and also:

- They engaged in useless, repetitive, often destructive activity, e.g., rocking, running endlessly, finger flicking at the walls (stereotypes). There was no interest displayed in social play or toys.
- They did not use or exchange language with others.
- The caretakers habitually stood or wandered around.
- The caretakers' only language and physical contact with children was to reprimand. The language environment came from constant television broadcasting.
- The caretakers 'did' for the children rather than encouraged independent attempts, e.g., feeding.

Specific behavioural and environmental objectives were established for developing an interactive spatial environment in the apartment living area.

Behavioural objectives. To facilitate altered social interaction between:

- Children
- Children and adults (vis-à-vis close, pleasant body contact and increased language from adults, through the medium of pleasant, simple play)
- Caretakers and specialist therapists (to improve information channels between the two, and to reduce caretakers' hostility).

Environmental objectives. To structure attention to achieve:

- Interactive sequences which would entail the minimum effort and would, therefore, enhance the likelihood of reward
- Generally elevated attention level to both non-social surrounding, and people
- Functional activities through enhanced attention levels.

Modifications had to be made rapidly, using available material and equipment as no funding was available.

Modifications were made in the experimental apartment overnight and plans were drawn up for a sequence of more sophisticated modifications. Figure 14.4 shows the modified apartment layout.

The modifications

Modifications were made to the physical environment as follows. Furniture was positioned to foster and reinforce certain patterns of social interaction, namely child–child

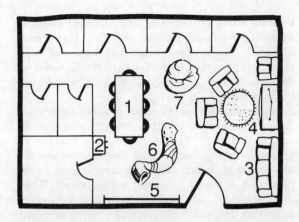

Key
1—Dining table and chairs
2—Buffet
3—Couch and lounge chairs
4—TV
5—Balancing bar
6—Crawling tunnel
7—Bean bag

Fig. 14.4 Experimental apartment after modification.
Figs. 14.3 and 14.4 from Clancy H G 1976 Integrating the
environment in therapy. Man–Environment Systems
6: 305–12. Reproduced with permission of the publisher.

face-to-face contact; adult contact involving touching,
and contact of a mutually rewarding type. Thus, placing
the couch close to the main entrance freed the cottage
parents from the need to patrol, and it also created a
semi-closed area promoting a feeling of comfort and
relaxation about sitting down. The cottage parents were
assured that they would not be judged as 'lazy', by sitting for lengthy periods. The psychiatrist set an example
by visiting each morning, sitting and playing with the
children, to reinforce the assurances. The single chairs,
excluding one, were positioned in a tight semi-circle
focused on the television. The rationale was that
children using these chairs were more likely to make
casual, or even intentional social contact with each
other. One chair was placed alone in a corner, but facing
into the room. Perhaps even solitary children occasionally need to retreat. Sitting in this chair, a child could
do so, but yet remain part of the group, at least visually.

Furniture was also re-arranged to promote learning of
a variety of socialization skills. For example, the dining
area was moved adjacent to the kitchen so that the
children could assist in serving and clearing away the
meals.

Versatile, self-exploratory play equipment was used to
turn the children's attention to different aspects of their

perceptual environment. The equipment comprised two
categories:

1. Equipment designed to encourage gross motor
   activity, for example, the soft crawling tunnel, and
   the balancing bars and boards illustrated in Figure
   14.3b
2. Some wall fixtures chosen to foster specific
   learning.

There were for example, very large texture boards; self-
rewarding busy boards with bells and buzzers, zip
fasteners, buttons and many other devices and active
pictures teaching specific concepts such as 'up', 'down',
'on' and 'off'. All wall fixtures were at the children's
height and were changed at intervals to avoid an
habituation effect. The possibilities of such equipment
are limited only by ingenuity.

Evaluation

The impact of the experimental programme on staff and
children is discussed descriptively. Data for analysis
were gathered by means of 16 mm movie record, and
time-sampled behavioural observations.

Within one week of full implementation of the
integrated treatment programme and the environmental
modifications, the following changes were readily observable in staff and children:

• All children looked more often, and for longer
  periods, at each other and at adults, that is to say,
  there was increase in social eye contact.
• Four previously non-talking children began using a
  few words, communicating — and quite
  spontaneously.
• Before the experimental programme the treatment
  unit had been a very noisy place. The noise quality
  was harsh, agitated and consisted largely of
  screaming sounds. Some doctors familiar with the
  unit, but unaware that the programme was in
  operation, passed through on several occasions and
  queried a change of noise quality. When asked,
  they described the altered sound environment as
  still being noisy but having a quality of
  'contentment' and 'relaxation'.
• There was an observable increase in the amount of
  smiling, both by children and adults.
• Cottage parents expressed eagerness to come to
  work, and pleasure in being in the environment.
• In the space of the three weeks of the project,
  there was not one act of destructive behaviour
  toward property by any child. This was reported

by the unit manager who had been initially most reluctant to agree to the range of proposed activities within the living apartments, because of the long history of destructiveness. It should be added that while elimination of destructive activity was an indirect benefit from the project, it was a very important one because it represented money — both in planning for capital outlay and environment maintenance.

Within the modified living apartments the social interactions between children, and children and adults did change in the directions planned. Undoubtedly there was a Hawthorne effect operating, but still it appeared that the modifications made to the physical environment were a facilitating factor in changing behaviour of all individuals. For example, it was found on the first morning of the environmental changes, that the children were using the cloth crawling tunnel and coming in contact with each other by doing so. The children were clearly alert to the changes and became increasingly exploratory, both of objects and people. Caretakers, on the other hand, altered their patterns of patrolling the apartment and by the end of the third week were sitting down and interacting with the children in an apparently comfortable way. A new range of interpersonal interaction experiences thus became available to the children.

Independent observers have suggested the following reasons for changes in the relationships between staff members involved in the programme described:

- There was increased attention of many kinds paid to children.
- The varied attention had an underlying consistency of intent, and was persistently intrusive on the child's isolated life. The quality of intrusion was essentially gentle, socially rewarding and intended to convey fun and excitement in living.
- There was designed variety and novelty of experience to which the children were exposed.

The inevitable effect of habituation by all individuals to the changes was considered. It was decided that criteria for further modifications would be, reappearance of bizarre behaviours toward the pre-programme levels, and a decrease in newly observed appropriate social behaviours, e.g., eye contact. These changes appeared about the fifth week after commencement of the programme and environment modifications. Minor compensatory changes were again made to the living apartments, for example, the large texture boards were repositioned on the walls. It was thought that by incorporating minor changes the same materials could be used over a considerable time (months), before being discarded because the children had exhausted every reasonable possibility for further exploration, and could therefore be assumed to have thoroughly habituated to the materials.

Full implementation of integrated treatment programming in one working month is probably unrealistic for most clinical teams. The point to be taken from this experimental programme in which the time available was one constraint, is that such programming must be implemented *as a total system* and not piecemeal. Where the latter is the case, each component or sub-system, establishes its own equilibrium and then negative feedbacks are applied to changes as they are attempted in other sub-systems. The total effectiveness of integrated programming is thereby lost, and the process of change lengthened to resemble the more conventional practices.

In conclusion, considerable effort is required to change any operating system. Yet this example illustrates that the effort can be justified in terms of the clearly observable gains to be had. To the clients, at least if they are children, the gains are rapid incremental movement in the direction of more normal development and thus potential participation in the open, though sheltered, society. For therapeutic specialists, the gains appear to be greater professional efficiency and motivation, with resulting job satisfaction and professional growth. For administrators of institutions the gains are economic ones.

Summary

The chief objective of any interactive environment is to design available physical space so that it exerts a therapeutic influence on individuals, specifically to engage their attention increasingly in interactions with their social and non-social environment, i.e., to alter the ratio of time spent in social and solitary activity. Once established, therapeutic effects result without the use of staff. This is an important consideration, particularly in large, understaffed institutions. Specific behavioural goals can be stated in the designing of the environment, and there is some evidence to suggest that there are sound economic reasons for its use

For example, destructive behaviour to property can be significantly modified. Patients become more socialized, even when the staff–patient ratio is quite unsatisfactory. This allows for altered patient–nurse relationships from basic caretaking and custodial supervision to involvement in useful therapeutic relationships.

Staff efficiency improves, as does morale and work commitment, and patients respond rapidly — more so when the interactive environment is linked with other therapeutic schemes, for example a token economy. Specialists should find their jobs facilitated by nurses' co-operation.

REFERENCES

Adler R 1986 Physical maltreatment of children. Australian and New Zealand Journal of Psychiatry 20: 404–412

Anthony E J, Cohler B J 1987 The invulnerable child. Guilford Press, New York

Axline V 1989 Play therapy. Churchill Livingstone, Edinburgh. First published 1947, Riverside Press, Cambridge, Massachusetts

Bakwin H 1942 Loneliness in infants. American Journal of Diseases of Childhood 63: 30–40

Balleu J R 1985 The role of natural helpers in prevention of child abuse and neglect. Social Work 30(1): 37–41

Barnes G 1988 Personal communication. Social Work Department, Monash University, Melbourne

Batdorf L, Krebill J 1983 Preventing parent burnout. Coalition for Child Advocacy, Bellingham

Bell J E 1969 The family in hospital: lessons from developing countries. Public Health Service Publication No 1933, Chevy Chase, Maryland

Bergmann T 1965 Children in hospital. Internation Universities Press, London

Blager R, Martin H 1976 Speech and language of abused children. In: Martin H P (ed) The abused child: a multidisciplinary approach to developmental issues and treatment. Ballinger, Cambridge

Bowlby J 1952 Grief and mourning in early childhood. Psychoanalytic Study of the Child 15: 8–52

Bowlby J 1973 Separation, anxiety and grief, volume II of Attachment and loss. Hogarth Press, London

Boss P C, Goddard C 1986 Child abuse — insight and understanding. In: Clements A(ed) Infant and family health in Australia. Churchill Livingstone, Melbourne

Brach field S, Goldberg S, Sloman J 1980 Prematurity and immaturity as influences on parent–infant interaction at 8 and 12 months. Infant Behavior and Development 3: 289–305

Brandon S 1976 Physical violence in the family: an overview. In: M Borland Ed. Violence in the family. Humanities Press, Atlantic Highlands, New Jersey

Bronfenbrenner U 1970 Two worlds of childhood. Sage Publications. New York

Brown R I 1966 The effects of varied environmental stimulation on the performance of subnormal children. Journal of child Psychology and Psychiatry 7: 251–261

Browning R M, Stover D O 1971 Behaviour Modification in Child Treatment. Adline, Chicago

Bullard D M, Glaser H H, Heagarty M C, Pivchick E C. 1967 Failure to thrive in the neglected child. American Journal of Orthopsychiatry 37: 680–690

Byrne D, London D, Reeves K 1968 The effects of physical attractiveness, sex and attitude similarity on interpersonal attraction. Journal of Personality 36: 259–271

Canter D 1975 Designing a therapeutic setting. New Behaviour 4: 374–375

Clancy H G 1976 Integrating the environment in therapy. Man–Environment Systems 6: 305–312

Clancy H, McBride G 1975 The isolation syndrome. Developmental Medicine and Child Neurology 17: 198–219

Cohn A H 1979 Effective treatment of child abuse and neglect. Social Work 24: 513–519

Committee for Children 1984a Physical abuse and neglect. Committee for Children Supplement, Seattle

Committee for Children 1984b Prevention of child sexual abuse: a trainer's manual. Committee for Children, Seattle

Cooke P 1982 A family service unit's approach to working with child abuse. Child Abuse and Neglect 6: 433–441

Crawford J W 1982 Mother–infant interaction in premature and full-term infants. Child Development 53: 957–962

Crnic K A, Ragozin A S, Greenberg M T, Robinson N M, Bashman R B 1983 Social interaction and developmental competence of preterm and full-term infants during the first year of life. Child Development 54: 1199–1210

Dimock R 1960 The child in hospital. Macmillan, Canada

Duberly J 1974 The role of nursing staff in helping the hospitalized child. In: Burton L (ed) Care of the child facing death. Routledge & Kegan Paul, London

Dunning H 1972 Environmental occupational therapy. American Journal of Occupational Therapy 28: 292–298

Egeland B, Sroufe A 1981 Developmental sequelae of maltreatment in infancy. New Directions for Child Development 11: 77–92

Elmer E, Gregg G S. 1967 Developmental characteristics of abused children. Pediatrics 40: 596–602

Esser A H 1971 Strategies for research in man–environment systems. In: Smith W M (ed) Ecology in human living environments. University of Wisconsin Press, Green Bay

Evans S L, Reinhart J B, Succop R A 1972 Failure to thrive: a study of 45 children and families. Journal of the American Academy of Child Psychiatry 11: 440–457

Ferguson D M, Fleming J, O'Neill D P 1972 Child abuse in New Zealand. Government Printer, Wellington

Finkelhor D 1986 A sourcebook of sexual abuse. Sage Publications, Beverley Hills

Garbarino J, Garbarino A. 1980 Emotional maltreatment of children. National Committee for Prevention of Child Abuse, Chicago

Garbarino J, Vondra J. 1987 Psychological maltreatment: issues and perspectives. In: Brassard M, Germain R, Hart S (eds) Psychological Maltreatment of children and youth. Pergamon, New York

Garrison E G 1987 Psychological maltreatment of children: an emerging focus for enquiry and concern. American Psychologist 42: 157–159

Geist H 1965 A child goes to hospital: the psychological aspects of a child going to the hospital. Charles C Thomas, Springfield, Illinois

Gil D G 1970 Violence against children: physical abuse in the United States. Harvard University Press, Cambridge

Groth A N, Burgess A W. 1977 Motivational intent in the sexual assault of children. Criminal Justice and Behavior: An International Journal of Correctional Psychology 4: 253–264

Heagarty M L, Boehringer J R, Lavigne P A, Brookes E G,

Evans M E 1973 An evaluation of the activities of nurses and pediatricians in a university outpatient department, Journal of Pediatrics 3: 875–879

Hart D 1976 The role of the play leader in the hospital. Australasian Nurses Journal 5(4): 30–32

Hart D 1979 Parents and professionals as partners. New Horizons in Education 61: 51–61

Hart S, Brassard M. 1987 A major threat to children's mental health: psychological maltreatment. American Psychologist 42: 160–165

Heinicke C M 1956 Some effects of separating two year old children from their parents. Human Relations 9: 105–176

Helfer R E 1978 Introduction — putting child abuse and neglect into perspective. In: Kalisch B J (ed) Child abuse and neglect – an annotated bibliography. Greenwood Press, Connecticut

Helfer R E 1980 Developmental deficits which limit interpersonal skills. In: Kempe C H, Helfer R E (eds) The battered child, 3rd edn. University of Chicago Press, Chicago

Howard A C 1986 Developmental play ages of physically abused and non-abused children. American Journal of Occupational Therapy 14: 691–695

Hoyle-Parent L 1978 effects of a low-stimulus environment on behavior. American Journal of Occupational Therapy 32: 19–25

Hutt C, McGrew W C 1967 Effects of group density upon social behaviour in humans. Unpublished paper. Symposium on changes in behaviour with population density. Association for the Study of Animal Behaviour, Oxford

James V L, Wheeler W E 1969 The care-by-parent unit. Pediatrics 43(4): Pt 1; 88

Jacob C G 1953 A study of the young child's contacts with staff members in a selected pediatric hospital. Nursing Research 2: 39–40

Jones D P, McQuiston M 1986 Interviewing the sexually abused child, 2nd edn. C Henry Kempe National Center, Colorado

Kashani J, Skekim W, Beck N 1987 Abuse as a predictor of psychopathology in children and adolescents. Journal of Clinical Child Psychology 16: 43–50

Kaufman J, Zigler E 1987 Do abused children become abusive parents? American Journal of Orthopsychiatry 57: 186–192

Kennell J, Jerauld R, Wolfe H, Chesler D, Kreger N C, McAlpine W, Steffa M, Klaus M H 1974 Maternal behaviour one year after early and extended post-partum contact. Developmental Medicine and Child Neurology 16: 172–179

Kielhofner G, Barris R, Bauer D, Shoestock B, Walker I 1983 A comparison of play behaviour in non-hospitalised and hospitalised children. American Journal of Occupational Therapy 37: 305–31

Klinzing D R, Klinzing D G, Schindler P D 1977 A preliminary report of a methodology to assess the communicative interaction between hospital personnel and the hospitalized child. American Journal of Public Health 67: 670671

Leonard M F, Rhymes J P, Solnit A J 1966 Failure to thrive in infants, a family problem. American Journal of Diseases of Children 111: 600–612

Lieberman A F 1977 Preschooler's competence with a peer: relations with attachment and peer experience. Child Development 48: 1277–1287

Light R J 1973 Abused and neglected children in America: a study of alternative policies. Harvard Educational Review 43: 556–598

Lindheim R, Glaser H, Coffin C 1972 Changing hospital environments for children. Havard University Press Cambridge

Lutkenhaus P, Grossman K E, Grossman K 1985 Infant–mother attachment at twelve mont and style of interaction with a stranger at the age of three years. Child Development 56: 1538–1542

McBride G, Clancy H 1973 The social properties of places and things. In: Rapoport A (ed) The mutual interaction of people and their built environment. Mouton, The Hague

McGrew W C 1972 An ethological study of children's behaviour. Academic Press, New York

Main M, Weston D 1981 The quality of the toddler's relationship to mother and to father: related to conflict behaviour and the readiness to establish new relationships. Child Development, 52: 932–940

Main M, Kaplan N, Cassidy J 1985 Security in infancy, childhood and adulthood: a move to the level of representation. In: Bretherton I, Waters E (eds) Growing points of attachment theory and research. Monographs of the society for Research in Child Development 50(1–2): 66–104

Mason E A 1965 The hospitalised child — his emotional needs. New England Journal of Medicine 272: 406–416

May G 1978 Understanding sexual child abuse. National Committee for Prevention of Child Abuse, Chicago

Morgan M K 1985 Safe touch. Rape Crisis Network, Oregon

Navarre E L 1987 Psychological maltreatment: the core component of child abuse. In: Brassard M, Germain R, Hart S (eds) Pychological matreatment of children and youth. Pergamon, New York

Newman O 1972 Defensible space. Architectural Press, London

Oates R K 1984 Parents who physically abuse their children. Australian and New Zealand Journal of Medicine 14: 291–296

Oates R K 1985 Child abuse and neglect: what happens eventually? Butterworths, Sydney

Oswin M 1973 The empty hours. Penguin, Harmondsworth

Parton N 1985 The politics of child abuse. Macmillan, London

Petrillo M, Sanger S. 1972 Emotional care of hospitalized children. Lippincott, Philadelphia

Plank E M 1962 Working with children in hospitals Lippincott. 2nd edn. Yearbook Medical Publishers, Chicago

Polansky N, Chalmers M A, Williams D, Buttenweiser E 1981 Damaged parents: an anatomy of child neglect. University of Chicago Press, Chicago

Provence S, Lipton R C 1967 Infants in institutions. International Universities Press, New York

Prugh D G, Straub E M, Sands H H, Kirschbaum M S, Lenihan E A 1953 A study of the emotional reactions of children and families to hospitalization and illness. American Journal of Orthopsychiatry 23: 70–105

Prugh D G 1965 Emotional aspects of hospitalisation of children. In: Shore M F (ed) Red is the colour of hurting:

planning for children in hospital. NIMH Bethesda, available from the Superintendent of Documents, Washington DC

Puchinger B, Zimprich H, Reiss Pateak E 1975 Empirical analysis of the behaviour of nursing staff in a children's hospital. Pediatrie und Padologie 10: 55–65

Queensland Centre for Prevention of Child Abuse 1986 Facts about child neglect. Department of Family Services, Brisbane

Reimer K 1984 The bruises don't always show: a child abuse and neglect training module. Minnesota Curriculum Services Center, White Bear Lake

Richer J, Hutchings V J 1973 Design for treatment. Health and Social Service Journal, June 23, 1425

Richer J M, Nichol S 1971 The physical environment of the mentally handicapped. British Journal of Mental Subnormality, 17: 1–12

Richmond J, Weinberger 1970 Programme implications of new knowledge regarding the physical, intellectual and emotional growth and development, and the unmet needs of children and youth. American Journal of Public Health 60: 23–28

Robertson J, Robertson J 1958 Young children in hospital. Tavistock, London

Rousseau O 1967 Mothers do help in paediatrics. American Journal of Nursing April: 798

Rutter M 1973 Maternal deprivation reassessed. Penguin, Harmondsworth

Salter A C, Richardson C M, Kairys S W 1985 Caring for abused preschoolers. Child Welfare 64: 343–356

Sandgrund A, Gaines R W, Green A H 1974 Child abuse and mental retardation: a problem of cause and effect. American Journal of Mental Deficiency 79: 327–330

Schaffer H R, Callender W M 1959 Psychologic effects of hospitalization in infancy. Pedriatrics 24: 528–539

Schultz D 1965 Sensory restriction: effects on behavior. Academic Press, New York

Sgroi S M 1984 Handbook of clinical intervention in child sexual abuse. Lexington Books, Massachusetts

Shope J 1970 Parental involvement programme. Nursing Outlook April: 32–34

Singer L M, Brodzinsky D M, Ramsay D, Stead M, Waters E 1985 Mother-infant attachment in adoptive families. Child Development 56: 1543–1551

Sommer R 1973 Personal space: the behavioral basis of design. Prentice-Hall, New Jersey

Soukup R, Wickner S, Corbett J 1984 Three in every classroom: the child victim of incest. Richards Publishing, Minnesota

Spitz R 1945 Hospitalism, an enquiry into the genesis of psychiatric conditions in early childhood. Psychoanalytic Study of the Child 1: 53–74

Springthorpe B J, Oates R K, Hayes S C 1977 Non-accidental childhood injury presenting in a hospital casualty department. Medical Journal of Australia 2: 629–632

Sroufe L A, Fox N E, Pancake V R 1983 Attachment and dependency in developmental perspective. Child Development 54: 1615–1627

Steele B F 1976 Violence within the family. In: Helfer R E, Kempe C H (eds) Child abuse and neglect – the family and the community. Ballinger, Cambridge

Steele B F 1980 Psychodynamic factors in child abuse. In: Kempe C H, Helfer R E (eds) The battered child 3rd edn. University of Chicago Press, Chicago

Steele B F 1986 Notes on the lasting effects of early child abuse throughout the life cycle. Child Abuse and Neglect 10: 283–291

Stout J 1988 Planning playgrounds for children with disabilities. American Journal of Occupational Therapy 42(10): 653–657

Thompson R A, Lamb M E 1983 Security of attachment and stranger sociability in infancy. Developmental Psychology 19: 184–191

Toro P A 1982 Developmental effects of child abuse: a review. Child Abuse and Neglect 6: 423–431

Wotton R Y 1979 Children's reactions to hospitalisation and disability. Australian Journal of Pediatric Monographs December 8–11

Young L 1986 Physical child neglect. National Committee for Prevention of Child Abuse, Chicago

Zubek J P ed. 1969 Sensory deprivation: fifteen years of research. Appleton-Century-Crofts, New York

RECOMMENDED READING

Azarnoff, Flegal 1979 A paediatric play programme. Charles C Thomas, Springfield

Cassel S, Paul M 1967 The role of puppet therapy on emotional responses of children hospitalised for cardiac catheterisation. Journal of Pediatrics 71: 233

Eckhardt L P, Prugh D G 1978 Preparing children psychologically for painful procedures. In: Gellert E (ed) Psychosocial apsects of paediatric care. Grune & Stratton, New York

Merrow D L, Johnson B S 1968 Perceptions of the mothers role with her hospitalised child. Nursing Research 17(2): 155

Peller L E 1972 The children's house. Man–Environment Systems 2(4): 221–232

Plank E M 1971 Working with children in hospitals, 2nd edn. Year Book Medical Publishers, Chicago

Seigel L J 1976 Preparation of children for hospitalisation: a selected review of the literature. Journal of Paediatric Psychology 4: 26

Showalter J E 1981 Preparation of children for hospitalisation in acute care hospitals in the United States. Pediatrics 68(3): 361–367

15. Applications for children with learning disabilities

READERS' OBJECTIVES

After reading this chapter, you should be able to:
1. Discuss the usefulness of the general term 'learning disabilities' as a clinical diagnosis.
2. Describe the typical behavioural characteristics of a learning disabled school child.
3. Describe the diagnostic evaluation process, and name two assessment procedures used by occupational therapists.
4. Discuss the theory and practice of major therapeutic and educational intervention approaches.

TERMINOLOGY AND DEFINITIONS

A child may fail in schoolwork because of the following reasons:

- A defect of sensory apparatus, e.g., deafness or visual defect.
- Intellectual subnormality and schoolwork beyond his/her capabilities.
- Minimal chronic brain syndrome which either produces (a) a limited attention span and distractability, and/or (b) perceptual difficulties involving the recognition of symbols (letters and/or words).
- A specific learning disability.
- Emotional disturbance to a degree which impairs his/her settling to a task. Such children may also not relate sufficiently well to teachers to be receptive to the learning situation.
- A home where negative attitudes to school are predominant. She/he repeatedly misses school, or truants.

Children with developmental motor disabilities face a number of difficulties over a wide range of learning tasks (Haskell et al 1977; Llorens 1970). For example, children with cerebral palsy may be restricted in ability to move or manipulate objects. The educational implications can mean that the child's ability to perform feeding, dressing, sitting, writing, and locomotion tasks is compromised.

Attempts to find or derive a precise and comprehensive definition of the term 'learning disability' are fraught with difficulty (Myers & Hammill 1982; Rie 1980). The difficulty results because we are dealing with a syndrome, that is to say, a collection of clinical manifestations or signs for which there is no known laboratory test. Learning disabilities have been referred

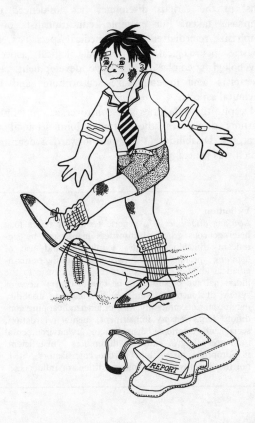

to by a variety of terms: the minimal brain dysfunction syndrome, clumsy child syndrome, psychoneurological learning disorders, and perceptual handicaps (Arnheim & Sinclair 1979; Francis-Williams 1976; Myers & Hammill 1982).

More recently, learning disabilities have been referred to as sensorimotor disorder, hyperactivity and sensory integration dysfunction. 'Hyperactivity' originates from a behavioural frame of reference, 'minimal brain dysfunction' from a neurological frame of reference and 'learning disability' from the educational framework. However, Schain (1977) suggests that in a clinical or practical sense, the terms refer to the same population. As a general rule, use of the term 'cerebral dysfunction' is preferable to cerebral damage. It helps reduce parental reaction to long past obstetrical events, and places the emphasis on functional issues rather than a damage/undamaged dichotomy. Often too, there is no clear evidence that damage has occurred, and problems are not detected until the child starts school, and mostly around the ages of 7–9 years.

Another reason for the variety of terminology is that workers in many disciplines have contributed to the field of learning disabilities, and each has highlighted particular aspects or approaches. Thus the 'conceptual lens' of the various disciplines has influenced the emphasis taken. For example, educationalists often emphasize remedial education, medical specialists emphasize neurological and pharmacological aspects, psychologists emphasize cognitive development, and therapists tend to emphasize sensorimotor and behavioural aspects.

Despite the difficulties and controversies in defining learning disabilities, the National Joint Council for Learning Disabilities (1981) put forward a definition which was generally accepted.

Definition

Learning disabilities is a generic term that refers to a heterogeneous group of disorders manifested by significant difficulties in the acquisition and use of listening, speaking, reading, writing, reasoning or mathematical abilities. These disorders are intrinsic to the individual and presumed to be due to central nervous system dysfunction. Even though a learning disability may occur concomitantly with other handicapping conditions (e.g., sensory impairment, mental retardation, social and emotional disturbance) or environmental influences (e.g., cultural differences, insufficient/inappropriate instruction, psychogenic factors), it is not the direct result of those conditions or influences

---

The child whose tested intelligence is normal, but who fails to progress in *one* area of schoolwork is usually described as suffering from a *specific learning disability* (Clements & Peters 1981). Reading disability or dyslexia or word blindness is the commonest specific learning disability and will be discussed further. Other handicaps may be dysgraphia (writing difficulty often associated with minor degrees of motor inco-ordination) and acalculia, difficulty with number concepts. If a child cannot read then she/he is unlikely to be able to spell.

A child is regarded as dyslexic, that is suffering from reading retardation when his/her reading age is two years or more behind his/her mental age. Dyslexic children may be grouped as follows:

1. Those in whom there is some demonstrable brain damage (minimal chronic brain syndrome).
2. Those in whom there is no demonstrable damage, or history of possible cerebral injury. However quite often there is a history of reading retardation in the males of the family.
3. Those children who have the capacity to read, but are unable to because of emotional or social factors, i.e., the reading disability is secondary to some other condition.

Children of the first two groups may suffer from *auditory* or *visual* perceptual difficulties. They commonly reverse letters or syllable, for example 'p' for 'q', 'saw' for 'was'. The child is unable to associate concepts with written symbols, and the syndrome may be part of a wider general *language* disability. There may be a history of delayed speech development. The WISC (Wechsler Intelligence Scale for Children) may show a verbal IQ 20 points or more below the performance IQ.

Many children who are dyslexic pass unrecognized at school, and are castigated by teachers, parents and peers for supposed 'stupidity' or 'laziness'. Schoolroom activities, such as taking turns in reading-out-aloud to class members can be very anxiety provoking to these children. Secondary emotional disturbance is extremely common, and these children may find their way to Child Guidance Clinics because of behavioural disturbance.

Incidence

Epidemiological studies of children with 'learning disabilities' are meagre, and the findings are conflicting (Walzer & Richmond 1973; Wender 1971). Lack of agreement stems from confusion in diagnosis (Nichols & Chen 1981; Swanson & Reinert 1979) and the absence of definitive, operational criteria for distinguishing between children who have problems learning, and those who are learning disabled per se (Myers & Hammill 1982).

It is estimated that between 5% and 10% of the school population suffer from minor neurological deficits which impair their efficiency, particularly in school achievement (Hayes 1979; Walzer & Richmond 1973). Boys are affected at least three times more than girls (Safer & Allen 1976; Weiss & Hechtman 1979; Wender 1971) with male first borns especially at risk (Solomon 1978).

Aetiology

Many aetiologies may give rise to the usually described clinical picture, namely:

a. Maternal factors

Abnormalities of pregnancy, prolonged and precipitous labour, multiple births, and prematurity can lead to brain damage in the infant. Additionally, maternal factors which affect the fetus, e.g., rubella, drugs including alcohol and smoking, toxaemia and RH incompatibility are other conditions which give rise to brain dysfunction.

Pasamanick and Knobloch (1966) suggest a continuum of reproductive casualty with obvious brain damage at one end (associated with such conditions as cerebral palsy and severe mental retardation) and minor defect at the other.

In Table 15.1 the varying manifestations of brain damage are represented as they have been reported in the literature.

Many children with minimal chronic brain syndrome do have a history consistent with cerebral insult, or an unfavourable intrauterine environment. (See Drillian & Drummond 1977)

b. Abuse to the child — 'the Forbes Syndrome' (See Chapter 14)

Prolonged abuse of a child either physically or by neglect, can result in neurological damage to the child which may result in 'learning disability'.

c. Minor congenital abnormalities

There may be a history suggestive of a hereditary basis in that some members of the patient's family suffer from the same defects.

d. Major cerebral dysfunctions

Included in this category are mental retardation; hyperkinetic behaviour disorder; cerebral palsy and all conditions where there is actual physical impairment in some part of the central nervous system.

e. Environmental factors

Sufficient environmental stress within a family, in the absence of any organic factor, may give rise to some of the features that characterize 'learning disorder syndrome'.

Table 15.1 Minor and major clinical and behavioural manifestations of brain damage

Defective System	Clinical and behavioural manifestations	
	Minor	Major
Motor	Clumsiness Tremor Inco-ordination Abnormal EEG — no clinical signs Over-/underactivity	Cerebral palsy syndromes Epilepsy Over-/underactivity
Sensory	Perceptual defects e.g., visuo-spatial, tactile, vestibular	Cortical blindness Deafness
Intellectual	Inconsistent developmental achievement	Severe intellectual disability
Language	Expressive/receptive language incompetence	Aphasia
Social skills	Developmental delay e.g., in ADL, in social interactive skills	Kanner's syndrome (autism)

Behavioural characteristics

A child who is designated as 'learning disabled' is typically described by adults, as one who:

— is failing in the formal school situation, and/or
— is clumsy with motor tasks, and/or
— cannot seem to get him/herself around his/her physical environment, and/or
— avoids/dislikes sport activities, and/or
— is messy, and/or
— attracts unwelcome attention from adults because of social behaviour.

On closer examination, the child may demonstrate:

1. Varying degrees of motor behaviour dysfunction.
2. Distorted perceptual functioning: about relationship of child's body to space, and about relationship between forms, i.e., between objects.
3. Impaired ability to deal with abstract conceptual thought.
4. Disturbed social behaviour — inattention, overactive behaviour, attention-seeking, lowered tolerance to frustration and demands, temper outbursts.

There is an implication that in the general syndrome of learning disability there is an information processing problem which stems from something other than specific neurological lesions, or from environmental experience. Disorders are related to thought, memory, speech/language, neuro-muscular co-ordination, reading and writing.

The behaviour characteristics will be examined in greater detail, and may be categorized as: motor defects, sensory and perceptual defects, hyperkinetic impulse disorders, intellectual difficulties, disorders of language function, electroencephalograph abnormalities (EEG), and secondary emotional disturbance.

Motor defects

— gross movements, e.g., walking or skipping
— fine movements, e.g., doing up buttons
— visual-motor integration, e.g., writing
— slight degrees of choreoathetosis
— synkinesis — that is, associated (minor) movements persisting at an age when they should have been outgrown. For example, the child brushes his teeth with his right hand, while his left hand replicates the movements.
— localised groups of muscles show spasticity or hypotonia, for example, squint is common.

Sensory and perceptual defects

Minor sensory defects may occur, and probably reflect cortical level dysfunction. A far more common finding is difficulties in perceptual processing. Sensory stimuli are transmitted normally but the child fails to organize meaningful patterns from the input. She/he has difficulty in abstracting, conceptualizing and generalizing. Auditory, visual, kinaesthetic, tactile and even social cues may be missed or misinterpreted. There is often:

— confusion with left/right discrimination
— poor body orientation in space and time
— a distorted body image (revealed by drawings)
— reading and writing difficulties — for example, the letter 'p' substituted for 'q', or 'd' for 'b', persisting beyond the normal age — about 7–8 years.
— delayed development of hand and eye dominance.

Hyperkinetic impulse disorder

Hyperkinesis is persistent purposeless motor activity, common especially in the early years of an affected child. Hyperkinesis is also typically associated with the following behaviour:

— great difficulty in attending to a task — the child is very readily distracted.
— the child attempts to gratify impulses instantly, and seems unable to wait. Attempts to prolong gratification lead to displays of 'explosive irritability'. If faced with major frustration, such as the adult insisting on prolonging need gratification, the child may react with what is called a 'catastrophic reaction' (Haskell et al 1977). The child is quite overwhelmed by emotion, and may cry uncontrollably, shout, scream, kick and throw objects if not restrained.
— the child exhibits a driving impulse to explore objects by handling and mouthing long after such behaviour has normally disappeared. One theory is that the child cannot maintain visual fixation long enough to explore in the more mature visual manner.

These behaviour patterns are associated with educational difficulties, accident proneness and tensions within the child's family.

Intellectual difficulties

There is no direct and inevitable link between intelligence and learning disability. It is of interest that a child who does not have any other obvious disability, such as cerebral palsy, will often have a testable IQ which is quite at variance in his or her family. This can often be accounted for by the child's failure on certain aspects of testing, which has a global effect on the test result. Solomon (1978) notes that learning disabled children tend to have near to average, or above average intelligence.

Language disorders

Disorders of language function may be manifest in spoken language, such as listening and speaking, and also in written language, such as reading and writing.

Children with congenital aphasia, or more properly dysphasia, may be included in the learning disability syndrome. However, it is important to differentiate between disorders of higher language function and poor language skills due to motor inco-ordination. That is to say that while speech impairments such as dysarthria, poor articulation and stuttering may lead to untelligible speech, these conditions do not effect the quality of ideas and grammar. Hence speech disorders per se are not considered language disorders.

Abnormalities of the electroencephalogram (EEG)

Though there is no history of clinical epilepsy, affected children frequently have EEG abnormality. About 35%–50% of children with a learning disability have an abnormal EEG compared with approximately 15% of the general population (Stevens et al 1968).

Secondary emotional disturbance

Because affected children mostly look quite normal, yet perform poorly, they receive little sympathy, and are frequently and inappropriately regarded as 'stupid' or 'lazy', or undisciplined, by parents and teachers. Mostly the child is intelligent enough to know that she/he should do better, and becomes extremely frustrated, demoralized, angry with self, or with others, for example parents and other siblings. Conflict between the parents and child, with secondary emotional disturbance is almost universal if the syndrome remains unrecognized during the early primary school years.

EVALUATION

The process

Following referral to a medical specialist the child will undergo:

— a comprehensive physical, neurological examination including an electroencephalogram (EEG). The major role of the EEG is to identify focal lesions and help diagnose underlying seizure diathesis such as petit mal.
— psychometric assessment, to establish a general intelligence quotient, and a learning skills behavioural profile.

The Wechsler Intelligence Scale for Children (WISC) is often used to identify: (a) a disparity between actual IQ and expected IQ. A verbal IQ of 20 or more points above performance IQ is a common finding. (b) a scatter in sub-tests, involving abstraction of information.
— specialist therapy evaluations

The psychologist may also demonstrate visual-perceptual difficulties (Frostig, Bender-Gestalt tests), visual-motor integration difficulties (Berry-Butenica test) and psycholinguistic difficulties (Illinois Test of Psycholinguistic Abilities). It has been found that many affected children show evidence of crossed laterality. For example, the child may have a left dominant eye yet be right handed and footed.

The occupational therapy component of evaluation will usually comprise:

— a general developmental assessment, e.g., the Gesell Developmental Appraisal, or the Griffiths Test of Mental Abilities 1970 (approved users) see Appendix VI.
— a screening test for specific learning disabilities, e.g., the Meeting Street School Screening Test.
— specific tests of skills needed·for effective formal learning. There are many available, and those chosen will reflect the particular theoretical orientation of the therapy facility. Some recommended examples are: The Pupil Readiness for Educational Behaviour (PREB), from the Teaching Resource Programmes Inc (see reference at the end of this chapter); The Ongoing Evaluation and Performance Scale (Knickerbocker 1980); the battery of sensory-integrative function tests (Ayres 1972, 1974, 1979); A Psycho-educational Evaluation of Basic Learning Abilities (Valett 1967, 1977); Frostig Evaluation Programmes (Frostig 1972; Frostig & Frostig 1969).
— observation of behaviour, specifically social interactions with peers, with adults, in structured task situations such as the school room, and in unstructured activity situations, such as the school playground and a fine motor play situation.

Together, the results from all assessments will provide a comprehensive picture of a child's developmental maturity, basic skills, and formal learning skills — both strengths and weaknesses.

INTERVENTION

Pharmacology

There is no global drug regime which is effective with children who have identified learning disabilities. If used at all, medication must be targeted at specific behaviour disorders, e.g. the control of epileptic seizures. The exception is in the case of a child with a diagnosis of hyperkinetic impulse disorder, where drugs play a very important part in management (Capute & Accardo 1980). The children often show idiosyncratic responses, both to the type of drug and its dose, and trial and error may be the only way of arriving at optimal treatment. This syndrome may require long-term administration of drugs, such as:

— Trial of phenothiazine tranquillizer, increasing the dose until the child responds, or adverse effects are noted. If unsuccessful, another phenothiazine may be tried, or a tranquilliser from a different group, e.g., haloperidol.
— The use of psychic energizers which have a calming effect in some children, and are used as the drug of choice by some workers in the United States.

Parental support, a regular routine with few distractions and limited demands on the child must complement drug treatment.

Diet

The most famous intervention approach using a special diet is the Feingold diet used with children displaying the hyperkinetic impulse disorder. Dr Ben Feingold (1976) of Kaiser Permanente Medical Centre, proposed that hyperactive children are allergic to natural salicylates, and to some artificial food colouring additives. Salicylates are found in a range of fruits, vegetables and cereals.

Dr Feingold found that when all food colourings and flavourings are removed from the diet of a hyperkinetic child, a noticeable change occurred in the child's behaviour. Initially observed changes are said to be loss of hyperactivity, aggression and impulsiveness. It is suggested that these changes are soon followed by improvement in muscular co-ordination as indicated by improved writing and drawing abilities, greater facility with speech and loss of clumsiness.

Disturbances in cognitions and perception are usually the last to respond. With an increased attention span which permits greater concentration, scholastic achievement improves rapidly.

Age seems to be an important determining factor in the degree and speed of response to dietary management. The younger the child, the more rapid and dramatic is the improvement.

Others have advocated the use of vitamins as a useful additive to diet (Cott 1972; Scrimshaw & Gordon 1968).

Special approaches

In the treatment of syndromes, it is common for specialists to promote their own theories about the causative factors and develop their own treatment plans. The particular theory and practical approach is, naturally enough, strongly influenced by the frame of reference of the individual.

An overview of the major theories and treatment interventions of learning disabilities is presented.

Educational

Until quite recently it was usually the child's teacher who recognized that the affected child was different. Those who have been highly influential in directing educational practice have taken the view that competent motor behaviour is the basis for all successful learning. Maria Montessori first expressed this idea and developed it in the context of a rich experiential curriculum which sought to deal with all aspects of a child's life — from doing up clothes to making complex decisions. Piaget's (1962) theoretical work about stages in the development of mature intelligence emphasized that the sensorimotor stage underlies all operational intelligence.

Skinner's studies on the control of behaviour through operant conditioning has contributed further to classroom practice (Lahey 1979).

Thus today, a teacher faced with a learning disabled child, is likely to lean heavily on the techniques of the physical education specialist teacher, and to combine motor activities with sensory learning approaches such as those of Montessori. These techniques may be used within the structured framework of behaviour modification.

Perceptual-motor

This framework has perhaps had the most pervasive and powerful influence on intervention approaches with learning disabled children.

The aim of perceptual-motor approaches is to make the participant (the child) a better learner. The theories of Hebb (1949) form the basis of this approach. Kephart (1960, 1963) regarded the 'slow learner' as one who has a breakdown in the ability to process information from the various sense channels. Posture is seen as the primary movement pattern, on which all other motor patterns are based. He conceived of learning as dependent on four basic movement generalizations:

— locomotion
— reaching and grasping objects
— balance and posture
— propelling objects

Kephart delineated the construct of laterality, that is, recognition of a right and left side of the body, and argued that these constructs are necessary for movement efficiency, and the ability to recognize symbols. Figure–ground discrimination was seen as necessary for reading, and body image was seen as necessary for a sense of relationship to surrounding space. Kephart's intervention relies on the practice of ritual motor movements, beginning with simple movements and graduating to more complex movements. Activities such as puzzles, pegboards, finger painting and dot-to-dot drawings are also used (Myers & Hammill 1982).

The Doman–Delacato method. The work of Delacato (1959, 1963) arises from the framework of perceptual motor training. The Doman–Delacato system rests on the concept of 'neurological organization'. The central theme is one of establishing normal patterns of motor behaviour by a system of passive or active movements, i.e., patterning, based on normal reflex behaviour. A multi-sensory approach is used and is said to re-establish normal integrative responses within the brain. Hebb's influence is seen in the emphasis on establishing 'memory traces' in the central nervous system. Kephart's influence is seen in the emphasis on motor behaviour as the basis of all other learning.

Although the original theory and practice was focused on children with relatively severe motor and other handicaps, it has become widely applied to children with learning difficulties, particularly reading problems (National Health and Medical Research Council 1977).

The Doman–Delacato approach is one which parents will enquire about, and may elect to try. It has been widely criticized for its theory (Kerschner 19683) Mc-Keith 1974), treatment methods (National Health and Medical Research Council 1977; Tannock 1976), restrictions on the child (Hudson et al 1978) and the demands on the family (for a detailed critique see Cummins (1988)). The major criticisms may be summarized:

• The claim that patterning affects the brain directly.
• The exclusion of the child from normal activity, and the need for vast manpower to implement the procedures.
• The lack of systematic research to back dogmatic claims for the system.
• The questionable validity of the Doman–Delacato neurological developmental profile.

Sensory integrative therapy. Ayres (1972), an occupational therapist, is another who has derived a theory and therapy system within the perceptual-motor training framework.

Ayres' approach derived from her clinical experience, and is based on general principles or theories of brain function. Like Rood (1954), Ayres held that integrative neural mechanisms link sensory input and motor output (Myers & Hammill 1982), and that the brain develops sequentially, with each new step dependent on the development of preceding skills (Ayres 1972, 1974, 1979). The prime objective of the sensory integrative approach is to enhance the ability of the brain to learn by modifying the impact of any neurological dysfunction. This approach differs in that the child is not instructed in routines, nor is an attempt made to eliminate *causes* of inadequate neurological organization (Price et al 1976). Ayres proposed three treatment principles, namely:

• The control of sensory input with emphasis on the convergence of sensory pathways, in particular tactile and vestibular pathways.
• Promotion of adaptive motor responses, mediated at the brainstem level.
• The replication of normal development sequence of skill acquisition.

Ayres' sensory integrative approach has stimulated a large amount of research, particularly in the areas of vestibular touch/tactile, proprioception and visual systems. While originally developed for use with children, it has also been used with adults.

Neurophysiological approaches

Neurophysiological approaches all rely on two propositions:

1. Ontogeny recapitulates phylogeny.
2. There is a relationship between proprioception and voluntary movement.

Neurodevelopmental treatment. This approach was developed by Karl and Berta Bobath, respectively a neurologist and physiotherapist (Bobath 1970, Wilcock 1986).

Neurodevelopmental treatment aims to normalize muscle tone and provide the sensation of normal movement patterns. The methods used involve inhibiting primitive phasic and tonic reflex activity, followed by immediate facilitation of righting and equilibrium reactions, according to a predictable development sequence.

The neurodevelopmental approach has been used with hemiplegic patients, those with Parkinson's disease, multiple sclerosis, cerebral palsy and other disorders of the motor system.

Proprioceptive neuromuscular facilitation (PNF). In the late 1940s Herman Kabat, a neurologist, devised a treatment approach based on the neurophysiological works of Sherrington, Gellhorn and Hellbrandt (Kabat & Knott 1953). Two physiotherapists, Knott & Voss (1968), expanded and refined the PNF approach.

As the name suggests, the techniques of PNF are aimed at promoting or hastening the response of the neuromuscular mechanism, by the stimulation of the proprioceptors (Knott & Voss 1968). Mass movement patterns which are spiral and diagonal are considered basic to all other techniques (Trombly & Scott 1977). Electrical stimulation and cold are used as adjuncts to treatment. Other techniques of PNF are:

— maximal resistance
— stretch
— stimulation of reflexes
— reversal of antagonists
— positioning and verbal command.

PNF has been applied to the treatment of a variety of conditions including rheumatoid arthritis, multiple sclerosis, amputee re-education, Parkinson's disease, spinal cord injury and brain dysfunction.

Rood. Rood (1954), an occupational therapist and physiotherapist, also developed an approach derived from clinical experience and based on neurophysiological and developmental theory. Rood's theoretical approach can be summarized as follows:

• Motor output is dependent on sensory input. Thus sensory stimuli can be used to activate and/or inhibit motor responses.
• Motor responses follow a developmental sequence.
• Movement is purposeful.
• Activity elicits desired movement patterns at a subcortical level, without the need for a patient's conscious or deliberate control.

Rood uses a variety of techniques to facilitate or inhibit muscle contraction and modify muscle tone. Some of the techniques include brushing, stroking, icing, warmth, vibration, pressure and tapping as well as olfactory, auditory and visual input (Pedretti 1981; Semans 1965; Trombly & Scott 1977). Rood's approach has been used with a variety of patients displaying developmental and neurological problems.

Conductive Education — Peto Method. Conductive education was devised by a Hungarian neurologist/educator, Professor Andras Peto, who established the Institute for Conductive Education in Budapest and directed it until his death in 1967. Conductive education is a structured training scheme for use with children who have sustained a central nervous insult, specifically cerebral palsied children. It is now used internationally as an intervention scheme.

The objective of conductive education is to prepare the handicapped child for normal education and home life, through a learning programme that integrates intellectual, linguistic and functional skills (Cotton 1965, 1975). Conductive education differs from other approaches in that the cognitive abilities of the child are stressed and incorporated into treatment. Some elements of the Peto method include the use of a 'conductor', 'rhythmical intention' groups, a designed physical environment and a long-term programme with complementary daily routine.

Although conductive education was originally designed for use with cerebral palsied children, it has also been used on other neurological conditions.

Myers & Hammill (1982) note that the treatment approaches of various professions tend to fall into two distinct and often conflicting camps, namely 'those who advocated the direct instruction of reading, writing, speaking and so on, and those who advocated the training of certain psycho-cognitive abilities presumed to underlie or greatly influence proficiency in reading, writing, speaking and so on.' Occupational therapists have mostly focused on those skills which underpin formal reading and writing activities, e.g., shape recognition and other perceptual competencies as well as motor skill competencies. Thus would probably be fair to say that occupational therapy intervention has tended to be in the latter 'camp' with the work of Rood and Ayres being particularly influential. However, it is our contention that the two approaches are complementary rather than competing. Cratty (1967) and Cratty & Martin (1969) summarize the state of the art about applications for children who fail at school.

1. Movement activities are helpful only to the extent that they enable a child to think about the sequence, variety and nature of the movements in which she/he is engaged.

2. Motor tasks may aid in the development of certain perceptual attributes. Visual-motor co-ordination is important to accurate hand movement for writing and drawing.
3. Improved motor task proficiency, reflected in better fitness and sport skills, may result in the increased academic performance of some children with learning problems, because their self-concept has been enhanced.
4. Movement experiences, if properly applied, may help some hyperactive children to place themselves under better control which will, in turn, lead toward increased competence in classroom tasks.
5. Visual training may aid those children who have demonstrated visual dysfunction. A careful visual examination must precede any such training and, the components of the training programme must be related to remediation of the identified specific deficits.
6. Structured movement programmes in which creeping and crawling are employed are of questionable value in the remediation of anything but severe motor ineptitude.
7. Helpful to the identification of children with potential reading problems are measures of (a) drawing; (b) scores obtained from measures of co-ordination tasks collected from preschool children; (c) evaluation of various visual attributes.

OCCUPATIONAL THERAPY

Occupational therapy approaches to children who display learning disabilities are focused on the development of functional competence (Brereton et al 1975). Broadly, the therapy is directed at the following areas:

— development of efficient motor behaviour
— development of efficient sensory-perceptual skill integration
— development of conceptual and body awareness skills
— development of mature social behaviour.

Efficient motor behaviour

Various authors have reported that 40–50% of children identified as having learning disabilities, with or without the hyperkinetic syndrome, have movement disorders (e.g., De Quiros 1976; Sevine et al 1975; Silver et al 1969). All treatment approaches have programme components directed at movement and motor behaviour. The difference is not so much in what is done to and

with the child, but in the beliefs about why it is being done, and what the activities will achieve.

The choice of programme and activities will, to some extent be determined by the severity of the child's movement dysfunction. For example, the Bobath and Peto methods are specifically designed for severely dysfunctional children who have cerebral palsy. On the other hand, the programmes of Valett (1967, 1977), Knickerbocker (1980), Cratty (1967) and Ayres (1972, 1974, 1979) are well suited to the child who shows only soft neurological signs, if any. A modern approach of considerable interest is that of Lazlo & Bairstow (1985) and Lazlo et al (1988). These authors focus specifically on the contribution of kinaesthetic perception to integrated movement and sensory functioning in the child with a learning disability. Lazlo and colleagues have developed an assessment and intervention programme, which is rationalized by reference to basic theory and experimental studies with young children, and focuses on the following:

— gross motor skill development, e.g., jumping, ball throwing
— fine motor skill, e.g., tying shoelaces
— spatial body awareness, expressed through body localization

A programme implemented in a normal school setting for a group of identified learning disabled children is presented in Example 15.1.

Watter & Bullock (1983) measured changes in academic scores, on the Milton Word Recognition Test over a 12-month period, as a function of a developmental physiotherapy programme with MCD and learning disabled children. These authors demonstrated positive gains by the children, and concluded that the most effective regime was that combining the experimental programme with remedial education. Other authors have also demonstrated gains in motor competency (e.g. Arnheim & Sinclair 1979).

Sensory-perceptual skill integration

The areas which are addressed include:

— directionality
— tactile discrimination
— laterality
— balance and body-spatial organization
— time orientation

Again, many programmes have been developed as remediation. Probably the one which has attracted most

---

Example 15.1: Programme for developing competent motor behaviour and body/spatial relationship awareness

Week 1

1. Roll like a log along a carpeted surface.
2. Lie on back, and curl up like a ball and rock in that position.
3. Ask children to assume the 'Superman' position, i.e., lying on tummy with head up, arms off the floor, and legs off the floor with knees straight.
4. Rub own body parts with different textures and feel the variations in textures. For example, hessian, towelling, silk, brushes, sandpaper, plastic, etc.
5. 'Make the room larger.' Ask the children if there is some way that they can make the room larger, e.g., move the walls out by pushing out or pushing the floor down. Get the children to collectively attempt to move a wall back by applying pressure with both hands, or lying on their back and pushing the wall with their feet. They may also attempt to push the floor down.
6. Walking heel-to-toe along a rope path, or a chalk line.
7. Obstacle course, e.g., getting the children to crawl over and under chairs and tables in varying positions.
8. Stand and throw a bean bag at a target.

Week 2

1. Rolling fast, then rolling slowly along a carpeted surface.
2. Curl up like a ball, and then roll along the mat, trying to stay curled up.
3. Assume 'Superman' position, and hold for as long as possible.
4. Separate children into pairs, then get them to rub their partners different body parts with a textured cloth, and identify the part.
5. 'Push me over'. Separate into pairs: one child remains in a fixed position and the other tries to push him over. Play this game in varying position, e.g., sitting, kneeling, lying down, and standing.
6. Walk heel-to-toe along thin line or a balance board, keeping a weight on the head (e.g., book).
7. Obstacle course. Add more components, e.g., between objects, through, around, etc.
8. Bounce and catch a ball.

---

attention in recent years is sensory integration therapy of Ayres (1972).

Ayres postulates that most rapid maturation of a child's nervous system occurs before eight years of age. Therefore, she urges that therapy be implemented as early as possible in a child's life.

Three types of sensory stimuli are considered most appropriate: vestibular; tactile; proprioceptive.

The theoretical rationale is that these stimuli have a pervasive effect on brain function, and enhance the general arousal level, thereby putting the child into a learning state of 'readiness'. Ayres postulates that visual and auditory perception training should follow a programme of vestibular, tactile and proprioceptive therapy

Specific evaluation has been designed as part of the approach, and comprises:

— SCSIT (Southern California Sensory Integration Tests) — 18 sub-tests, 4–8 years 11 months
— Motor accuracy test, now available to 10 years
— Clinical observations — 17 sub-tests
— Post Rotatory nystagmus test.

Reliability of the motor accuracy test is said to be very acceptable, but that does not appear to hold true for other sub-tests.

Examples of sensory integrative therapy activities are well described by Ayres (1972, 1974, 1979), Price et al (1976), Knickerbocker (1980). Ziviani et al (1982) reported changes associated with a 13-week therapy programme based on neurodevelopmental and sensory integrative procedures. Positive changes were noted in motor skill performance of children in learning disabled classes. Specifically, the limb functions of speed, dexterity, visual-motor control and co-ordination were most altered. These skill areas are essential to, for example, competent reading, writing, using scissors. The study by Ziviani et al is a valuable indicator of the potential of the sensory integrative approach for controlled experimental evaluation of therapy effects.

Conceptual and body awareness skills

'Self-concept' is a generic label to describe the way in which a person views him or herself, for example, as 'good', 'bad', 'attractive', 'unattractive', 'worthy', 'worthless', 'competent', and so on. Some of the child's feelings of self relate to and/or are influenced by his or her ability to perform motor tasks. For a boy, the ability to play sports and his physique are important factors influencing self-confidence and popularity; while for a girl, particularly during adolescence, her figure is important to her feelings of self. Body build may also influence personality (Kagan 1966).

An important component of self-concept is body image. Body image involves the ability to discriminate between right and left, up and down, position in space, body size, location of bodily parts, etc. Verbal-cognitive and movement training influence and enhance the development of body image. In respect to the influence of movement on the development of body image, children often know their right hand because that is the hand they write with.

Cratty & Martin (1969) provide some useful guidelines for helping in the training of body image. These guidelines are graded in degree of complexity and make use of verbal-cognitive factors and movement components.

Social behaviour

It is well recognized that children with learning difficulties often have secondary behavioural problems and this will be an area of intervention by the occupational therapist. Some children may present as openly anxious or aggressive whilst others may present as withdrawn or defeated. It is essential to structure tasks so that children experience success. A fuller discussion on managing behaviour problems, is presented in Chapter 16.

SUMMARY

There are many reasons why children fail to learn at school, and a brief review has been provided in this chapter. The confusion in terminology applied to children with learning disabilities has impeded our understanding of the aetiologies, especially for those children who do not display frank, or extreme signs and symptoms of cerebral dysfunction. Some of the older diagnostic labels are still in use, e.g., the minimal cerebral dysfunction syndrome, the clumsy child syndrome. However, the modern emphasis has shifted to examining and directing remedial action at functional disabilities which interfere with the affected child's ability to achieve full potential, both developmentally, and specifically at school.

The diagnostic process brings together medical and educational specialists, perhaps more closely than in any other area of intervention with children. Drugs may have a small role to play. However, the most influential

intervention yet available to us, are approaches which seek to shape and refine emerging developmental skills. These approaches also provide compensatory ways to assist the affected child minimize interference of specific motor, sensory and perceptual disabilities.

There is no experimental evidence to support a view that any one of the many intervention approaches available is more effective, or to be preferred over all others (Wilcock 1986). Myers & Hammill (1982) even question whether the approaches which address sensory, motor and perceptual skill development and remediation are not, in fact, merely variations on a theme. Thus, at our present stage of research and objective evaluation, therapists and other specialists are justified in selecting pragmatically among the many excellent practical programmes available, with one proviso. There is no evidence that there is any validity in those programmes which claim a causal link between movement activity, increased measurable intelligence and improved academic (schoolwork) scores.

Occupational therapists have been very active in clinical research about the possible reasons underlying learning difficulties. One area of research has received considerable attention both inside and beyond the profession. Namely, the role of sensory integration and dysfunction in the production of learning difficulties.

Sensory integration therapy is still experimental, and for that reason exciting. The objectives are to take data about a given child's sensory perceptual and motor functions, as discovered on standardized tests, and systematically design treatment measures to deal with the problems discovered by the tests. The accompanying therapy is important as an example of the profession seeking to be more systematic and rational in treatment designs. Data is being amassed to allow objective evaluation of the theory and arguments. Whatever the verdict proves to be about this one approach, and its attendant therapy practices, occupational therapists have established themselves as valuable and economically sound members of the educational team in the normal school system.

REFERENCES

Arnheim D D, Sinclair W A 1979 The clumsy child: a program of motor ability, 2nd edn. C V Mosby, St Louis

Ayres A J 1972 Sensory integration and learning disorders. Western Psychological Services, Los Angeles

Ayres A J 1974 The development of sensory integrative theory and practice. Kendall Hunt Iowa

Ayres A J 1979 Sensory integration and the child. Western Psychological Services, Los Angeles

Bobath B 1970 Adult hemiplegia: evaluation and treatment.

William Heinemann Medical Books, London

Brereton L G, Sattler J, Ironside M 1975 Cerebral palsy: basic abilities. Spastic Centre New South Wales, Mosman, Sydney

Capute A J, Accardo P 1980 The minimal cerebral dysfunction/learning disability syndrome complex. In: Gabel J, Erickson M T (eds) Child Development and developmental disabilities. Little Brown, Boston

Clements S D, Peters J E 1981 Syndromes of minimal brain

dysfunction. In: Black P (ed) Brain dysfunction in children: etiology, diagnosis and management. Raven Press, New York

Cott A 1972 Megavitamins: the orthomolecular approach to behavioural disorders and learning disabilities. Academic Therapy 7: 245–258

Cotton E 1965 The Institute for Movement Therapy and School for Conductors, Budapest, Hungary. Developmental Medicine and Child Neurology 17: 437–446

Cotton E 1975 Conductive education and cerebral palsy. The Spastics Society, London

Cratty B J 1967 Movement behaviour and motor learning (2nd ed). Lea & Febiger, Philadelphia

Cratty B J, Martin M M 1969 Perceptual-motor efficiency in children. Lea & Febiger, Philadelphia

Cummins R A 1988 The neurologically impaired child: Doman–Delacato techniques reappraised. Croom Helm, London

Delacato C H 1959 The treatment and prevention of reading problems. Charles C Thomas, Springfield

Delacato C H 1963 The diagnosis and treatment of speech and reading problems. Charles C Thomas, Springfield, Illinois

De Quiros J 1976 Diagnosis of vestibular disorders in the learning disabled. Journal of Learning Disabilities 9(1): 50–58

Drillien C M, Drummond M B, 1977 Neurodevelopmental problems of early childhood. Blackwell, Oxford

Farnham-Diggory S 1978 Learning disabilities. Harvard University Press, Cambridge

Feingold B 1976 Hyperkinesis and learning disabilities linked to the ingestion of artifical food colors and flavors. Journal of Learning Disabilities 9: 551–559

Francis-Williams J 1978 Early identification of children likely to have specific learning difficulties. Report of a follow up. Developmental Medicine and Child Neurology 18: 71

Frostig M 1972 Visual perception, integrative function and academic learning. Journal of Learning 5: 1–15

Frostig M, Frostig M G L 1969 Move-grow-learn, movement education activities by Marianne Frostig. Follett, Chicago

Griffiths R 1970 The abilities of young children. Child Development Research Centre, London

Haskell S H, Barrett E K, Taylor H 1977 The education of motor and neurologically handicapped children. Croom Helm, London

Hayes U 1979 A developmental approach to casefinding among infants and young children. US Department of Health, Education and Welfare, DHEW Publicaton, Rockville

Hebb D O 1949 The organisation of behaviour. Wiley, New York

Hudson A M, Murphy A C, Clunies-Ross A A 1978 Research into the Doman–Delacato Method: implications for special educators. Australian Journal of Special Education 2(1): 17–10

Kabat H, Knott M 1953 Proprioceptive facilitation techniques for the treatment of paralysis. Physical Therapy Review 33: 53–63

Kagan J 1966 Body build and conceptual impulsivity in children. Journal of Personality 34: 118–128

Kephart N C 1960 The slow learner in the classroom. Merrill, Columbus

Kephart N C 1963 The brain injured child in the classroom. National Society for Crippled Children and Adults, Chicago

Kershner J R 1968 Doman–Delacato theory of neurological organisation applied with retarded children. Exceptional Children 34: 441–450

Knickerbocker B M 1980 A holistic approach to the treatment of learning disorders. Charles B Slack, Thorofare NJ

Knott M, Voss D 1968 Proprioceptive neuromuscular facilitation: patterns and techniques, 2nd end. Harper & Row, Hagerstown

Lahey B B 1979 Behaviour therapy with hyperactive and learning disabled children. Oxford University Press, Oxford

Lazlo J I, Bairstow P J 1985 Perceptual motor behaviour: developmental assessment and therapy. Holt Rinehart & Winston, Eastbourne

Lazlo J I, Bairstow P J, Bartrip J 1988 A new approach to treatment of perceptual-motor dysfunction — previously called clumsiness. Support for Learning 3: 35–40

Llorens L A 1970 Facilitating growth and development: the promise of occupational therapy. American Journal of Occupational Therapy 24(2): 93–101

McKeith R 1974 Questions and answers about Doman–Delacato. Intellectually Handicapped Child Sept/Nov 22–25

Myers P I, Hammill D D 1982 Learning disabilities. Proceedings — Education, Austin

National Health and Medical Research Council 1977 Report of the therapeutic methods sub-committee to investigate the methods used by the institute for the achievement of human potential. Australian Government Publishing Service, Canberra

National Joint Committee for Learning Disabilities 1981 Learning disabilities: issues of definition. In: Myers P L, Hamill D D (eds) Learning disabilities. Proceedings — Education, Austin

Nichols P L, Chen T 1981 Minimal brain dysfunction: a prospective study. Lawrence Erlbaum Associates, Hillsdale

Pasamanick B, Knobloch H 1966 Retrospective studies on the epidemiology of reproductive casualty: old and new. Merrill-Palmer Quarterly 12: 7–26

Pedretti L 1981 Occupational therapy: practice skills for physical dysfunction. C V Mosby, St Louis

Piaget J 1962 Play, dreams and imitation in Childhood, Norton, New York

Price A, Gilfoyle E, Myer C (eds) 1976 Research in sensory-integrative development. American Occupational Therapy Association, Rockville

Rie H E 1980 Definitional problems. In: Rie H E, Rie E D (eds) Handbook of minimal brain dysfunctions: a critical view. Wiley, New York

Rood M S 1954 Neurophysiological reactions as a basis for physical therapy. Physical Therapy Review 34: 444–449

Safer D J, Allen R P 1976 Hyperactive children: diagnosis and management. University Park Press, Baltimore

Schain R J 1977 Etiology and early manifestations of MBD. In: Millichap J G (ed) Learning disabilities and related disorders: facts and current issues. Year Book Medical Publishers, Chicago

Scrimshaw N S, Gordon J E (eds) 1968 Malnutrition, learning and behaviour. MIT Press, Cambridge

Semans S 1965 Treatment of neurological disorders: concepts and systems. Physical Therapy 45: 11–16

Sevine M, Rasch J, Levine C, Rubenstein J 1975 Adolescents with developmental disabilities: a survey of their problems and their management. Clinical Paediatrics 14(1): 25–32

Silver A, Hagin R, Hersch M S 1969 Reading disability: teaching through stimulation of deficit perceptual areas. American Journal of Orthopsychiatry 27: 774–752

Solomon G E Minimal brain dysfunction. In: Wolman B B, Egan J, Ross A O (eds) Handbook of treatment of mental disorders in childhood and adolescence. Prentice-Hall, Englewood Cliffs, New Jersey

Stevens J R, Sachdev K, Milstein V 1968 Behaviour disorders of childhood and the electroencephalogram. Archives of Neurology 18: 160–177

Swanson L H, Reinert H R 1979 Teaching strategies for children in conflict. Mosby, St Louis

Tannock R 1976 Doman–Delacato method for treating brain injured children: an assessment. Physiotherapy Canada 28: 203–209

Teaching Resources Programs Inc, 100 Boylston Avenue, Boston

Trombly C A, Scott A D 1977 Occupational therapy for physical dysfunction. Williams & Wilkins, Baltimore

Valett R E 1967 The remediation of learning disabilities. Fearon Publishers, Palo Alto

Valett R E 1977 Humanistic education. C V Mosby, St Louis

Walzer S, Richmond J 1973 The epidemiology of learning disorders. Pediatric Clinics of North America 20: 549–598

Watter P, Bullock M I 1983 Developmental Physiotherapy for children with both minimal cerebral dysfunction and learning difficulties. Australian Journal of Physiotherapy 29(2): 53–59

Weiss G, Hechtman L 1979 The hyperactive child syndrome. Science 205: 1348–1354

Wender P H 1971 Minimal brain dysfunction in children. Wiley–Interscience, New York

Wilcock A A 1986 Occupational therapy approaches to stroke. Churchill Livingstone, Melbourne

Ziviani J, Poulsen A, O'Brien A 1982 Effect of a sensory-integrative neurodevelopmental programme on motor and academic performance of children with learning disabilities. Australian Occupational Therapy Journal 29(1): 27–33

16. Applications for children with clinical behaviour disorders

READERS' OBJECTIVES

After reading this chapter, you should be able to:
1. Describe the factors which contribute to clinical behaviour disorders in children.
2. Name and discuss three types of intervention with children with clinical behavioural disorders.
3. Compare and contrast the principles and procedures of behaviour therapy and non-directive play therapy.

DESCRIPTION AND INCIDENCE

Clinical behaviour disorders in children are, for the most part, not discrete disease entities in the way, for example, that measles or mumps are. Rather, psychiatric or behaviour disorders are syndromes, representing a collection of signs and symptoms which are not always clearly related to each other. The clinical syndrome reflects the child's reaction to a complexity of factors which interact. These factors are (Barker 1979):

- Factors within the child
  — constitutional
  — temperamental
- Environmental
- Effects of physical disease and injury.

Constitutional and temperamental factors. Of themselves, constitutional factors are not known to cause psychiatric disorders, but they give rise to conditions in the child which may then lead to behaviour which requires psychiatric intervention. Some examples are genetic and metabolic abnormalities (Graham et al 1973; Thomas et al 1968).

Environmental factors. Chapter 14 specifically examined some of the impacts that the external environment may have on a child. However, the concept of 'environment' can also be applied to intra-uterine life.

For example, maternal diseases during pregnancy — rubella, syphilis, toxoplasmosis, and more recently AIDS — may give rise to conditions in a child which will be associated with clinical behaviour disorder.

Effects of physical disease and disability. The psychological effects associated with various physical diseases and disability processes have already been examined in other chapters.

Nurcombe (1972) has defined differences between psychiatric practices with children and adults as follows:

- The child is a chronologically immature individual in a fluid state of incomplete physical development. She/he is both more flexible and more vulnerable.
- Organic defect has a more profound, far-reaching effect.
- The child is usually passive in the process of referral for investigation.

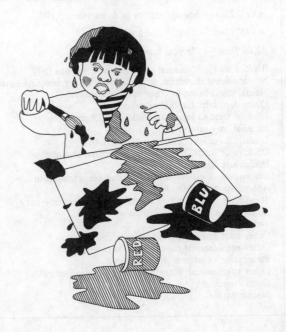

Origins

The United States Joint Commission on Mental Health of Children 1970 proposed that when emotional and mental disorders in children are viewed in terms of their origins, five major categories can be distinguished:

1. Faulty training and faulty life experiences,
2. Surface conflicts between children and parents, at school, and arising in the course of sexual development.
3. Deeper conflicts which become internalized — and lead to the so-called neuroses.
4. Difficulties associated with physical and mental handicaps.
5. Difficulties associated with severe mental disorders, such as the psychoses.

Incidence

There are no accurate international figures for the incidence of clinical behaviour disorders in children and adults, though the trend does appear quite strongly to be that boys are significantly more affected than girls. At least, boys come to attention for diagnosis and intervention more commonly than do girls. Past studies in the United Kingdom, the United States and Australia suggest that the incidence may be in the range of 6%–10% of population head (Henderson et al 1971; Leslie 1974; Prugh & Kinsley 1970; Rutter 1973).

Classification

A number of systems have been developed for classi-

Example 16.1: The 5-Axis scheme for classification of clinical psychiatric syndromes (based on the WHO International Classification of Diseases 1977)

AXIS One (Clinical psychiatric syndrome)
Psychoses (290–299)
Psychoses specific to childhood (299)
Neurotic disorders, personality disorders and other non-psychotic mental disorders (300–316)
Neurotic disorders
Special symptoms or syndromes not elsewhere classified
Acute reaction to stress
Adjustment reaction
Specific non-psychotic disorders following brain damage
Depressive disorders not elsewhere classified
Disturbances of conduct not elsewhere classified
Disturbances of emotions specific to childhood and adolescence
Hyperkinetic syndrome of childhood
Psychic factors associated with diseases classified elsewhere

AXIS Two — Specific delays in development (400)

AXIS Three — Intellectual level

AXIS Four — Medical conditions

AXIS Five — Abnormal psychosocial situations (500)
No significant distortion or inadequacy of psychosocial environment
Mental disturbance in other family members
Discordant intra-familial relationships
Lack of warmth in intra-familial relationships
Familial over-involvement
Inadequate or inconsistent parental control
Inadequate social, linguistic or perceptual stimulation
Inadequate living conditions
Inadequate or distorted intra-familial communication
Anomalous family situation
Stresses or disturbance in school or work environment
Migration or social transplantation
Natural disaster
Other intra-familial psychosocial stress
Other extra-familial psychosocial stress
Persecution or adverse discrimination
Other psychosocial disturbance in society in general
Other (specified)
Not known

fying psychiatric and behaviour disorders in children and adults. The one that is universally accepted and in general use is the 5-Axis scheme based on the International Classification of Diseases (ICD) (Rutter et al 1975, WHO 1977). In this multi-axial system, every disorder is classified along an axis, from a point reflecting normality (e.g., 'no abnormality') to a point allowing for inadequate information or understanding (e.g. 'information unavailable').

The 5-Axis Classification Scheme is presented in Example 16.1, with the sub-classifications shown only for those axes relevant to this discussion of psychiatric behaviour disorder. Such a classifactory system allows for a holistic picture of the child to be assembled, by reference to the child's position in relation to each of the axes. Nurcombe also produced a more detailed classification of the psychoses of infancy and childhood.

A classification of the psychoses of infancy and childhood (Nurcombe 1972)

1. Psychoses of infancy and early childhood
   a. Psychoses of infancy (Reiser)
      Terms which are synonymous, co-terminous or co-extensive:
      Symbiotic psychosis (Mahler)
      Interactional psychotic disorder (GAP) characterized by unusual sensitivites, precocious ego-development, regression often at time of change or trauma; with panic, tantrum, bizarre reality testing, inability to separate from mother, autistic withdrawal
      Childhood schizophrenia (Bradley, Despert, Bender, Goldfarb)
      Early infantile autism (Kanner)
      Atypical child (Rank, Putnam)
   b. Psychosis secondary to sensory deprivation, e.g. blindness
   c. Psychosis secondary to emotional deprivation
      Anaclitic depression — hospitalism (Spitz, Bowlby)
   d. Psychosis secondary to organic brain dysfunction
      i. acute
      ii chronic brain damage, metabolic disease (phenylketonuria, lipoidosis, demyelinating disease)
2. Psychoses arising during later childhood
   a. Psychoses arising from gross stress
   b. Psychoses occurring in a sibling — sibling, parent-child Dyad (e.g. twin, gross infantilization, folie à deux)
   c. Schizophreniform regression
   d. Severe depression
   e. Psychosis arising from organic states
3. Borderline states (Geleerd, Ekstein)
   a. States of severe ego deviance (Beres)

Reproduced by permission from Nurcombe B 1972 An outline of child psychiatry. N.S.W. University Press, Kensington NSW 2033

Signs, symptoms and manifestations

A comprehensive picture of the developmental problems which present in children appears in Example 16.2
Broadly, the symptoms may be grouped.

Aggression

Either direct or indirect, excessive, uncontrolled or uncontrollable.
— Temper tantrums, disobedience, destructiveness, biting, kicking, scratching, screaming, attacks on siblings. Bullying others, cruelty to animals.
— Hypersensitivity, restlessness, poor concentration.
— Habit tics and spasms.

Inwards retreat
— Fearfulness: ready tears; specific fears, e.g. of dark; inability to enjoy social relationships with contemporaries; inability to go to school; excessive day dreaming; wandering away from home.
— Disturbed sleep: e.g. the child is slow to fall asleep; nightmares and terrors; sleep walking; wakefulness during night.
— Disturbed appetite: little desire for food; excessive food fads; compulsive eating; pica.

Abnormal behaviour
— Sexual: precocity; exhibitionism; excessive and public display of masturbation.
— Mood: states of elation or depression; attempted suicide.
— Bizarre behaviour: mannerisms; ritualistic or stereotypical behaviour.

Eysenck (1960) presents a model, showing the grouping of symptoms in children into personality problems and conduct problems, along the continuums of introversion–extroversion and neuroticism. This appears in Figure 16.1.

DIAGNOSIS

Diagnosis must involve more than simply finding a technical label in child psychiatry since:

— Clinical syndromes are often not clear cut.
— Syndromes may change or blur in the process of development or after environmental change.
— A diagnosis such as 'conduct disorder' is no more precise that 'headache'. Both lack specificity.
— A single symptom (e.g., eneuresis) may be associated with a wide variety of psychological disorders in different patients and at different developmental levels.

Example 16.2 Developmental problems commonly requiring diagnosis and intervention by a paediatric psychiatry team (after Prugh & Kisley 1970)

Age	Developmental problems
Birth – 3 months	Birth defects
	Feeding disorders: colic, regurgitation, vomiting, failure to thrive, marasmus, pylorospasm, feeding refusal, atopic eczema
6–9 months	Extreme stranger anxiety
	Early infantile autism
1 year	Physiologic anorexia
	Sleep disturbances: resistance or response to over-stimulation
	Extreme separation anxiety
	Interactional psychotic disorder
	Bronchial asthma
	Pica
	Teeth grinding
	Pseudo-retardation
	Temper tantrums, negativism
2 years	Toilet training disturbances: constipation, diarrhoea
	Excessive feeding
	Bedtime and toilet rituals
3 years	Speech disorders: delayed, elective mutism, stuttering
	Petit mal seizures
	Nightmares, night terrors
	Extreme separation anxiety
	Excessive thumb sucking
	Phobias and marked fears
	Developmental deviations: lags and accelerations in motor, sensory, and affective development
4–5 years	Food rituals and fads
	Sleepwalking
6–8 years	School phobias
	Developmental deviations: lags and accelerations in cognitive functions, psychosexual, and integrative development
	Tics
	Psychoneuroses
	Enuresis, soiling and excessive masturbation
	Schizophreniform psychotic disorder
	Nail biting
	Learning problems
	Psychophysiologic disorders
9–11 years	Personality disorders: compulsive, hysterical, anxious, overly dependent, oppositional, overly inhibited, overly independent, isolated and mistrustful personality, tension discharge disorders, sociosyntonic personality disorders, and sexual deviations
	Pre-linquent patterns
12–18 years	Legal delinquency
	Anorexia nervosa
	Dysmenorrhea
	Sexual promiscuity
	Excessive masturbation
	Pseudopsychotic regressions
	Suicidal attempts
	Acute confusional state
	Schizophrenic disorders (adult type)

— The diagnosis may be formulated in terms of:
  a. clinical entity (e.g., Kanner's syndrome)
  b. developmental diagnosis
  c. dynamic reactive proposition (e.g., response to separation from the family).

The process

After referral, data is collected by a number of methods such as taking a history from adults familiar with the child, observing the child in several contexts, and by formal testing.

The emphasis presented in the reported problems is likely to reflect the concerns of the person taking the referral initiative. Thus, if it is a teacher, the problem behaviour reported is likely to be that which disrupts the classroom, or interferes with the child's learning process. On the other hand, parents will most likely em-phasize different concerns.

Examination of the child should include:

— a developmental history
— a general physical and neurological examination
— psychological testing
— assessment of the child and family by relevant specialist, e.g., occupational therapist.

INTERVENTION

Psychopharmacology

The use of drugs with children displaying clinical behaviour disorders remains empirical, and on the whole, unsatisfactory. The field generally lacks in the application of modern, sophisticated research techniques required for, and applied to drugs administered to adults. Specifically, the role of dosage and the necessity

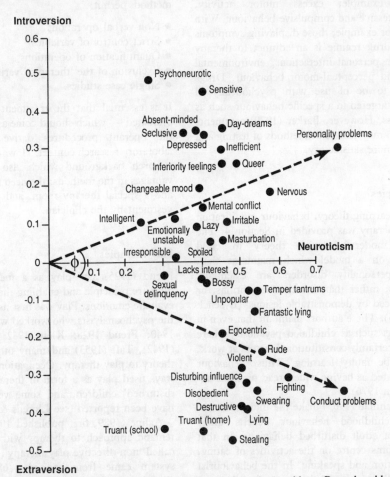

Fig. 16.1 Grouping of symptoms in children into personality problems and conduct problems. Reproduced by permission from Eysenck H J 1960 The structure of human personality. Methuen & Co., London

for maintenance therapy with children is poorly studied and documented; adverse and toxic reactions in children are poorly examined and understood; the longer term effects on the neurological, biochemical and metabolic systems of immature and developing individuals are not understood.

The paucity of our knowledge about drug therapy efficacy with children appears to stem from a number of factors. Not least of these factors is the diagnostic problem of dealing with a complex syndrome — a potpouri of clinical signs and symptoms, which may reflect a constellation of interactive, intrinsic and extrinsic precipitating factors. Further confusion is added by the question of whether there is organic brain damage.

At present the main use of drugs is in the treatment of hyperactive children, some depressed children, and possibly some anxious children. With the hyperactive child, drug regimes are aimed directly at target behaviours, for example, excess motor activity, restlessness, aggressive and compulsive behaviour. With other children, for example, those displaying symptoms of anxiety, the drug regime is an adjunct to therapy which focuses on personal interactions, environmental manipulation, and perceptual-motor behaviour. Drugs do not appear to be of use with psychotically ill children, unless targeted to a specific behaviour such as motor restlessness. However, Barker (1979) comments that this situation may change as methods of testing and trialing become more satisfactory.

Behaviour therapies

A discussion of learning theory, behaviour modification and behaviour therapy was provided in Section 4. The application of modern learning theory to child psychiatry rests on a model which maintains that, 'neurotic and personality disorders are essentially learned reactions, rather than inherited conditions, or conditions produced by demonstrable lesions' (Eysenck & Rachman 1965). These authors maintain that even in clinical conditions such as childhood psychosis, where there are almost certainly consititutional factors at work, there will still be faulty learning. Thus, behaviour therapy is postulated as having widespread practical application (Norman 1976)

Eysenck & Rachman (1965) make the interesting observation that childhood behaviour deficits differ dramatically from adult disturbed behaviour, in that children's symptoms centre on the activities of eating, sleeping, elimination and speaking. In the behaviourist model, the child's problem behaviour arises because she/he fails to develop an adequate way of responding, and thus may develop the clinical symptoms related to bodily activities, e.g., enuresis, anorexia, dyslexia. Whereas the aim of therapy with adults is to break down a developed behaviour pattern (e.g., phobia), with children the behaviour therapist's aim is to build up an adequate behaviour pattern. Behaviour therapy was in its heyday in the 1960s and 1970s, and still continues to be an important and influential approach to treatment. Some notable programs have been reported with children displaying enuresis (wetting) and encopresis (soiling) (Jones 1960; Wolfe 1961; Yates 1959) with autistic children (Ferster 1961, Lovaas 1967) and children exhibiting school phobias (Eisenberg 1958).

In summary, the exponents of learning theory see this theory as applying to clinical conditions. They maintain that operant conditioning methods can be used to generate and/or sustain stable behaviour patterns. The advantages when used with children are that the methods permit:

- Non-verbal operations
- Strict control of variables
- Quantification of operations
- Exclusion of the 'therapist' variable
- Single case studies.

It is essential that the treatment can be studied and evaluated — which should come as no surprise, because the operant procedures derive from a controlled laboratory research context. However, it is precisely this research background which also accounts for disadvantages in the methods: the need for special equipment and a special therapy room; and considerable time investment by the clinician.

Play therapies

Freud (1925) saw play as a means of fulfilling the pleasure principle and enabling the child to express and evaluate emotions. Play was first used therapeutically by the psychoanalyists who worked with children (Erikson 1940; Freud 1928; Klein 1932; Rank 1945). Allen (1942), Taft (1953) and many others applied Rankian theory to play therapy. Occupational therapists have always used play as a form of therapy with 'emotionally disturbed' children, and some very fine programmes have been reported (see Llorens & Rubin 1967).

Axline (1989, first published 1947) developed a systematic approach to therapy with children which she called 'non-directive play therapy'. The impetus for her system came from the idea of therapy which is client-centred, that is, which embodies the principle of non-direction from the therapist. This approach was first described by Carl Rogers (1942) with adults and came to be known as 'Rogerian Techniques'. Rogers' main assumption has been that 'the individual has a sufficient capacity to deal constructively with all those aspects of his life which can potentially come into conscious awareness'.

Axline's work has had a powerful and long lasting impact on therapy with emotionally, or behaviourally disordered children. Other workers have recorded their own refinements of the 'non-directive' therapy approach (e.g., Ginott 1959, 1961, 1964; Hindmarsh 1979; Moustakas 1959). It is the approach of choice for occupational therapists, and for that reason a detailed discussion and critique is provided in this chapter.

OCCUPATIONAL THERAPY

Observing play behaviour

In all areas as occupational therapy with children, but especially in paediatric psychiatry, a therapist will be asked to comment on the child's behaviour in a play situation. There are two aspects that must receive comment — the child's social behaviour, and task behaviour. However, both social and task behaviour occur in an environmental context, and it can have a powerful influence on the child's responses. Therefore, it is essential to report on the context in which the reported behaviour occurred. A detailed discussion about observing behaviour has been provided in Chapter 8, and the reader is urged to review that chapter in association with this specialized discussion.

Play as evaluation

Information may be collected by report, or directly by observation (Lowe & Costello 1976). There are several very useful evaluation tools which are available for occupational therapy use. For example, there is the Symbolic Play Test (Lowe & Costello 1976), and the Imaginative Play Predisposition Interview proforma (Singer 1973). Takata's Play History (1974) is also widely used.

What to observe.

In order to define what questions you seek answers to, it is helpful to draw up a sheet of paper into two columns, head one 'what to look at', and the other column 'why'. Then jot down what you think you should look at, and attempt to answer 'why'. This planning device can save you the frustration of collecting inappropriate information (data) and too much or not

enough of it. As a general rule, you will always need to gather information about:

1. What the child does — the pattern of play or other behaviour.
2. The physical context.
3. Social interaction.

The simplest level of observing and reporting about play is to note the class or category of play, in order to establish a level of play maturity, and to detect any pattern.

Alternatively, and especially in a group situation, you could use an open ended descriptive checklist of the kind shown in Example 16.3.

A simple playchart like this one provides a useful means for sharpening parents' awareness of their child's behaviour. The mother and/or father can be encouraged to keep a diary of the child's activities over one or two days. The therapist then interprets this information in terms of play behaviour.

Non-directive play therapy

Rationale

Non-directive play therapy is a therapeutic experience, based on the theory that the individual has the capacity to be self-directed, and to solve problems, if given a suitable opportunity in which to do so. Sheehy (1976) summarized the main points of Axline's theoretical model:

- A child needs the permissiveness to be himself.
- A child has an internal drive towards self-realization.
- Each child has the ability to solve his own problems and direct his own life.
- Mature behaviour is more satisfying than immature behaviour.
- A child learns to control or abandon feelings when these are brought to the surface. In a permissive situation the child is able to look at problems realistically, and eventually resolve them.
- The non-directive method
  — results in the child's self-acceptance and self-respect
  — allows a child the personal permissiveness to use all capacities
  — results in the child realizing self-responsibility
  — allows the child to apply this philosophy to relationships outside therapy.

Munro (1952), in an article apparently unrelated to non-directive therapy, commented 'In one sense I let the

Example 16.3: Categories of play behaviour and a simple checklist format

Description of play	Solitary	Parallel	Onlooking	Being Sociable	Simple co-operating	Complex co-operating
1. Plays apart from others						
2. Plays with different things from others						
3. Absorbed in own play, shows no interest in activities of others.						
4. Plays alongside others but talk is not directed to anyone in particular.						
5. All playing same role or with same things but without sharing or taking turns — at most may defend own playthings.						
6. Shows great interest in the activities of others but without attempting to join in.						
7. Tries to join in with the group play, either to get accepted or to get others to play own game.						
8. Sociable talk with others, often not about the content of the play activity.						
9. Shares toys, takes turns, divides play simply.						
10. Talk largely concerned with the content of play.						
11. Playing at games with definite roles (e.g. hospitals) or with rules about what to do (e.g. lotto).						

group do the work. I wait for them to play the active role, to comment, criticize, and it still delights me how often they do just what has to be done, and at the right time.' In a similar vision, Macnamara (1963) in describing her experience with a group of mothers, concluded that, 'There is undoubtedly great value in accepting the thoughts and feelings of group members, and thus allowing the development of an atmosphere in which emotional growth can take place.' This is precisely what is asserted to happen in non-directive play therapy.

The term 'non-directive' is perhaps rather misleading for it implies that the therapist, although physically present in the treatment room, does not intervene in any way regardless of the child's actions or vocalizations, i.e., that the therapist is present in the role of recorder and observer only. This idea is diametrically opposed to the actual practice of non-directive play therapy.

A situation wherein a child is left to use a wide variety of materials, without purpose, or a goal, is not therapeutic. This type of situation can only result in frustration and confusion and subsequent aggression on the part of the child. To be successful, non-directive play therapy depends primarily on the therapist's skill in developing a relationship of trust and mutual respect.

Treatment is usually undertaken on an outpatient basis, as it is long term and hospitalization is unnecessary. However, the occasion does arise where it is thought that play therapy will be of benefit to a child who is already in hospital. Usually, the child commences in an individual setting and at a later stage is introduced into a group.

Principles

Axline (1989, 1964a,b,c 1966, 1979) outlined various principles which serve to guide the therapy. Summarized, they are:

— That there be acceptance of the child by the therapist, in a treatment setting consisting of the patient, the therapist, and a selected quantity of materials. According to the Oxford Dictionary 'acceptance' means to take or receive what is offered with consenting mind. Axline distinguishes acceptance from approval.

— The therapist establishes a feeling of permissiveness in the relationship so that the child feels free to express his feelings completely. The term 'permissiveness' has been defined by Ginott (1959) as 'the acceptance of all symbolic behaviour, be it destructive or constructive, as it appears in therapy, and without censure or restriction'.

— The therapist is alert to recognize the feelings the child is expressing and reflects back those feelings in such a manner that the child gains insight into his behaviour. The term 'reflection' means to throw back or reproduce an image as seen in a mirror, of certain essential features or qualities of another thing.

Non-directive play therapy has emphasized reflection over interpretation of a child's play. However, the two concepts often intertwine, especially when a child uses play rather than speech to convey his emotions (Clancy 1963).

— The therapist maintains a deep respect for the child's ability to solve his own problems if given the opportunity. The responsibility to make choices and institute change is the child's.

— The therapist does not attempt to direct the child's actions, or conversation, in any manner.

— The therapist does not attempt to hurry the therapy along. It is a gradual process, and is recognized as such by the therapist.

— The therapist establishes only those limitations that are necessary to anchor the therapy to the world of reality and to make the child aware of

responsibility in the relationship (Dorfman 1951, Ginott 1964). From a review of the literature the most commonly used limits are:

a. Insistence on adhering to time constraints, for example, keeping therapy appointments, and finishing sessions on time.
b. Not allowing the child to destroy the materials or furnishings.
c. Not allowing physical harm to another person.

Apprehension is often expressed by parents and others unfamiliar with the rationale of treatment. The question frequently posed is — if the child is allowed to indulge in a socially or otherwise unacceptable behaviour during treatment — and this is accepted — then will the behaviour carry over at home and school? Or similarly, will correction in one place and not another be confusing? This seems not to be the case. The child, recognizing a genuine effort to help him, and it must be genuine, will not violate the bounds of the therapeutic relationship. Care must be exercised to discover whether such behaviour elsewhere, if it does occur, has been in evidence before therapy commenced. If it has, then continuation is obviously not the result of therapy. However, if it is linked with therapy then the therapist should reappraise all aspects of his/her handling. Although parental counselling is not considered vital to the success of non-directive play therapy, Axline (1989), Slavson (1952), and Ginott (1961) are all in agreement that it is a desirable adjunct to therapy for the child.

Roles

The child. Originally Axline's approach applied only to emotionally disturbed children, and the child was seen as the focus of all change. However, therapy has been conducted with the mentally deficient (Bernhardt & Bernard 1975), handicapped children, and normal children. Non-directive play therapy does not seem to be a suitable treatment medium to use with either the brain injured child or the psychotic child. The treatment plan with a brain injured child is essentially one of training and it employs a maximum degree of direction and supervision from the therapist. The problem of treatment in any form with a psychotic child is well recognized. In the early stages of treatment when the patient—therapist relationship is being established, the principle of non-direction may be used. However, it cannot logically continue throughout the entire course of treatment, as often the psychotic child's language is unintelligible to the therapist, and therefore verbal reflection is not possible. Again, the therapist must penetrate the child's defence of withdrawal from contact with other people, and non-directive play therapy does not offer the appropriate means for doing this.

The literature has discussed a variety of suitable age ranges for the application of Axline's model. Axline herself identified no particular suitable age group, however, Dorfman (1951) has used the approach with 11-year-olds, while Clancy (1963) set a limit of eight or nine years. Lower age limits have not been discussed in the literature.

The therapist. Research has demonstrated the successful use of a variety of people as play therapists. They have included nurses (Morrison & Newcomer 1975; Newcomer & Morrison 1974), parents (Guerney 1979), occupational therapists (Clancy 1963), teachers, as well as psychologists and psychiatrists (Axline 1989).

Inevitably, the personality of the therapist enters into the therapy situation. She/he must be sufficiently mature and secure in his/her own interpersonal relationships never to use the patient—therapist relationship for personal ends. One must be aware at all times that this is a possibility. The personal demands made on the therapist are emotionally and physically exhausting. Within the play therapy situation she/he must be prepared to accept behaviour and language which may elicit in her, horror, even disgust, outside the treatment room. She/he is no longer the authority figure who can reject and punish such expression. Therefore, she must be confident in her own mind that what she is doing is valid and will help the child. Apprehension may be aroused in the therapist by mess and aggressive behaviour. Tolerance of this behaviour will sometimes draw questioning appraisal of the therapist's methods from her colleagues. These are all issues which must be raised, addressed and resolved by each therapist.

The parent or significant adult. Parental counselling has been seen by Axline as important but not essential to successful treatment. Concurrent counselling and play therapy were seen to speed up the overall process. However, Axline believed primarily in the child's ability, through therapy, to overcome the problems in his or her life.

Environment and media

Axline (1989) outlined the ideal characteristics of the playroom. These included soundproofing, a one-way mirror, washable floors and walls, a sink, and a 'stage' at one end. The size of the room is also important. If it is too large it will be easy for the child to disassociate him/herself from the therapist, and difficult for the therapist to establish and maintain good rapport with the child. Conversely, if too small, the child may find the atmosphere claustrophobic and too intense, and anxiety may increase. Lee & Hutt (1964), Hutt & Hutt (1965) and McGrew (1972) have developed and described such a playroom.

Clancy (1963) categorized suitable play media into two groups:

1. unstructured media (such as clay or sand), and
2. representative media (such as dolls or puppets).

Axline (1989) advised that all materials should be simply constructed, durable, easily accessible and easily used. Forward (1957) suggests exclusion of all mechanical type toys such as walking animals and quacking ducks, from the treatment room, on the basis that they give no scope to the child's imaginative powers, and are therefore of no value as a diagnostic or therapeutic medium.

Therapy process

The depth of feeling that the child shows is only made possible by the degree of permissiveness shown by the therapist. The child's role is the dominant one: she/he directs the play hour, selects from the variety of materials the things that are meaningful, and therefore important. She/he should not be forced to conform to a social or artistic standard in the chosen activity. Whether she/he shall even take the opportunity to play, is left to him/her. The treatment session is the child's probing ground. When outright guidance is sought by the child the therapist's approach could be, 'You want me to tell you what to make — you can make anything you want', thereby giving reassurance to the child. Nor should the therapist set out a pre-arranged selection of toys hoping that these will be taken over by the child, as in the example of the therapist setting out the doll's house and family of dolls for the child to play with, because she surmises that there are problems in the family relationships.

This attitude of relying on the child's ability to make decisions should be maintained throughout therapy. This experience in itself is a step forward in emotional growth, and once achieved, further problems and situations will be easier for the child to handle. Example 16.4 presents one way by which the therapist can introduce non-directive play therapy.

Reflection versus interpretation. The therapist should avoid giving interpretation to the child of the symbolism involved in his/her play. If it is the wrong interpretation, that is, one which does not coincide with that intended by the child at the particular moment, anxiety may be heightened, and a whole chain reaction of disturbance may follow. However, the therapist is

---

Example: 16.4 Introducing non-directive play therapy

When the child first enters the room the therapist usually says, 'You may play with these toys however you like — the time is yours and you may do whatever you wish while you are here.' It is necessary to explain how to use some of the materials, for example how to make dough, or mix paints. During the initial contact the child is very alert to the therapist's attitude, and consistency is most important.

---

free to, and indeed must, reflect back the child's own vocalisations, thereby bringing the emotional component of the child's thought and gesture to notice.

There is a difference between reflection and interpretation which is sometimes rather difficult to explain. Indeed, occasions arise when the therapist can offer a simple interpretation to the child (see Example 16.5).

Example: 16.5 Interpretation versus reflection

A child declared his intention of smashing a piece of furniture. The therapist replied, 'You want to smash that chair because you are angry with your mother.' This could be a fact, but it would be surmise, *i.e., interpretation*, on the therapists part. Even if correct, the child might not be ready to accept feelings expressed in such a straightforward manner at that time. *Reflecting* the child's feeling in the same situation, the therapist would say, 'You feel angry enough to break the chair.'

When a child is ready to express feelings in front of an adult, she/he will do so. She/he cannot be hurried. Any attempt to force him/her to do so causes retreat. Some children are very slow to make use of the time in what the therapist may call 'a therapeutic manner'. However, the child may be going through a period of gaining confidence to express self. Such a period calls for patience and understanding on the part of the therapist. If she/he can let the child take time, she/he will be rewarded for restraint.

The therapist should try to see things through the child's eyes, to develop the feeling of empathy — change is a gradual process.

Group therapy. Although the child must be regarded primarily as an individual, she/he forms a unit within a group in society. It is within this group that she/he has failed to mature, and it is to such a situation that she/he must return. Therefore, therapy includes situations which are symbolic of wider society in that there are others present to whom she/he must relate in some way. Thus the child has an opportunity to develop and ex-

periment with new patterns of response to other people. Again, the group experience brings out problems of adjustment that are not always evident in an individual situation. The principles which apply to the individual treatment session also apply to the group session.

It is advisable that the group be kept small. The recommended size is three to six members, including the therapist. If possible, the children should have similar needs or problems. A very useful practice, where possible, is to include one or more of the patient's siblings as members of the group. However, when a therapist wishes to include any member of the patient's family in the treatment session, she/he must first gain the child's permission. Quite often the child will ask if his brother(s) or sister(s) could come to therapy.

If the group exceeds six members, it is very likely: that the shy, withdrawn child may become 'submerged' and overlooked; and when difficulties rise to the surface, the therapist will be unable to deal with the many problems arising simultaneously. The purpose of the group will thus be defeated.

The group will always consist of children in varying stages of treatment, as it is a continuous procedure. There will be those children new to the group, those who have been participating for some time, and those ready for discharge. The latter child is important as she/he provides stability for the rest of the group.

In addition to having this opportunity to test experiences against those of others, the child is often greatly relieved to discover that problems are not unique.

Evaluation of non-directive play therapy

One of the major criticisms of Axline's (1989) model has been her lack of research, especially experimental research (Ginott 1964; Lebo 1964, 1979). Axline provided very little experimental support for her work. Of her own papers, most have used the single case study design, supplemented by follow-up studies (Axline 1989, 1950).

These are obstacles to conducting research in the field of non-directive play therapy. The time, effort and money required to obtain records of therapy sessions have been a major obstacle (Dorfman 1951). Confounding variables such as method of transport to the clinic (Sheehy 1976) or the placebo effect (Lebo 1964), and lack of accurate, reliable tools for analysis or evaluation have also been a problem (Howe & Silvers 1981). Other methodological flaws have made research in the field questionable (Fleming & Snyder 1947, Ginott 1964). Despite these obstacles a number of studies have been conducted. These have focused on the process of therapy, outcomes of therapy, and comparisons between various treatment approaches.

The process. Landisberg & Snyder (1946) demonstrated an increase in physical activity and expression of feelings in the latter three-fifths of therapy sessions. Emotions have been more commonly expressed through actions than verbally (Finke 1947; Landisberg & Snyder 1946). Finke (1947) also found that therapy could be divided into three stages, which corresponded closely with six phases outlined by Axline (1989).

Outcomes. Studies evaluating the outcomes of play therapy have displayed conflicting results. Follow-up studies have been predominantly supportive of the effectiveness of non-directive play therapy (Axline 1950; Clay 1956; Rexford et al 1956). Studies using mentally deficient children with emotional problems have demonstrated little support (Johnson 1953, Leland et al 1959, Subotnik 1975). Elliot & Pumfrey (1972) hypothesized that non-directive play therapy was more effective with children who have above average intelligence, and higher socio-economic status. Certainly, most supportive studies have used children who were emotionally disturbed, maladjusted or with behaviour problems (Cox 1953; Dorfman 1951; Fleming & Snyder 1947).

Comparison with other approaches

Few studies have evaluated non-directive play therapy in comparison with the other approaches in the field. Morrison & Newcomer (1975) conducted a study using moderately intellectually handicapped children who were treated with directive and non-directive therapy. They found no significantly different effects between the two approaches. Subotnik (1975) compared non-directive play therapy with behaviour modification techniques for controlling poor classroom behaviour. No significant results were demonstrated, but the play therapy group children displayed a greater degree of improvement than either of the behaviour modification groups. A study by Sheehy (1976) also supported the benefits of non-directive play therapy compared with other eclectic approaches.

Many authors have criticized Axline's (1989) use of limits (Rhoden et al 1981) and the permissive principle during therapy. In particular, some have been concerned for the therapist, and his or her ability to cope with emotional abuse from the child and the suppression of natural emotional reactions (Peoples 1979).

Axline's preoccupation with the emotional development of children has also been criticized. Harter (1977)

advocated combining Piagetian and psychoanalytical views of play in order to recognize the role which cognitive development might play in therapy. Singer (1973) also believed that some children needed to be taught how to play symbolically if they were to benefit from play therapy.

Jeffrey (1981), after surveying 20 child psychiatry units, found that non-directive play therapy was the most favoured approach used by occupational therapists in this field. However, in many centres, occupational therapists have modified Axline's approach without proper research into the effectiveness of their new approach (Hindmarsh 1979), thus sometimes bringing play therapy into disrepute. Again, most therapists have tended to 'accumulate' materials without evaluating their therapeutic value (Lebo 1979).

Many authors have believed that personality rather than training was the criterion for a successful play therapist. Ginott (1961), while supporting this view, also advocated careful supervision and training in certain techniques. Certainly occupational therapy training provides the necessary background in child psychology and pathology, counselling skills and use of various play materials, along with a theoretical basis for therapeutic value of play (Reilly 1974).

As an outcome of Axline's work, others have been stimulated to develop different approaches. Some examples include Filial Therapy (Guerney 1979), therapy with the intellectually handicapped (Leland & Smith 1965) and group play therapy (Ginott 1961).

Case illustrations

This chapter concludes with examples of children in non-directive play therapy implemented by an occupational therapist. Example 16.6 Ann, aged seven years, illustrates the therapy applied in the conventional setting. Ann attended the hospital as an outpatient.

In contrast, the case history of Darryl (Example 16.7), aged six-and-a-half years at the time of treatment, illustrates the success of non-directive play therapy when used in a hospital ward.

Example 16.6: Ann
Ann was born one year after her parents' marriage which followed a stormy three month's courtship. The marital situation was far from tranquil as the husband was a heavy drinker. Ann grew up in an atmosphere of parental discord, insecurity and distrust. She had always been a 'difficult baby' according to her mother. Toilet training presented a crisis between mother and child, and Ann was finally trained at four years of age. Nocturnal enuresis had continued up to the time of treatment.

Two years after Ann's birth, a boy was born. The patient was totally unprepared for the birth of this second child. At this juncture the husband deserted the family, leaving them without financial aid. At first Ann reacted to this altered situation by manifesting bewilderment. Later, as her understanding increased, she reacted with extreme jealousy towards the baby. On several occasions she was found in the act of attempting to strangle him. She constantly sought attention, was disobedient, aggressive, and subject to temper tantrums.

The mother was forced to return to work, Ann was placed in an orphanage, and a babysitter employed to care for the baby at home. In the orphanage Ann quickly became so uncontrollable that her mother was requested to remove her, as she was proving a constant source of disturbance to the other children. She was placed in a smaller foster home, and from here referred to the hospital outpatient clinic.

The social worker at this home reported that Ann was destructive, negativistic, bullied all the boys younger than herself, and displayed temper tantrums and screaming fits in a range of situations. She commenced school and appeared to behave in the same manner. Two months after Ann's admission to the foster home, her mother had not visited her.

A two-fold plan of treatment was instituted:

Parental counselling. It was not possible for Ann to leave the foster home, and so efforts were directed at encouraging closer contact between Ann and her mother.

Discussion with mother aimed to help her gain some understanding of Ann's behaviour, and also to help her develop a tolerant supportive attitude towards the child while the difficult behaviour persisted.

Non-directive play therapy. Therapy was implemented twice weekly, and was later tapered off to one hour weekly, then fortnightly, until treatment ceased.

In spite of her history, there was no difficulty in establishing a good rapport with this child. She entered and used the playroom with the same forthrightness that she had shown in reacting to her environment. During the initial sessions she found and used the feeding bottle which was in the room. After several sessions, she discarded the bottle and ignored it thereafter. She expressed her aggressive feelings, at first self-directed, but later vented upon the therapist (verbally), and objects in the room. This behaviour lessened in intensity, until eventually the child was able to direct her expression of these feelings into more appropriate play activity. Her regressive toilet habits were at first fully tolerated. As the therapeutic relationship developed, the opportunity for more socialized habits was provided, and toilet habits became normal for her age.

The child brought to the therapist some of her problems in relationship to her environment — notably her awareness that her temper tantrums were unacceptable. She expressed, in primitive terms, her wish to be assured that she was loved by the therapist, however asocial her behaviour. She showed jealousy of the therapist's attention to other children, in a group situation. This was interpreted as a result of the close relationship with the therapist, and because of feelings of maternal deprivation.

Gradually, she came to accept the therapist's reassurance that she was loved, even when not having direct attention. With more mature social behaviour, a favourable change occurred in Ann's mother's attitude toward her, and this itself bore fruit. Ann was able to take her place in a school, and therapy was tapered off with the reassurance that she could return, but this was not necessary.

Example 16.7: Darryl
Darryl had been hospitalized in a large city children's hospital on many occasions with osteomyelitis of the left femur, existing for three years. He was referred to the Hospital Child Guidance Clinic because of his outbursts of extreme aggression, and disruptive behaviour in the ward. He had no previous history of emotional disturbance, either at home, or on previous admissions. His difficult behaviour appeared to coincide with this period of hospitalization and deprivation of family contact.

He was the eighth child in a family of ten living siblings. On each occasion his admission to hospital was arranged through a country children's health scheme, as his home was in the country. The only contact that Darryl had with his family during these extended periods in hospital was by letter.

Some contact had been made with this child before commencement of treatment, as the therapist was treating another child in the ward. Darryl appeared to be an alert child, with a very engaging manner. Medical treatment included immobilization of the left lower limb and traction. He did not tolerate the necessary physical restraint at all, and his behaviour became increasingly aggressive. He ripped his blankets to shreds and completely removed his traction apparatus. The predominant attitude of the nursing staff towards this child was hostility. Non-directive play therapy with the child presented difficulties, namely:

- He was confined to bed and his ability to move around was severely limited.
- The ward was not a suitable place to initiate treatment. This problem was overcome by wheeling his bed into an adjacent room for the duration of therapy sessions.
- Adequate contact with his parents was not possible. The only solution to this problem seemed to be to establish contact through letters with his mother, and to encourage her to write frequently to Darryl.

Response to therapy. The child was given one hour each day, because of the severity of the problem behaviour. A selection of the suggested materials was taken to Darryl, and once he was familiar with the range, he was encouraged to select specific material for the following session. Finger and brush paints, puppets, plasticine, building bricks, recorded stories and music were the most frequently requested materials.

It was soon obvious that Darryl's aggressive behaviour was his outward manifestation of extreme apprehension and bewilderment. He, like Ann, expressed to the therapist his awareness that his behaviour was unacceptable to the hospital personnel, together with his desire for acceptance.

Darryl followed closely the same progress in therapy that Ann had done. He had unfortunately earned a bad reputation by the time treatment was commenced, and the attitude of rejection and hostility was passed from one member of staff to another, not always with good reason. The co-operation of the nursing staff was sought in maintaining as tolerant and accepting an attitude toward the child as possible.

Darryl appeared to find the most satisfactory means of release and communication through finger paint, and would often close the session with the comment, 'That's enough, I feel better now.'

In addition to his regular therapy, the therapist accompanied him whenever it was necessary for him to leave the ward, for example, to go to X-ray, and have an application of plaster in theatre. Once he was with the therapist he would take an interest in the proceedings, whereas before participation in play therapy, he had been so apprehensive that heavy sedation for all procedures had been necessary. His contact with the therapist continued throughout his entire period of three months in hospital. The treatment times were gradually tapered off to a regular individual session two days a week, with participation in an activity group with another therapist three days a week.

At the close of therapy Darryl made an illuminating remark to the therapist. 'At first I didn't really know who you were, you were just someone who came each day, but now I really know you.'

Both children were reacting to their environment in an aggressive manner, with extreme behaviour. Ann's problem arose in her immediate family circle. Darryl's problem arose in an institutional setting, the hospital, while he was without contact with his family.

SUMMARY

This chapter provides an overview of approaches taken to the description and classification of childhood disorders of behaviour. The 5-axis classification is reviewed as a point of reference, and clinical manifestations related to it. Intervention through drug use, the behavioural approaches based on learning theory and psychoanalytic approaches are briefly described.

The origins, treatment method, and application of non-directive play therapy in occupational therapy received detailed examination and the following points were made:

1. Play is used as a means of communication with the child who is the patient.
2. The therapist does not make any demands on the

child. Tolerance, love and complete acceptance dominate the treatment program.
3. The therapist reflects the emotion contained in the child's actions, gestures and vocalizations, but does not attempt interpretation.
4. The most important component of non-directive play therapy is *empathy* existing between the child and the therapist.
5. Discipline is maintained within practical limits of time and physical damage to people and objects.

The importance of this special child—adult relationship within non-directive play therapy is that the therapist, while knowing satisfactory solutions to the child's problems, guides the child to the point where she/he discovers these answers. Thus the therapy experience is more meaningful for the child.

REFERENCES

Allen F H 1942 Psychotherapy with children. W W Norton, New York
Axline V M 1950 Play therapy experiences as described by child participants. Journal of Consulting Psychology 14: 53–63
Axline V M 1964a Non-directive therapy. In: Haworth M R (ed) Child psychotherapy. Basic Books, New York, pp 34–39
Axline V M 1964b The eight basic principles. In: Haworth M R (ed) Child psychotherapy. Basic Books, New York, pp 93–94
Axline V M 1964c Recognition and reflection of feelings. In: Haworth M R (ed) Child psychotherapy. Basic Books, New York, pp 239–242
Axline V M 1966 Dibs in search of self. Cowe & Brydone, London
Axline V M 1979 Play therapy as described by children. In: Schaefer C (ed) The therapeutic use of child's play. Jason Aronson, New York
Axline V M 1989 Non-directive play therapy. Churchill Livingstone, Edinburgh First published 1947, Riverside Press, Cambridge, Massachusetts
Barker P 1979 Basic child psychiatry. Granada, London
Bernhardt M, Bernard M 1975 The use of play therapy with the mentally retarded. Journal of Special Education 9: 409–414
Clancy H 1963 The application of non-directive play therapy in occupational therapy. Australian Occupational Therapy Journal 10: 4–19
Clay C O 1956 A follow-up study of eight mothers and eight children served by a child guidance clinic of Jacksonville, Florida. Unpublished Master's thesis, Florida State University
Cox F W 1953 Sociometric status and individual adjustment before and after play therapy. Journal of Abnormal and Social Psycholgy 48: 354–356
Dorfman E 1951 Play therapy. In: Rogers C R, Client-centred therapy. Houghton Mifflin, Boston, pp 235–277

Eisenberg C 1958 School phobia. American Journal of Psychiatry 114: 712–718

Elliot C, Pumphrey P 1972 The effects of non-directive play therapy on some maladjusted boys. Educational Research 14: 157–161

Eysenck H J 1960 The structure of human personality. Methuen, London

Eysenck H J, Rachman J 1965 The application of learning theory to child psychiatry. In: Howells J G (ed) Modern perspectives in child psychiatry, Oliver & Boyd, Edinburgh

Erikson E 1940 Studies in the interpretation of play. Genetic Psychological Monographs 22: 557–671

Ferster C B 1961 Positive reinforcement and behavioural deficits of autistic children. Child Development 32: 437–456

Finke H 1947 Changes in expression of emotionalized attitudes in six cases of play therapy. MA Thesis, University of Chicago

Fleming L, Snyder W 1947 Social and personal changes following non-directive group play therapy. American Journal of Orthopsychiatry 17: 101–116

Forward G 1957 The disturbed child. British Journal of Occupational Therapy 20(9): 14–19

Freud S 1925 Formulations regarding the two principles in mental functioning. In: Freud S Collected Papers. Hogarth Press and The Institute of Psychoanalysis, London, Vol IV pp 13–21

Freud A 1928 Introduction to the technique of child analysis. Nervous and Mental Disease Monographs 48

Ginott H G 1959 The theory and practice of 'Therapeutic Intervention' in child treatment. Journal of Consulting Psychology 23: 160–166

Ginott H 1961 Group psychotherapy. McGraw Hill, New York

Ginott H G 1964 Research in play therapy. In: Haworth M H (ed) Child psychotherapy, Basic Books, New York, pp 431–435

Graham P, Rutter M, George S 1973 Temperamental characteristics as predictors of behaviour disorders in children. American Journal of Orthopsychiatry 43: 328–339

Guerney L F 1979 Play therapy with learning disabled children. Journal of Clinical Child Psychology 8: 242–244

Harter S 1977 A cognitive-developmental approach to children's expression of conflicting feelings and a technique to facilitate such expression in play therapy. Journal of Consulting and Clinical Psychology 45: 417–432

Henderson A S, Krupinski J, Stoller A 1971 Epidemiological aspects of adolescent psychiatry. In: Howells J G (ed) Modern perspectives in adolescent psychiatry. Oliver & Boyd, Edinburgh

Hindmarsh W A 1979 Play diagnosis and play therapy. American Journal of Occupational Therapy 33: 770–775

Howe P, Silvers L 1981 Behavioural observation of children during play therapy: preliminary development of a research instrument. Journal of Personality Assessment 45: 168–182

Hutt C, Hutt S J 1965 Effects of environmental complexity on stereotyped behaviours of children. Animal Behaviour 13: 1–4

Jeffrey L I 1981 Exploration of the use of therapeutic play in the rehabilitation of psychologically disturbed children. Fellowship Thesis, University of Newcastle on Tyne

Johnson E Z 1953 The clinical use of Raven's Progressive matrices to appraise potential for progress in play therapy: a study of institutionalized mentally and educationally retarded children. American Journal of Orthopsychiatry 23: 484–851

Jones H G 1960 The behavioural treatment of enuresis nocturna. In: Eysenck H J (ed) Behaviour therapy and the neuroses. Pergamon Press, Oxford

Klein M 1932 The Psycho-analysis of children. Hogarth Press, London

Landisberg S, Snyder W U 1946 Non-directive play therapy. Journal of Clinical Psychology 2: 201–214

Lebo D 1964 The relationship of response categories in play therapy to chronological age. Child Psychiatry 2: 330–336

Lebo D 1979 Toys for non-directive play therapy. In: Schaefer C (ed) The therapeutic use of child's play. Jason Aronson, New York, pp 435–477

Lee D, Hutt C 1964 A play-room designed for filming children: a note. Child Psychology and Psychiatry 5: 263–265

Leland H, Smith D E 1965 Play therapy with mentally subnormal children. Grune & Stratton, New York

Leland H, Walker J, Taboado A, 1959 Group play therapy with a group of post-nursery male retardates. American Journal of Mental Deficiency 63: 848–851

Leslie S A 1974 Psychiatric disorders in the young adolescents of an industrial town. British Journal of Psychiatry 125: 113–124

Llorens L A, Rubin E Z 1967 Developing ego functions in disturbed children. Wayne State University Press, Detroit

Lovaas O I 1967 A behaviour therapy approach to the treatment of childhood schizophrenia. In: Hill J P (ed) Minnesota Symposium on Child Psychology, Vol 1. University of Minnesota Press, Minneapolis

Lowe M, Costello A J 1976 Symbolic play kit. AFER Publishing, Windsor

McGrew W C 1972 An ethological study of children's behaviour. Academic Press, New York

Macnamara M 1963 Helping children through their mothers. Journal of Child Psychology and Psychiatry 4:29–46

Morrison T, Newcomer B 1975 Effects of directive vs non-directive play therapy with institutionalized mentally retarded children. American Journal of Mental Deficiency 79: 668–689

Moustakas 1959 Children in play therapy. McGraw-Hill, New York

Munro D M G 1952 An Experiment in the use of group methods with parents in a child guidance clinic. British Journal of Psychiatric Social Work 6: 16–20

Newcomer B I, Morrison T L 1974 Play therapy with institutionalized mentally retarded children. American Journal of Mental Deficiency 78: 727–733

Norman C W 1976 Behaviour modification: a perspective. American Journal of Occupational Therapy 30(8): 491–497

Nurcombe B 1972 An outline of child psychiatry. New South Wales University Press, Sydney

Peoples C 1979 Fair play therapy: a new perspective. The Journal of Psychology 102: 113–117

Prugh D, Kisley A 1970 Emotionally disturbed and mentally ill children and youth. In: Crisis in child mental health a challenge for the 1970s. Report of the Joint Commission on Mental Health of Children, Harper & Row, New York

Rank O 1945 Will therapy. Knopf, New York

Reilly M 1974 Play as exploratory learning. Sage Publications, Beverley Hills

Rexford E N, Schleifer M, Amerongen S T 1956 A follow-up of a psychiatric study of 57 antisocial children. Mental Hygiene 40: 196–214

Rhoden B L, Kranz L, Lund K 1981 Current trends in the use of limits in play therapy. The Journal of Psychology 107: 191–198

Rogers C 1942 Counselling and psychotherapy. Houghton Mifflin, Boston

Rutter M 1973 Why are London children so disturbed? Proceedings of Royal Society of Medicine 66: 1221–1225

Rutter M, Shaffer D, Shephard M 1975 A Multi-axial classification scheme for psychiatric disorders in childhood and adolescence. The Institute of Psychiatry, Department of Child and Adolescent Psychiatry, London

Sheehy R 1976 A critique of non-directive play therapy. Unpublished paper, University of Queensland

Singer J L 1973 The child's world of make-believe. Academic Press, New York

Slavson S R 1952 Child psychotherapy. University Press, New York

Subotnik L S 1975 Client-centred group therapy compared with behaviour modification in changing inappropriate behaviour of elementary school children. Psychotherapy and Psychosomatics 24: 138–141

Taft J 1953 The dynamics of therapy in a controlled relationship. Macmillan, New York

Takata N 1974 The play history. In: Reilly M (ed) Play as exploratory learning. Sage, Beverley Hills

Thomas A, Chess S, Birch H G 1968 Temperament and behaviour disorders in children. New York University Press, New York

Wolfe J 1961 The systematic desensitisation treatment of neuroses. Journal of Nervous Mental Disorders 132: 189–203

World Health Organization 1977 International classification of diseases. Geneva

Yates A 1959 The application of learning theory to the treatment of tics. Journal of Abnormal and Social Psychology 56: 175–182

17. Preparing the child and family for death

READERS' OBJECTIVES

READERS' OBJECTIVES

After reading this chapter, you should be able to:

1. Discuss the implications of current medical management of the terminally ill child for occupational therapy intervention.
2. Demonstrate understanding of the ways in which children perceive death, as they grow and develop.
3. Describe the predictable responses of parents to a diagnosis of terminal illness for their child.
4. Define the general objectives of occupational therapy with a terminally ill child and the family.
5. Discuss the intervention role of an occupational therapist in relation to the child's mother.

One of the most difficult professional activities is working closely with a family who must face the death of their child through illness. Our natural feelings of tragedy and injustice when a child dies before fulfilment make dealing with the dying person even more difficult. In past generations, childhood death was commonplace, and there were few families who did not lose an infant or toddler (Kubler-Ross 1974). There was an inevitability and acceptance of that situation, and the general community provided some understanding and support to grieving families. However, with medical, technological advances, child mortality has been reduced dramatically. Moreover, medical science has enabled us to prolong life, even when the outcome is still death at an early age. The community, in particular parents, does not accept childhood death as one of life's inevitabilities, nor are families psychologically prepared to deal with it.

The major causes of childhood death are accidents, and the cancers, notably leukemia, which represents one-third of all childhood cancers (Parker & Mauger 1979). Most children who sustain injuries which prove to be fatal, for example, through car accidents, or burns,

typically die in hospital, and death is commonly preceded by unconsciousness. Usually there is little time for the parents to be emotionally prepared. The picture is markedly different where children have cancer, or another chronic disease or illness. The diagnosis of a life threatening disease has major social, psychological and economic impacts on the child and the family. When the patient and the family are acquainted with the diagnosis of malignancy, its implications and management, their expectations of a normal life pattern changes suddenly to one of possible or imminent death of the child (Ekert 1983). Their realization of the loss of control over their destinies and of mortality become the paramount concerns. Despite current advances in treatment of childhood malignancy the best the physician can offer is hope, expressed as a probability based on statistics for cure or death (Ekert 1983).

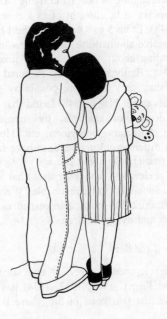

Insecurity is introduced into the daily lives of the family once the child is diagnosed as having cancer. The multidisciplinary team in the oncology unit must aim to restore the family's feeling of security (Ekert 1983).

The concept of care for the terminally ill is comparatively new in our health care system and is a non-traditional setting in which the occupational therapist has begun to practise. It is new in that little has been researched, documented or published with respect to occupational therapy intervention. It is non-traditional in that a new perspective has been added to the occupational therapy belief in the restoration of function and maximal independence.

CHILDREN'S PERCEPTIONS OF DEATH

The way that children understand and represent death has traditionally been examined and explained in terms of developmental age linked to acquisition of cognitive skills. The theoretical approach of much of the research has been strongly influenced by a Piagetian framework (Kane 1979; Koocher 1973, 1974). Furman (1970) believes that to understand how a child perceives death can give insight into how the child will respond to death. From a therapy viewpoint, such understanding will assist the therapist to design intervention which is developmentally appropriate.

Most theorists agree that children probably pass through general stages in the acquisition of perceptions of death, and three or four stages are generally postulated. Notably, up to 5 years the child is thought to have little understanding of death and dying (Anthony 1940). Death appears to be thought of as a reversible process (Nagy 1948). From 5 to 9 years, the child becomes more knowledgeable about death, and begins to have gained understanding about the causes and finality of death (Nagy 1948; Reilly et al 1983). Personal death is still seen as being only a remote possibility (Kane 1979). During this stage, Nagy (1948) found that children personified death, for example, by representing it as ghost-like characters, bogeymen, etc. However, other studies in different cultural settings have failed to replicate this finding. By about the age of 9 years, children begin to understand and articulate that death is permanent, inevitable, and irreversible (Weininger 1979). Let us examine the particular responses of normally developing and dying children.

Infants and toddlers

Several developmental theorists such as Gesell & Ilg (1971) and Piaget (1951, 1952, 1954) have stated that during the first two years of life, there is little under-standing of complex concepts such as death. Games such as peek-a-boo, and daily activities such as sleeping and wakefulness may assist the child to appreciate the difference between 'being' and 'non being' (Maurer 1961). Maurer suggests that 'throwing away' or 'casting' games are play about 'early flirtations with death' as they reinforce the notion that some objects do not return. Clearly such an approach is difficult to evaluate because of the child's limited language skills. Kastenbaum (1967), in reviewing literature in this field, states that researchers are limited to observing behaviour and 'guessing'.

Schowalter (1970) observes that the younger the child the more responses to dying are shaped by adults. Schowalter maintains that infants under six months of age cannot separate themselves from their environment, and therefore only suffer the physical deterioration of their illness. The effects of hospitalization and separation on infants are well documented.

For the infant and toddler, separation from closely bonded loved ones, the feeling of abandonment and loneliness are key sources of anxiety. Thus, in treatment of very young, dying children it is crucial that they remain in close proximity to their parents, either at home or in the hospital.

Preschool aged children

While the preschool child has usually had some firsthand experience with the death of a pet, insect, flower or relative (Schowalter 1970), the death concept is still vague and not yet conceived as permanent (Nagy 1948). Fairy tales and cartoons tend to reinforce notions that death is not permanent. The child of this age has some understanding of limited aspects of time, such as today and tomorrow, but is still grappling with concepts such as months, seasons, and years.

Studies by Safier (1964) and Gartley and Berasconi in 1967 (in Schowalter 1970) concluded that the dying pre-school child is not as vulnerable to separation as the toddler, and is less anxious when questioned about death than at any other age.

At this age, the child may see his illness as a deserved punishment for a real or imagined misdeed. Hospitalization tends to reinforce illness as a punishment for the child by separating him from his parents and subjecting him to painful tests and medical procedures. Schowalter (1970) described two different reactions to feelings of guilt. The child may respond with 'good' behaviour, compliant, and overobedient characteristics. The second reaction is one of rebellion and antagonism, with the child projecting his anger onto parents and staff. In both situations the child must be aided to work through his feelings. Parents, too, must be supported and reassured to handle their child's behaviour and not to withdraw.

School-aged children

There is much dissension about the awareness of death of the child of 5 to 11 years. Spinetta (1974), and Yudkin (1967) considered that the child under 10 years of age lacks the intellectual ability to conceptualize death and thus will experience little anxiety if it is not discussed. These authors noted that even desperately ill children seemed unable to conceive that they would not recover.

However, an alternative view is that ill children of this age are aware that something very serious is happening to them even if they are not aware of their approaching death. Waechter (1971), Spinetta (1974) and Kubler-Ross (1974) maintained that children with a fatal prognosis were not only aware that they were dying but were able to express that awareness by actual death related words.

Fear of death becomes apparent at this age, bringing with it mixed reactions of horror, confusion, and anger from the child (Ingoldby 1980). A growing body of literature suggests that children in the age group 6 to 10 years are fearful and anxious about their impending death, despite not being told directly the fatal nature of the illness (Spinetta et al 1974; Waechter 1971).

Several authors have written about the child's ability to diagnose his or her own illness (Spinetta 1974; Spinetta et al 1974; Vernick 1973). Children with a terminal illness tend to be more anxious, than children with a chronic disease (Spinetta & Maloney 1975; Waechter 1971). Moreover, the study of children's drawings suggests that they are more aware of their condition than they articulate (Bach 1974, 1975, cited in Eiser 1979). Vernick (1970) maintains that regardless of the children's age, they appear to be aware that they may die from their illness.

Adolescent children

By the age of around 10 or 11 years, the preadolescent child comprehends the universality and permanency of death (Anthony 1940; Melear 1973; Nagy 1948; Safier 1964). The adolescent with a terminal illness is faced with particular problems. Not only does she/he have to cope with the normal social, emotional and physical growth changes, but she/he also has to cope with chronic illness and diminishing functional ability.

Schowalter (1970) sensitively points out that it is during this stage of development that physical beauty becomes highly valued, thus making the physical and psychological ravages of cancer all the more difficult to cope with. Moreover, just as the child is beginning to experience real independence, she/he is faced with loss of control, and the need for assistance in many personal daily living functions. Children of this age group are prone to feelings of disgrace and shame (Schowalter 1970). While younger children experience the problem of physical separation, the adolescent faces emotional separation. While the young child and adults can turn to others for support, the adolescent with his/her new found independence may not accept support and understanding from significant others, as she/he approaches death (Pakes 1977). The young person may harbour resentment toward unaffected peers who are a constant reminder of his or her own lack of future (Ingoldby 1980).

The 'half-child/half-adult' has a mature, or almost adult-like understanding of death, and the response to death is similarly more adult-like (Schowalter 1970). Thus denial and depression are quite common. Robertson (1978), when looking at management of the dying adolescent advocated the need to treat them openly and honestly allowing them to as much independence as possible, a role in decision making, and an opportunity to act as persons in their own right.

DYING CHILDREN AND THEIR FAMILIES

The impact of a fatal disease on the child depends on a number of factors:

- The age of the child
- The level of cognitive functioning
- The nature of the illness
- Personality traits
- The child's experience with death and emotional adjustment
- Available type and quality of support systems.

Each family responds to situations in its own characteristic way (Kyriacou 1983; Pakes 1977). Consequently, some families faced with the impending death of a child, will be thrown into utter despair, and will see no joy in life. Others, despite being anxious and sad, will try and get the most out of each day. Some family members will blame each other, while others will rally and support each other. The threat of losing a child is one of the most stressful occurrences that a family can experience. Broad ranging problems can become manifest, and can include jealousies, guilt, unresolved grief reactions in siblings, divorce and mental illness (Binger et al 1969,

Friedman 1967, Marstein 1960). In *General Systems Theory*, Von Bertalanffy (1968) explains and predicts such behaviour, in holding that change in one part of the system affects change in the other parts, as well as the whole system. Elfer (1979) draws the analogy between the family network of relationships and a straw mobile. When one straw is removed or changed, the whole mobile becomes initially unstable, but later settles down, with each straw having both a new position and a new role. There can be a period of initial instability, followed by a period of adjustment when family members may acquire new roles and expectations. Of course, if the family structure is already weak, it may not be able to withstand the strain of serious illness.

Reactions to the news of impending death

Kubler-Ross (1974) outlined the emotional reactions to death, identifying that the individual and family will move through the stages in their own unique way, with some individuals never achieving acceptance of impending death. She counsels that the stages are artificial, but helpful to our own understanding, and people approaching death oscillate between the various stages. The stages are discussed in some depth.

Shock and denial. Often when parents are first told of the diagnosis, they react with a variety of defence mechanisms such as denial, dissociation, regression and repression (Freedman et al 1980, cited in Ekert 1983), and emotions such as shock, grief and thoughts or words to the effect 'it can't be true'. Kubler-Ross (1974) suggests that denial is a perfectly normal and adaptive behaviour. It allows the reality of illness to be suppressed so that positive plans can be made and painful interventions endured (Geist 1979, O'Malley et al 1979). Kubler-Ross refers to this process as a 'functional buffer'.

Initially parents react with feelings of guilt and question their ability as parents; for example, they may question whether they sought medical treatment early enough. For many parents, this initial period is followed by increased levels of activity, where they search for information on the illness (Eiser 1979). Families then pass into a phase of angry protest.

Anger and protest. The reaction is typified by words to the effect 'why me?'. This stage can be disruptive to relationships, and anger can be directed towards family, friends, loved ones, God, hospital staff, as well as the community at large.

Bargaining. The child patient and parents may try to make a deal with God, the family, or any one who will listen, in order to get relief or respite from the situation. The rationale appears to be that, if God or parents do not respond to angry pleas and protest, then perhaps 'nice' behaviour may gain some reward or respite. When the bargain does not work, the affected adult and child may experience anger, or despair.

Depression. When the child patient and family can no longer deny the illness, depression occurs. Kubler-Ross describes two kinds of depression:

- Reactive depression occurs because of loss.
- Preparatory depression occurs because of impending loss or death in the future.

Acceptance. Many parents of dying children can never 'accept' impending death, but rather become resigned to it. During times of remission the parents try and lead as 'normal' a life as possible, however, many parents are prone to overindulge the child (Parker & Mauger 1979; Vernick 1973). As the child enters the terminal stage of the illness, the parents enter into a stage of preparatory mourning which is a stage of grief before to the final loss, when the inevitability of death is acknowledged (Aldrich 1974). During this period of time, parents may also relinquish some of the emotional bond with the child (Richmond & Waisman 1955). Not only are there enormous emotional demands and stresses placed on the parents of a terminally ill child, but there are also enormous physical demands. For example, there are medical appointments to be kept, visits to outpatient clinics; time with the child when she/he is hospitalized; discussions with school teachers, social workers and other professionals; continuing to nurture and care for their other children; coping with personal sleep interruption, and undertaking the extra tasks associated with the sick child's activities of daily living. Often many of these responsibilities fall on the mother (Eiser 1979, Futterman & Hoffman 1973, Maguire 1983, Van Dongen-Melman & Sanders-Woudstra 1986).

Siblings

Fear, regression, and jealously are three typical responses by siblings to a dying or chronically sick brother or sister (Elfer 1979). The extra attention afforded the terminally ill child is usually at the expense of the other children in the family. In fact, Spinetta (1981) found that in terms of family relationships the siblings have their needs met least of all. A recurring theme in the literature, is the disruption in interpersonal relationships, particularly the parent-child relationship (Cairns et al 1979, Iles 1979). Disorders in siblings reported by parents have included poor school performance, school phobia, depression, enuresis, headaches and abdominal pains (Binger et al 1969).

Parents, and others should be aware of practical issues that need addressing, for example:

— the age of the siblings
— their relationship with the sick child
— the likelihood that siblings might feel that the sick child is favoured.

Siblings should be prepared for the death of a brother or sister and should continue to visit the child in hospital, to the terminal stages (Ekert 1983). During crisis situations, such as the death of a family member, children require parental support, but their need comes at a time when the parents also need support. Parents may inevitably communicate confusion, grieving, and ambivalence (Weber & Fournier 1985), which can place stress and confusion on the children. A child may become 'overwhelmed' by excessive parental grief or breakdown, unless the child is given adequate explanation (Salladay & Royal 1981). Ekert (1983) also suggests that siblings attend the funeral, as a ritual way of bringing their relationship with the dead child to a close.

Parents

Kubler-Ross (1974) emphasizes the importance of maintaining 'hope' in order to support a family coming to terms with the terminal nature of an illness. Hope should never be unrealistic, for example, by implying that a child will recover. Rather, it can be expressed to parents by talking about all that can be done for the child's condition and symptoms. Kubler-Ross puts the proposition that telling a family or child that she/he is dying is 'to deprive him/her of the glimpse of hope that she/he may need in order to live until she/he dies.' However, many would not agree with her.

Talking about death

When faced with questions about death, parents and professionals can experience frustration and anxiety (Banus 1971; Lornetto 1980; Pakes 1977; Travis 1976). Kavanaugh (1972) and Parker & Mauger (1979) maintained that children who have been told the truth and were allowed to talk about it openly responded with honesty and maturity. They pointed out that the child kept in ignorance will feel guilty and responsible for the behaviour of those around them, will fail to grow beyond the stages of denial and isolation, and will be deprived of peace and dignity. Schowalter (1970), however, was more cautious and advocated not telling the school age child of the prognosis because of the child's emotional immaturity.

Very little escapes the notice of children, even in the preschool years. Children quickly learn the names and functions of various pieces of hospital equipment, and have been observed to monitor the condition of other patients by looking into rooms. Children know that moving a patient to a private room or to a more highly staffed area can mean a deterioration in a patient's condition (Spinetta et al 1974; Vernick 1973). Children will, for example, check the name plates on doors to see if anyone died during the night. Natterson & Knudson (1960) identified three main sources of stress in hospitalized dying children, one of which is the death of another child. The other two sources of stress are traumatic procedures, and separation from their mothers. Banus (1971) provides some practical suggestions for the therapist about what to tell children about impending death. The therapist needs to establish:

— the policy of the hospital
— the policy of the child's physician
— the decision of the parents
— what the child has been told already
— the child's understanding of the meaning of death.

Ultimately, it is the parents' decision what is to be told to the child (Parker & Mauger 1979), but they may ask for the assistance of medical staff or other professionals, including the occupational therapist.

INTERVENTION

The family

The place of the family in the treatment team can be depicted in diagrammatic form as a central nucleus of intermediaries between the child and all other members of the team. It is vital to ensure that help for the child is channelled through the family members. When provided by others the message communicated may be that the family cannot cope with the problem themselves (Mott 1982).

The aims of intervention with the family are:

1. To allow parents to express some of their feelings, of guilt, anxiety and apprehension about dealing with a disease beyond their control.
   Communication skills of specialists become particularly crucial. Some hospitals have found that in addition to individual counselling, parent self-help groups provide opportunity for venting frustration and shared anxiety.
2. To nurture the parent–child bond. Families should be involved as much as possible in the daily care of their child. The aim of the team is to enhance the parents' contribution, rather than usurp it. A

common parental response is an all-embracing care of the child, which stems from a desire to protect the child from the rigours of the world, and thus to compensate for their responsibility for the disease. This response frustrates the development of independence of the child — an aim of the therapist.

3. To interpret the child's behaviour to the parents. Cancer can cause emotional problems in almost any child. Frequent trips to the hospital, missing school, feeling sick or tired can all make the child anxious and difficult to handle. Parents may misinterpret their child's behaviour and feel rejected. Hints on behaviour management may be beneficial, reinforcing the child's need to be treated as normally as possible with no fuss, presents or concessions.

4. To nurture the parent–sibling relationships. It is more important to offer support to the siblings of the dying child, than perhaps at any other time in their young lives. Parents should have a frank and honest discussion with them, giving medical advice should the children wish. The siblings should be prepared for the child's death, visit the child in hospital and be included in treatment activities (Ekert 1983).

The child

Willetts & Sperling (1983) postulate that if the dying child's needs for reassurance, support, acceptance and understanding are not met, the illness process may be intensified. It is generally accepted that admission to hospital for children is stressful (Barker 1974, see also Chapter 14). The child with a life threatening disease suffers the additional burden of an uncertain prognosis and the real threat of having to contend with death. It is possible for the hospital situation to become excessively impersonal, with a great deal of attention being paid to the child's illness, and too little to his feelings (Plank 1971). Possible explanations are that staff may simply be too busy, or may feel very guilty about simply sitting and talking to a child. They may be inclined to feel that they are only achieving something for their patients if they are actively doing something.

While the importance of effectively communicating with hospitalized children has been recognized and accepted, few attempts have been made to describe or assess such communicative interactions. Klinzing and colleagues (1977) described interactions, but made no attempt to determine what factors influence the occurrence of these interactions.

Goffman (1963), Bryne et al (1968), Alessi & Anthony (1969) and Richardson (1971) have suggested that physical unattractiveness predisposes individuals to impoverished inter-personal relationships. These workers also found a negative effect for unattractiveness. Another factor which appears to have an impact on interactions between the child and his caretaker is the severity of his illness. When a child is seriously ill, caretakers appear to give less supportive attention to that child. Such caretaker behaviour must compound the stress of hospitalization and separation from the family for the child. Such effects have been carefully studied and documented in literature and films by Bowlby (1973) and Robertson (1952).

Perhaps one explanation is that a personal approach may be difficult for the first few days of hospitalization especially with the unhappy, negativistic or seriously ill child. A situation exists in which complete devotion to a helpless patient is demanded of the nurse, while the child regards him/her with hostility, and rejects efforts at giving comforts. The quiet child, who may be very unhappy, frequently has the greatest need for attention, but is often neglected.

Further investigation is needed to determine more clearly which factors influence the attention a child will receive in hospital.

Occupational therapy

One of the problems that professionals face when confronted with the needs of the dying child, is that they themselves often do not have the psychological resources for fulfilling these needs (Forbes 1984). It becomes an emotional burden to establish open, empathetic communication with every such patient — too much grief, too much sadness, too great a sense of futility and failure (Epstein 1975). Dying children and their families need to discuss sensitive and traumatic subjects, requiring the occupational therapist to be skilled and attuned to communication skills crucial to the therapeutic process (Whitley et al 1979).

It is essential for the therapist to examine personal attitudes toward grief and dying thoroughly, and resolve these issues at some private level in order to be helpful rather than destructive (Crawford 1980, Grammage et al 1976).

The goals of occupational therapy with dying children are related to holistic areas of the child's development — social and emotional, physical and educational.

The occupational therapist's role

Picard & Magno (1982) when reviewing hospice care

said, 'The presence of an occupational therapist in the hospice array of services points to a continued meaning in life, even if that life is measured in days.'

Tigges & Sherman (1983) demonstrated how quality of life was improved by enhancing skill areas important to the patient, 'The occupational therapist must concentrate on making the most of the patient's capacity and independence in self-care, work and play within the constraints of their physical limitations.'

Treatment with the dying child requires a 'day-at-a-time' approach — to provide for the maximal quality of life from each day despite how few these may be. The occupational therapist in oncology must consider the child and his family to develop the child's maximal capacity. Often the occupational therapist is one of the few people in the treatment centre whom the child does not associate with pain, and unpleasant medical treatment. The therapist can explain hospital procedures to children and the parents, in a relaxed, calm way, taking the time that medical doctors often cannot afford. People often have minimal knowledge of anatomy and physiology, so the therapist can explain these concepts in understandable terms. Vernick (1970) states that one of the most important things that staff and parents can do is to let the child know what is happening to his or her body, and what is likely to happen in the future. She/he can also systematically provide the physical contact and attention that may be avoided by others.

The need to consider the psychosocial aspects of cancer cannot be understated. Cancer treatment produces a high degree of stress, and anxiety can occur for a number of reasons:

- Anxiety and pain from medical procedures such as bone marrow aspirations, lumbar punctures and injections
- Nausea and vomiting from the chemotherapy and conditioned responses associated with the treatment
- Loss of hair
- Disfigurement
- Skin reactions
- Tiredness
- Suppressed immunity.

Even as an outpatient, the child can be faced with many trips to hospital, painful and unpleasant treatment procedures, missing school, and feeling sick and tired. Even optimal care at home or in hospital can interfere with social and developmental skills. The child can become very dependent on the parents and regress due to psychological, or physical factors, for example, decreased strength, or lack of experience and practice.

Objectives

1. Encourage mobility and independence in self-care, leisure and daily activities.

This may require aids, prostheses and training, slings, splinting, for accomplishment of daily tasks to keep the child at home as long as is possible, and maintain physical strength. The child should be encouraged to continue participation in schooling, social events and usual activities within limitations. The principle of family involvement should be maintained as much as possible, so that they reinforce skills learned. The family's involvement is also a gentle indirect way of showing parents what can realistically be expected from the child (Banus 1971).

2. Provide a permissive and relaxed play situation in which children can express and work through their anger and anxiety.

Therapeutic play gives opportunity for medical procedures to be explained, and for children to prepare themselves by acting out fear, anxiety and aggression (Adams 1976). Many researchers have highlighted the finding that children often misinterpret or fantasize that illness and medical treatment is punishment for some past 'bad' behaviour (Schowalter 1970). This type of therapy intervention allows the therapist to explain the rationale and procedures of various medical procedures and thus reinforces reality (Ingoldby 1980, Willets & Sperling 1983).

3. Teach the child various coping skills in order to reduce or relieve stress, anxiety and pain.

Some of the techniques which have been used include fantasy exploration, graded imagery experiences, positive memory recall, hypnosis, meditation, biofeedback, breathing exercises, reinforcement and systematic contraction and relaxation of muscle groups (Hilgard & LeBaron 1982; Jay et al 1985; Schultz 1980).

The occupational therapist can also act as a role model for the child, and therapy sessions allow development and practice of skills and coping techniques, to deal with 'curious onlookers' or others who may tease, torment, or ask sensitive questions. Taking the child to a shopping centre, playground or 'McDonalds' is particularly useful as it gives the child the opportunity to practise coping strategies, in the company of a supportive adult. Support should similarly be offered to the siblings and parents.

4. To help the child to understand, integrate and feel more in control of what is happening to him/her.

Like many adults, children may be unable to talk about dying, or more likely may be unable to find anyone who is willing and able to listen to their subtle cues and expressions of fear. So children may die lonely, with people all around them.

When children are hospitalized, they lose control over their environment. This applies particularly to the adolescent who has reached the age where it is appropriate to have some independence. Adolescents can feel most indignant about being placed in a children's ward which has policies such as lights out at 7.30 pm. The modern trend towards establishing separate places for adolescent people allows for more flexible policies. Through the tasks associated with occupational therapy, the child or young adult continues to exercise control and mastery over the abnormal environment of hospital. Bluebond-Langner (1978) speaks of the depersonalizing way we as a society have come to deal with people who cause us to feel uncomfortable — as do dying children. We ignore them, turn away, treat them as 'objects' — we deprive them of rights over their bodies. As an example, she records that no adult on the hospital staff in which she conducted research asked the dying children's permission to be interviewed, or engage in simple procedures. But the adults gave permission on the children's behalf.

All specialists must convey respect toward the child to help facilitate a true perception that she/he indeed does continue to have some areas of control over his/her daily life. Respect can be conveyed in many ways, for example, asking the child's opinion, giving choices for selection, giving the authority or leadership role to the child in activities and games. As Bluebond-Langner puts it, the therapist has an important and special role, 'being there for him/her', no matter what the children's behaviour. Axline's (1989) non-directive personal interaction style is a most useful style for a therapist working with dying children. It is dynamically interactive, yet the therapist is like a mirror to the child, reflecting for him or her what is crucially and personally important — to the child, not the powerful adult. Involvement of the family can also facilitate a feeling of control. At times parents themselves feel helpless or inadequate when the child is in hospital, undergoing complex technical procedures.

5. To promote the child's optimal social development. The honey-pot model described in Chapter 4 has particular application to the terminally ill child. It is so important to design and promote experiences and situations which overcome the natural reluctance of others — peers, siblings, nursing and caretaker staff — to interact with the child. The kitchen and social activity centred on food provide a most facilitating social context, and this suggestion reinforces applicability of the honey-pot model.

Therapeutic activities should be provided to generally maintain, and foster developmentally appropriate behaviours and skills. Parents should be counselled about the expected norms of behaviour and achievement for the child's age, and suitable activities for them and other children at home.

Evaluation of occupational therapy

Despite the large amount of literature pertaining to the problems of the dying there is little dealing with the contribution of the occupational therapist in this area. There appear to be several reasons (Forbes 1984, 1988):

— Society has built up a taboo around death and the dying person. Hence, it may be that therapists have avoided addressing the area for this reason.
— Medicine traditionally focused on the preservation of life, and terminal illness and death have been seen as a dismal failure of medical knowledge.
— Occupational therapy involvement in paediatric oncology is relatively recent, and further literature will take some time to amass.
— The major difficulty in evaluating the efficacy of treatment methods in oncology is in delineating the indicators of successful intervention. Generally the eradication or improvement of the presenting problem is seen as the measure of success or failure. The terminally ill child defies this yardstick as his/her condition leads ultimately to his/her demise. So what does constitute effective treatment of the terminally ill child? How can we measure successful and fulfilled death, quality of life, or acceptance of dying? The subjectivity of these factors renders evaluation difficult.

Whitley et al (1979) have provided one of the few guides so far that has attempted to evaluate efficacy of occupational therapy intervention with dying children. However, small sample size, lack of control group, observer bias and the subjectivity of interview data render it difficult to draw firm conclusions from the study. There is scope for further research in this area, to ensure that service delivery is appropriate and effective in dealing with the dying child.

AFTER DEATH: PLANNING FOR THE FUTURE

When it becomes clear that the child is in the last stages of the illness process, the focus of the therapist's attention should shift from the child/family unit, to the family/child unit, with special attention to the mother. By this time the child's mother will be spending long hours each day with her dying child, and her life will be centred on the child's needs. If such a pattern is maintained up to the child's death, then the mother must suddenly face another disruption of gigantic proportions in her own life. She will have lost not only her child, but also her normal daily routines at home, or in her workplace. The child's death will remove her major, if distorted, daily activity base, and the major gap in her life will not be quickly or easily replaced or restored. Her losses are thereby multiplied, placing her at grave risk for personal emotional trauma. Mothers are much more vulnerable than other family members, because our society believes that it should be the mother who adopts the major nurturing role (Oakley 1972).

We suggest that effective therapy systematically plans a bridge for the child's mother, in particular, across the period of death into her and her family's new future. Practically, this should entail helping the mother disengage herself physically from her child. Instead of spending more hours, she should slowly but gradually spend less hours with the child. At the same time, she should be assisted to redevelop her familiar pre-illness life patterns, and/or begin to extend herself by taking on some new and personally satisfying activities. It really does not matter what these are — gardening, an educational course, a new challenge at her workplace, exotic cooking. The principles are that the activity absorbs her attention and physical energy, and leads her to *plan* for future developments. Mother can bring her own occupations back to the child's world so that the pair can share and plan together on the mother's behalf. This way of looking toward the future is another way of engaging in 'hopeful' behaviour. It is a positive way of helping the mother build memories of the child's participation which she can carry over the inevitable dark weeks ahead of her. For example, if mother takes up 'fitness', she and her child can make and keep a log, which the child monitors. It is something to talk about day — each how far she ran, how she is improving, what it is doing to her figure, appetite — ordinary things — and funny incidents that all runners encounter in public places! It gives the child reasons to anticipate her visits with pleasure, and both have positive goals in being together. The *quality* of time together can be enhanced.

Naturally, a mother will feel very guilty, or at least feel that she should be guilty about 'abandoning' her child in this way. The therapist is an important representative of authority, who can give the necessary emotional permission to the mother, and the social support necessary to achieve the healthy step of reintegrating her and her family's life. We do not suggest that this will be an easy task for the therapist. Many mothers and colleagues may initially view this approach as heartless and selfish.

The occupational therapist ought to initiate and maintain contact with the child's family after death. Mothers, in particular may find great comfort in simply talking over those times, and thus resolving the painful grieving problems.

SUMMARY

Children's perceptions of death appear to occur in stages, somewhat reminiscent of developmental and cognitive stages of growth and development. While there is little agreement in the literature as to how many stages there are, three or four stages are usually discussed.

The impact of a terminal illness on each member of a family unit is immense. Parents experience the full range of physical, psychological, emotional and financial stress. The siblings can experience an array of emotions, such as feeling neglected, jealous, fearful and confused. The dying child may experience pain, side effects from medical treatment, separation anxiety, when hospitalized, and fear of mutilation and death. The occupational therapy contribution is a life affirming rather than a death denying one.

This book began with a statement of occupational therapy philosophy which expressed as its first tenet, that there is healing value in occupation. This assertion holds true for the dying child and his or her family. The occupational therapist's particular contribution is to emphasize that the dying child is still a living person with feelings, abilities and capacity for development. The occupational therapist can enhance the quality of life of both the child and family, and aid them to cope and grow through one of life's greatest traumas.

We conclude this book with a re-affirmation of this philosophy, for all child clients, their families, and you their therapist — expressed through an ancient Sanskrit poem.

Look to this day for it is life,
The very life of life.
In its brief course lie all the realities and truths of existence;
The joy of growth; the splendour of action;
The glory of power.
For yesterday is but a memory and tomorrow only a vision,
But today well lived makes every yesterday a memory of
    happiness and every tomorrow a vision of hope.
Look well, therefore, to this day.

REFERENCES

Adams M A 1976 A hospital play program: helping children with serious illness. American Journal of Orthopsychiatry 46(3): 416–424

Aldrich C K 1974 Some dynamics of anticipatory grief. In: Schoenberg B, Carr A C, Kutscher A H, Peretz D, Goldberg I K (eds) Anticipatory grief. Columbia University Press, New York

Alessi D E, Anthony W A 1969 The uniformity of children's attitudes towards physical disabilities. Exceptional Children 35: 543

Anthony S 1940 The child's discovery of death. Harcourt Brace, New York

Axline V M 1989 Play therapy. Churchill Livingstone, Edinburgh. First published 1947, Riverside Press, Cambridge, Massachusetts

Bach S R 1974/1975 Spontaneous pictures of leukemic children as an expression of the total personality, mind and body. In: Eiser C (ed) 1979 Psychological development of the child with leukemia: a review. Journal of Behavioural Medicine 2(2): 141–157

Banus B S 1971 The Developmental therapist. Charles B Slack, Thorofare

Barker P 1974 Psychological effects on children of admission to hospital. Update October: 1019–1024

Binger C M, Ablin A R, Feuerstein Q C, Kushner J H, Zoger S, Mikkelson C 1969 Childhood leukemia: Emotional impact on patient and family. New England Journal of Medicine 280: 414–418

Bluebond-Langner M 1978 The private worlds of dying children. Princeton University Press, Princeton

Bowlby J 1973 Attachment and loss, Vol 2: Separation, anxiety and anger. Hogarth Press, London

Bryne D, London D, Reeves K 1968 The effects of physical attractiveness, sex and attitudes similarity on interpersonal attraction. Journal of Personality 36: 259–271

Cairns N U, Clark G M, Smith S D, Lansky S B 1979 Adaptation of siblings to childhood malignancy. Journal of Pediatrics 95: 484–487

Crawford M 1980 Psychosocial aspects of death, dying and bereavement. Australian Occupational Therapy Journal 26: 116–120

Eiser C 1979 Psychological development of the child with leukemia: a review. Journal of Behavioural Medicine 2(2): 141–157

Ekert H 1983 Long term needs of children and parents with chronic life threatening diseases. Australian Family Physician 12(4): 237–241

Elfer P 1979 Social work with children with leukemia and their families. In: Lonsdale G, Elfer P, Ballard R Children grief and social work. Blackwell, Oxford

Epstein C 1975 Nursing the dying patient. In: Freedman A H, Kaplan J H, Sadcock B J (eds) Comprehensive book of psychiatry. Williams & Wilkins, Baltimore

Forbes F 1984 Unpublished manuscript, University of Queensland Department of Occupational Therapy, Brisbane

Forbes F 1988 Personal communication

Freedman A M, Kaplan H J, Sadock B J (eds) 1980 Comprehensive textbook of psychiatry. In: Ekert H (ed) Long term needs of children and parents with chronic life threatening diseases. Williams & Wilkins, Baltimore

Friedman S B 1967 Care of the family of the child with cancer. Pediatrics 40: 498–507

Furman R 1970 The child's reaction to death in the family. In: Schoenberg B, Carr A, Peretz D, Kutscher A (eds) Loss and grief: psychological management in medical practice. Columbia University Press, New York

Futterman E H, Hoffman I 1973 Crisis and adaptation in the families of fatally ill children. In: Anthony E J, Koupernik C (eds) The child and his family: the impact of disease and death. John Wiley, New York, pp 127–143

Geist R A 1979 Onset of chronic illness in children and adolescents: psychotherapeutic and consultative intervention. American Journal of Orthopsychiatry 49: 4–23

Gesell A, Ilg A 1971 The first five years of life. Methuen, London

Goffman E 1963 Stigma. Prentice-Hall, New Jersey

Grammage S L, McMahon P S, Maher P 1976 The OT and terminal illness: learning to cope with death. American Journal of Occupational Therapy 30(5): 294–299

Hilgard J R, Le Baron S 1982 Relief of anxiety and pain in children and adolescents with cancer: quantitative measures and clinical observances. International Journal of Clinical and Experimental Hypnosis 30: 417–442

Iles J P 1979 Children with cancer: healthy siblings' perceptions during the illness experience. Cancer Nursing 2: 371–377

Ingoldby H 1980 Reactions to the dying child to his illness. Australian Occupational Therapy Journal 27(3): 148–151

Jay S M, Elliott C H, Ozolins M, Olson R A, Pruitt S D 1985 Behavioural management of children's distress during painful medical procedures. Behavioural Research Therapy 23: 513–520

Kane B 1979 Children's concepts of death. Journal of Genetic Psychology 134: 141–153

Kastenbaum R 1967 The child's understanding of death: how does it develop? In: Grollman E A (ed) Explaining death to children. Beacon, Boston

Kavanaugh R E 1972 Facing death. Penguin, New York

Klinzing D R, Klinzing D G, Schindler P D 1977 A preliminary report of a methodology to assess the communicative interaction between hospital personnel and the hospitalised child. American Journal of Public Health 67(7): 670–671

Koocher G 1973 Childhood, death and cognitive development. Developmental Psychology 9: 369–375

Koocher G P 1974 Talking with children about death. American Journal of Orthopsychiatry 44(3): 404–411

Kyriacou C B 1983 Differences in cultural attitudes toward death and dying. Australian Family Physician 12(4): 257–258

Kubler-Ross E 1974 On death and dying. Tavistock, London

Lornetto R 1980 Children's conceptions of death. Springer, New York

Maguire G P 1983 The psychological sequence of childhood leukemia. In: Duncan W (ed) Paediatric Oncology Springer Verlag, Berlin, pp 47–56

Marstein B 1960 The effects of long-term illness on children on the emotional adjustment of parents. Child Development 31: 151–171

Maurer A 1961 The child's view of death. Journal of Existential Psychiatry 6: 193–212

Melear J 1973 Children's conceptions of death. Journal of Genetic Psychology 123: 359–360

Mott M 1982 Caring for children with cancer. In: Wilkes E (ed) The dying patient. MTP Press, Lancaster

Nagy M 1948 The child's theories concerning death. Journal of Genetic Psychology 73: 3–27

Natterson J, Knudson A 1960 Observations concerning fear of death in fatally ill children and their mothers. Psychosomatic Medicine 22: 456–465

Oakley A 1972 Are husbands good housewives? In: Barker P (ed) One for sorrow, two for joy. George Allen & Unwin, London

O'Malley J E, Koocher G, Foster D, Slavin L 1979 Psychiatric sequelae of surviving childhood cancer. American Journal of Orthopsychiatry 49: 608–616

Pakes E 1977 The Dying Child and his family. In: Stienhauer P D, Rae-Grant Q (eds) Psychological problems of the child and his family. Basic Books, New York

Parker M, Mauger D 1979 Children with cancer. Cassell, London

Piaget J 1951 Play, dreams and imitation in childhood. Norton, New York

Piaget J 1952 The origins of intelligence in children. International Universities Press, New York

Piaget J 1954 The construction of reality in the child. Basic Books, New York

Picard H B, Magno J B 1982 The role of occupational therapy in hospice care. American Journal of Occupational Therapy 36: 597–598

Plank E N 1971 Working with children in hospitals. Western Reserve Press, Illinois

Reilly T P, Hasazi J E, Bond L A 1983 Children's conceptions of death and personal mortality. Journal of Pediatric Psychology 8: 21–31

Richardson S A 1971 Children's values and friendships: a study of physical disability. Journal of Health and Social Behaviour 12: 253

Richmond J B, Waisman H A 1955 Psychological aspects of management of children with malignant diseases. American Journal of Disturbed Children 89: 42–47

Robertson J 1952 Film: a two-year old goes to hospital. Tavistock Child Development Research Unit, London

Robertson, S 1978 Adolescents and dying. Medical Journal of Australia 1: 419–421

Safier G 1964 A study in relationships between the life and death concepts in children. Journal of Genetic Psychology 105: 283–294

Salladay S A, Royal M E 1981 Children and death:

guidelines for grief work. Child Psychiatry and Human Development 11(4): 203–213

Schowalter J E 1970 The child's reaction to his own illness. In: Schoenberg B, Larr A, Peretz D, Kutschor A H (eds) Loss and grief: psychological management in medical practice. Columbia University Press, New York

Schultz E W 1980 Teaching coping skills for stress and anxiety. Teaching Exceptional Children. Fall: 12–15

Spinetta J J 1974 The dying child's awareness of death. Psychological Bulletin 81: 256–260

Spinetta J J 1981 The siblings of the child with cancer. In: Spinetta J J, Deasy-Spietta C P (eds) Living with childhood cancer, Mosby, St Louis, pp133–142

Spinetta J J, Maloney L J 1975 Death anxiety in the outpatient leukemia child. Pediatrics 56: 1034–1037

Spinetta J J, Rigler D, Karon M 1974 Anxiety in the dying child. Pediatrics 52: 841–845

Tigges K N, Sherman L M 1983 The treatment of the hospice patient: from occupational history to occupational role. American Journal of Occupational Therapy 37(4): 235–238

Travis G 1976 Chronic illness in children, its impact on child and family. Stanford University Press, Palo Alto

Van Dongen-Melman J E W M, Sanders-Woudstra J A R 1986 Psychological aspects of childhood cancer: a review of the literature. Journal of Child Psychology and Psychiatry 27(2): 145–180

Vernick J 1970 Meaningful communications with the fatally ill child. In: Anthony E J, Koupernick C (eds) The child and his family: the impact of disease and death, Vol 2. John Wiley, New York

Von Bertalanffy L 1968 General system theory. George Brazelton, New York

Waechter E H 1971 Children's awareness of fatal illness. American Journal of Nursing 71: 1168–1172

Weber J A, Fournier D G 1985 Family support and a child's adjustment to death. Family Relations 34: 43–49

Weininger O 1979 Young children's concepts of dying and dead. Psychological Reports 44: 395–407

Whitley S B, Branscomb B V, Morena H 1979 Identification and management of psychosocial and environmental problems of children with cancer. American Journal of Occupational Therapy 33(11): 711–716

Willetts H C, Sperling A 1983 The role of the therapeutic recreationist in assisting the oncology patient to cope. In: Wiernick P H (ed) Support care of the cancer patient. Futura Publishing, New York

Yudkin S 1967 Children and death. Lancet 1: 37–41

Appendix I: Summary of prenatal development

Age (weeks)	Structural development	Functional development (weeks)
2.5	Neural groove indicated	
3.5	Primitive blood vessels and heart; neural crest formed	Heart beat begins
4	All somites present; limb buds form; neural tube closes; optic cup and lens pit forming	
5	Premuscle masses in head, trunk and limbs	
6	Limbs recognizable; semicircular ducts become outlined	
7	Muscles differentiate rapidly — assume final shapes and relations; cerebral hemispheres becoming large; eyelids forming	Contralateral neck flexion (7.5)
8	Digits well formed; first ossification in middle of long bones; cerebral cortex begins to get typical cells; well-represented, definitive muscle in trunk, limbs and head; olfactory nucleus appears	Contralateral neck and trunk flexion (8.5) Spontaneous movement (9.5) Mouth opening (9.4) Stretch reflex (9.5)
10	Limbs nicely modelled; ossification spreading; spinal cord attains definitive internal structure; eyelids fused	Eyelid squint (10) Ventral head flexion (10) Incomplete finger closure (10.5) Plantar flexion of all toes (11)
12	Sex determined by external inspection; brain attains general structural features; spinal cord shows cervical and lumbar enlargements; internal ear formed; some bones well outlined; taste buds appear	Lip closure and swallowing (12) Dorsiflexion of big toe and toe fanning Flexion at foot, knee, hip (12) Elevate angle of mouth (13) Complete finger closure (13) Contralateral resonses established (13) Vestibular and proprioceptive influence on responses (13)
16	Face looks 'human'; hair on head; most bones distinctly indicated; joint cavities appear; cerebellum assumes some prominence; general sense organs differentiating (cutaneous)	Muscular movements can be detected in utero; reciprocal innervation in movements (16) Diagonal responses (16) 'Scowl' combined with head extension (16) Temporary diaphragm contraction (17) Effective but weak true grasp (18.5)
20	Myelination of cord begins; nail plate begins	Side-to-side head turning (22) Weak vocal sounds (22)

Age (weeks)	Structural development	Functional development (weeks)
24	Cerebral cortex layered typically	Sucking (24) Sneezing (24) Tendon reflexes (24) Palpebral reflex (25) Permanent respiration if delivered (27)
28	Cerebral fissures and convolutions appearing rapidly; eyelids reopen	Synergic muscle action (28) Corneal reflexes (28) Audible sucking (29)
32		Taste sense present; olfactory present
36	Most general sense organs completed	
40	Myelination of brain begins	Iris reflexes

Source: Based mainly on data presented by Humphrey T 1964. Some correlations between the appearance of human fetal reflexes and the development of the nervous system. In: Purpura D P, Schade J P (eds) The growth and maturation of the brain, Elsevier Publishing, New York.

Appendix II: Significant developmental milestones

Compiled by M. C. O'Leary

The summarized ages for each developmental stage are approximate and drawn from a range of sources. This compilation is intended to provide a composite view of the child at each developmental level, to give a better background for understanding and treatment of the child, and give insight into the relationship between different aspects of overall child development.

1 MONTH

Motor development	Eye-hand co-ordination	Communication	Social development
Prone: Lifts head slightly. Assumes fetal position. *Supine:* Holds head to side. Fixed posture, symmetrical bilateral flexion. Large jerky movements, arms more than legs. Legs kick between flexion and semi-flexion. Rolls part way to side. Pushes with feet against adult hand. *Sitting:* Back rounded. Marked head lag. Complete head lag when pulled to sit. *Standing:* Stepping, placing, and walking reflexes. *Reactions:* Primary reflex domination: Moro, Galant, grasp, extensor thrust. Ventral suspension: head and legs flexed.	*Eye movement:* Stares at walls and windows. Looks at toy or person momentarily. Follows moving light to midline only. Visual field 15–20 cm *Hands:* Hands held fisted. Hand clenches on contact (grasp reflex). One hand to mouth. Immediately drops rattle placed in hand. Does not look at hands.	Impassive face. Some vocalization other than crying (small throaty noises when content). Startled by sounds Responds to bell with generalized physical movements. Quieted by voice. **Performance adaptation** Can feel a touch but cannot look. Paper on face: generalized physical movements. Hand to mouth. Opens and closes mouth in response to food stimuli. Reacts to sounds.	Quieted when picked up. Sleeps 4/5 of the day. Enjoys a bath. **Feeding** Two night feeds. Co-ordinates sucking, swallowing, breathing (2 weeks). Positive suck, bite, gag, rooting, and tongue thrust.

2 MONTHS

Motor development	Eye-hand co-ordination	Communication development	Social
Prone: Holds head erect for a few seconds. Head mostly midline. Rolls side to prone. Hips low — frog position	*Eye movement:* Follows moving bell-ring, horizontally past midline. Follows ring vertically. Eye to eye contact. Delayed midline regard.	Listens to bell. Searches for sound with eyes. Vocalizes in response to touch and voice. Chuckles and coos (single vowel sounds). Alert face. Eye to eye contact.	Smiling (6 weeks). Visually recognizes mother. **Feeding** One night feed. Recognizes bottle or breast visually.
Supine Kicks vigorously and reciprocally. Energetic arm movements. Head still mostly to side.	*Hands:* ATNR causes involuntary hand regard and visual fixation. Fingers fan out during extension movements. Retains ring put in hand.	**Performance adaptation** Holds ring placed in hand. Searches for sound visually.	Hands on bottle or breast while feeding. Rooting disappearing. Positive suck, bite, and gag reflexes.
Sitting: Back rounded. Head bobbingly erect. PTS — some head lag.			
Standing Walking reflex disappearing.			
Reactions ATNR strong. Moro present. Ventral suspension: head compensates, legs still flexed.			

3 MONTHS

Motor development	Eye-hand co-ordination	Communication	Social development
Prone: Sustained lifting of head to 45°. Supports weight on forearms. Pelvis flat.	*Eye movement:* Follows bell-ring moved in a circle. Prompt midline regard. Glances from one object to another. Follows moving object 15 to 25 cm away.	Makes 2 or more different sounds. Listens to music. **Performance adaptation** Paper on face: vigorous head turning. Massed cubes: regards, arms activate, contact. Sensory exploration with hands in mouth.	Spontaneous social smile. Follows moving person with eyes. Returns examiner's glance with smiling and cooing. Laughs when head covered with cloth. Enjoys repeating activities.
Supine Head held near midline. Symmetrical arm and head movements predominate. Movement smoother and more co-ordinated. Rolls side to supine. Prefers suppine.	*Hands:* Hand regard. Hands mostly open. Hands to midline. Plays with own fingers clasping hands. Pulls at people's clothing. Holds rattle and sometimes regards at same time. Hits objects accidentally.		**Feeding** Anticipates feeding on sight with increased activity. Fixes eyes on mother's face while feeding. Mature swallow. Swallows strained foods.
Sitting: Head mostly up when supported in sitting. Back firmer. PTS — only slight head lag.			
Standing Takes small fraction of weight.			
Reactions ATNR diminishing. Moro still present. Ventral suspension: head up, some hip extension. Labyrinthine righting.			

4 MONTHS

Motor development	Eye-hand co-ordination	Communication	Social development
Prone: Lifts head to 90° continuously. Lifts head and chest. Props on forearms with tendency for one arm flexed, one extended. Legs extended.	*Eye movement:* Visually explores new range of vision 180°. Looks at rattle when grasped, shakes it.	Searches for sound with head movement. Laughs aloud and squeals. 'Babbles' to people and toys. Two or more different sounds. Listens to tuning-fork.	Frolics when played with. Resists adult who tries to take toy. Friendly to strangers. Smiles and vocalizes at mirror. Pulls clothes over face in play.
Supine: Symmetrical arm and head postures. Hands engage in midline. Rolling prone to supine.	*Hands:* Grasp — primitive voluntary clutch. Grasps ring or cube when given. Takes toys to mouth if given. Fingers scratch at table top. Sucks fingers. Reaches for objects. Resists withdrawal of toy. Drops one cube for another.	**Performance adaptation** Grasps cube placed in hand. Resists withdrawal of toy held. Localizes tactile stimulation by touching part of body just touched. Finds partially hidden object.	**Feeding** Pats bottle or breast. Mouths and swallows strained foods.
Sitting: Head erect continuously. When supported, back firm. Lumbar curve. PTS — slight head lag. Sits propped 25–37 cm.			
Standing Bearing some weight on legs.			
Reactions ATNR occasionally. Moro and other primitive reflexes mostly inhibited. Ventral suspension: head up, hip extension incomplete. Parachute reaction present for arms and legs. Labyrinthine Righting Response (LRR) present.			

5 MONTHS

Motor development	Eye-hand co-ordination	Communication	Social development
Prone: Props on extended arms. Weight on forearms, reaches for toy. Pivots. May try swimming movements.	Reaches for ring and grasps. Bilateral hand approach. Tries to get toy which is out of reach. Stops hand regard. Mouths objects. Anticipates movement of objects visually. Reaches for second object purposefully. Controls elbow extension (grasps toes). Palmar grasp on ulnar side. Sucks fist and finger.	Turns head deliberately to bell. Turns head to speaking. Coos or stops crying on hearing music. Interested in sounds of objects. Loves playful tease. Grunts, growls.	Anticipates being lifted. Turns to person talking. Discriminates strangers. Recognizes mother when she enters the room. Enjoys repeating activities. Splashes in the bath.
Supine Hips flexed, legs extended. Plays with toes. Feet to mouth. Raises hips. PTS — no head lag, assists to lift head. Roll — prone to supine, side to side.		**Performance adaptation** Eyes and hands combine in joint action. Reaches for toy and grasps. Pulls at paper placed over face. Shows interest in a box. Plays with toys.	**Feeding** Gums or mouths solids. Chewing begins. Holds own bottle.
Sitting: Sits erect when supported. No head wobble when body swayed. Sits momentarily leaning forward on hands.			

(continued)

5 MONTHS

Motor development	Eye-hand co-ordination	Communication	Social development
Standing Bears most of weight when held. *Reactions* Primitive reflexes inhibited. LRR, plus optical righting present. Parachute reaction — arms and legs. Ventral suspension — positive Landau (head & hips extend).			

6 MONTHS

Motor development	Eye-hand co-ordination	Communication	Social development
Prone: Light progression on tummy. Draws up knees. Pivots in a circle. Lifts head and chest well up, weight on hands. *Supine* Lifts head from lying. Kicks strongly, legs alternating. Moves arms in brisk purposeful fashion. Roll — sometimes supine to prone. *Sitting:* Sits with slight support. Sits alone for 30 seconds. Can turn head to look around when secure. PTS — lifts head by self. *Standing* Supported standing: bounces actively. *Reactions* Landau present. Postural fixation reactions (body righting), LRR and optical righting. Forward protective extension in sitting. Equilibrium reaction in prone position.	*Prehension:* One handed approach. Radial palmar grasp. Reaches in pronation. No voluntary release. Begins to transfer hand to hand. *Fine motor:* Secures and plays with toys, shaking, banging. Manipulates objects attentively. Takes and plays with toy from table. Holds one cube in each hand. Still takes everything to mouth. Contacts and rakes at small objects. *Vision:* Precise vision 15–30 cm. Follows fast moving objects. Looks vaguely for toy when dropped. Visually insatiable. Eyes move in unison, (any squint now definitely abnormal).	Babbles to people. Makes more than 4 different sounds. Single consonant as well as vowel sounds. Imitates sounds e.g. cough, tongue click. Displeasure by sound other than crying. Screams with annoyance. Responds when called. Laughs, chuckles, and squeals aloud in play. **Performance adaptation** Holds 2 cubes. Looks vaguely for dropped toy. Manipulates objects.	Pulls at adult face. Pats mirror image. Plays peek-a-boo. Stretches arms to be picked-up. Turns immediately to mother's voice across the room. Responds to facial expression and tone of voice. Some initial shyness with strangers. Works for toy out of reach. Resists toy being pulled. **Feeding** Drinks from a cup held by adult. Takes solids well. Chewing and biting. Teething begins. Dribbling plentiful. Chews rusk. Tastes and smells different things.

7 MONTHS

Motor development	Eye-hand co-ordination	Communication	Social development
Prone: Creeps, especially backwards. Weight on abdomen and hands. Can lift one hand toward toy. *Supine* Does not like supine for long. Lifts head to sit up. Pulls head to sitting. *Sitting:* Back straight, weight on hands. Can recover balance when leans forward. Sits unsupported. Roll — supine to prone. *Standing* Supported standing, takes almost full weight. Bounces actively, stepping reaction. Stands, hands held. *Reactions* Landau, body on body, optical, and LRR present. Forward protection in sitting. Equilibrium reactions in supine and prone.	*Prehension:* Small objects — inferior scissor grasp (thumb adducted). Radial palmar grasp. Grasp in half supination. Transfers objects hand to hand. Immediate one-handed approach. *Fine motor:* Strikes one object with another. Objects to mouth. Reaches for and picks up string. Bangs objects on table. *Vision:* Looks for dropped toy.	Two syllable babble. Responds to simple requests accompanied by gesture. Responds to no-no and different tones of voice. Babbles to self when alone. **Performance adaptation** Looks for fallen object. Transfers objects. Drops one cube for a third. Strikes one object with another.	Knows strangers from familiar friends. Imitates familiar gestures. Manipulates cup and spoon in play. Bites and chews toys. Loves to play with paper. **Feeding** Feeds self biscuit. Drinks from a cup. Still dribbling.

8 MONTHS

Motor development	Eye-hand co-ordination	Communication	Social development
Prone: Creeps forward on abdomen . Arms and legs more co-ordinated. Can go onto hands and knees. *Supine* Rolls over and sits up. *Sitting:* Sits unsupported with little overbalancing. Goes sitting to prone, prone to sitting. *Standing* Stands holding onto furniture. Takes full weight. *Reactions* Protective extension, forwards and sideways in sitting. Equilibrium reactions in supine, prone, and developing in sitting.	*Prehension:* Inferior pincer grasp, Thumb presses on proximal interphalangeal joint of forefinger. Ambidextrous. Release of objects beginning. *Fine motor:* Pulls string to get toy. Manipulates two objects at once. Index finger approach (pokes objects).	Babled phrases — (4+ syllables). 'Mama' or 'Dada' as babbles. Listens to conversation. Singing tones. Imitates 'nursery tricks'. **Performance adaptation** Manipulates two objects at once. Paper over face — plays with and crumples. Pulls string to get toy. Holds own bottle.	Obtains toys out of reach. Displeased if toy taken away. Prompt reactions to situations. Pats doll. **Feeding** Holds own bottle. Helps hold cup for drinking. Munches food (lateral chewing).

9 MONTHS

Motor development	Eye-hand co-ordination	Communication	Social development
Crawling: Rocks on all fours. Attempts to crawl, sometimes succeeds.	*Prehension:* Neat pincer grasp with slight wrist extension. Can release toy against firm resistance but cannot yet drop voluntarily. Grasps string scissor fashion.	Babbles in long repetitive string of syllables. One word clear. 'Mama' or 'Dada' (but not always appropriately). Listens to stopwatch. Performs tricks on verbal request (repeated for applause). Understands 'no' and 'bye'. Begins to imitate sounds. Responds to simple verbal requests. Shouts to attract attention.	Reacts to (plays with) mirror image. Shows toy held in hand. Clings to known adult. Pulls off hat. Throws body back and stiffens in annoyance or resistance. Loves peek-a-boo. Shakes bell.
Sitting: Can be left sitting on the floor. Can change position and reach for toys without overbalancing. Prefers to sit.	*Fine Motor:* Dangles ring by the string. Shows toy held in hand but cannot give. Manipulates objects with lively interest.		**Feeding** Finger feeds. Beginning to use spoon. Helps to hold cup.
Standing: Pulls self to stand. Cannot lower himself. Lifts and replaces foot when standing at rail.	*Vision:* Visually very attentive. Concentration span increasing. Watches people and moving objects at 3 metres with sustained interest.	**Performance adaptation** Lifts inverted cup in search of toy. Rattles box. Looks at pellet inside bottle. Degree of concentration in playing with toys and getting objects.	
Reactions: Protective extension reliable — forwards and sitting. Equilibrium reactions in supine, prone, sitting, and developing in crawling.			

10 MONTHS

Motor development	Eye-hand co-ordination	Communication	Social development
Crawling: Crawls on hands and knees.	*Prehension:* Thumb opposition in pincer grip. Can extend index finger and poke. Can release objects voluntarily in crude manner. Wrist extension when extending fingers.	Shakes head for 'no'. One or two clear words. Imitates sounds.	Gives affection, returns kiss or hug. Drops objects to have them picked up, and watches where they go. Puts necklace around neck. Offers and gives toy to adult. Clasps hands and waves goodbye.
Sitting: Pivots and twists around to pick up objects. Sits well in chair. Usually plays in straight-legged sitting position (i.e., long sitting) with toys between legs.	*Fine Motor:* Throws objects. Can ring a bell. Pulls pull-along toy by string. Pulls ring stack apart. Unwraps a toy.	**Performance adaptation** Clicks 2 bricks together. Lifts lid off box. Pulls pull-along toy by string. Form board — removes round form. Unwraps a toy.	**Feeding and ADL** Finger feeding — often all 8 incisors are cut. Still dribbles and chews on objects. Holds arm out for sleeve or foot for sock when dressing.
Standing: Pulls up and stands holding on to furniture. Can stand holding on with one hand. Lowers self from standing. Can lift foot sideways.	*Vision:* Anticipates movement of a rolling ball.		
Reactions: Protective extension — forwards, backwards, and sideways. Equilibrium reaction in supine, prone, sitting, and crawling.			

11 MONTHS

Motor development	Eye-hand co-ordination	Communication	Social development
Crawling: Rapid crawling with good reciprocal pattern. Can 'bear-walk' with extended legs. *Sitting:* Does not turn over completely when sitting up from supine. *Standing:* Cruises sideways at rail. May walk if both hands held. *Reactions:* Landau and body on body righting still present. Protective extension backwards in sitting well established.	*Prehension:* Neat pincer to tip of index. Can pick up small objects. with neat pincer. *Fine Motor:* Points at objects. Stacks rings. Drops objects one after another into container. *Vision:* Begins to look at books.	Says two clear words. Uses 'Mama' and 'Dada' with meaning. Jargon begins. Short babbled sentences of 6+ syllables. Calls attention to needs or interesting events by pointing or vocalizing. Imitates speech sounds. Follows simple verbal commands. Responds to own name. **Performance adaptation** Finds toy under cup. Covers own face in peek-a-boo. Puts objects in and out of containers.	Plays interpersonal games like pat-a-cake. Interested in toy car. Plays with cup, spoon, and saucer. Puts objects in and out of container. Throws and picks up object again. Moves to rhythm. **Feeding & ADL** As for 10 months.

12 MONTHS

Motor development	Eye-hand co-ordination	Communication	Social development
Crawling: Crawls onto low ledge or step. *Standing:* Stands alone momentarily. *Walking:* Walks around cot or playpen. *Reactions:* Equilibrium reactions developing in standing.	*Prehension:* Prehension fully developed. Wrist extended with ulnar deviation on pincer grip. Difficulty releasing small objects. *Fine Motor:* Holds pencil as if to mark paper. Likes holding little toys. Rolls a ball. Ambidextrous. *Vision:* Recognizes familiar person 6 metres away. Brisk response to peripheral vision test.	Says 2 or 3 clear words. Babbled monologue when alone. Reacts vocally to music. Identifies objects by use (comb, hanky, etc.). Looks at named objects. Gives named objects on request. Responds suitably to everyday familiar sounds. Jargon in conversational cadences. **Performance adaptation** Accepts third cube without dropping Manipulates box, lid and cubes. Formboard — inserts round piece. Beginning awareness of colour, shape, size.	Gives objects on request. Likes to be constantly in sight and hearing of familiar adult. Co-operative ball play. Enjoys messy activities. Casts objects in play or rejection. Hugs doll or animal. Likes repetitive play. **Feeding & ADL** Can hold cup for drinking. Uses spoon but spills. Ceases dribbling and mouthing. Co-operates and helps with dressing. Beginning to refuse food. Responds appropriate to hot, cold, sweet, sour.

15 MONTHS

Motor development	Eye-hand co-operation	Communication	Social development
Walks alone well, wide base, arms and hips abducted). Likes pushing trolley etc. Can carry a toy when walking. Stoops and recovers. Lets self down from standing by collapsing. Kneels unaided. Sitting to standing unaided. Crawls up stairs safely.	Begins to show preference for one hand. Picks up crumbs with precise pincer grasp. Pegboard — removes all pegs, places 1 or 2 pegs. Uses pencil on paper a little — scribbles. Builds tower of 2 blocks after demonstration. Can hold 4 cubes in hand at once. Will put many objects into container without removing any. Plays rolling a ball. Plays pushing little cars along. Turns pages of a cardboard book. *Vision:* Looks at book with interest — pats pages. Watches happenings outside window with interest. Follows with eyes the path of small toy moving past 4 metres away.	Uses 2 to 6 clear words in correct context. Definitely tries to sing. Loves rhymes and jingles. Jargon — loudly and freely, large range of tones and sounds. Imitates vocal tones just heard. Demands objects by imperious finger pointing. Expresses wants by gesture. Points to familiar people and objects when named. Understands and obeys simple instructions. Gets named object from another room. Says 'no' meaningfully. **Performance adaptation** Builds tower of 2 cubes. Pulls cloth to get toy. Tries to get toy with a stick. Puts many objects into container without removing any. Explores properties and possibilities of objects.	Imitates ball games or social games. Explores properties and possibilities of objects with lively interest. Physically restless and intensely curious. Emotionally labile and dependent on adults' re-assuring presence. Needs constant supervision for protection. Casts objects in play or refusal. No longer mouths toys. **ADL** *Feeding* Drinks well from one-handed cup. Uses spoon alone but spills some (lacks full control of supination). Responds to meal preparation and participates in meals. Refuses some foods. *Dressing:* Helps — extends arm or leg when needed. Brings shoes on request. *Toileting:* May indicate wet or dirty pants.

18 MONTHS

Motor development	Eye-hand co-ordination	Communication	Social development
Walks for long distances without falling. Able to stop and turn suddenly. Stands stiffly, with little knee flexion and eyes to the ground. Arms and legs abducted. Can walk backwards. Stands pulling a toy on a string. Walks up and down stairs safely. Walks upstairs with hand held. Pushes or pulls large boxes or objects around walks 20 cm forward on beam on floor Climbs into adult chair and turns around to sit. Seats self in small chair without turning around. Squats to play. Walks into ball when kicking. Hurls ball while standing, keeping good balance.	*Fine motor*: Picks up pin, thread etc. Hand preference beginning. Scribbles deliberately and spontaneously. Holds pencil in primitive tripod grasp or palmar grasp. Tower of 3 bricks. Places 6 pegs in holes. Throws a ball overhead. Constructive play with boxes and other materials. Tries to turn door knob. Turns pages a few at a time. *Vision*: Fixes eyes on pendulum at 3 metres, watches briefly. Points to distant object out of doors.	Long babbled sentences — some words clear. Uses 6 to 10 words clear, appropriately. Echoes prominent on last word in sentences. Tries to join in nursery rhymes. Knows 1 or 2 body parts, points to on self and others. Says 'thank you' or equivalent Matches sounds to animals. Understands most nouns. **Performance adaptation** Tower of 3 bricks. Formboard — inserts square piece. Lid back on box. Dumps raisin from bottle when shown. Gets toy with stick. Matches 2 objects in box.	Imitates everyday activities and household tasks. Climbs onto chair to reach things. Remembers where objects belong. Likes adult to show book, points at objects. Plays contentedly alone, but likes to be near familiar adult. Alternates between clinging and resistance. Explores environment energetically. Enjoys messy play. Attempts to make mechanical toy work. **ADL** *Feeding:* Feeds self well. Hands cup or empty plate back to adult. *Dressing:* Can take off shoes, socks, hat, or nappy. Puts hat on head. *Toileting:* Asks for attention.

21 MONTHS

Motor development	Eye-hand co-ordination	Communication	Social development
Walks up stairs alone, holding a rail, 2 feet to a step. Walks down stairs, one hand held. Seats self at small table. Descends from adult chair alone. Tries to jump. Walks a few steps on 50 cm balance beam on floor. Can kick a ball, unsteadily. Squats to play for long periods.	*Fine motor*: Enjoys vigorous straight scribble. Imitates circular scribble. Tower of 5+ bricks. Can pour water from one cup to another.	Points to any 3 body parts. Vocabulary of 20+ words. Discriminates 2 actions using the one object, e.g. point to the ball, give me the ball. Uses two-word sentences. Tries to tell experience using babble and recognizable words. Asks for food and drink by name. Responds to 'what's that' by labelling. Calls playmates by name. Names 2 pictures. Eight objects in box identified, by pointing. Understands personal pronouns. **Performance adaptation** Builds tower of 5+ bricks. Completes circle and square placement on formboard. Removes raisin from bottle without prompting.	Tries to tell experiences. Alternately clings to, and pushes away adult. Cries when activity is blocked. Pretends to feed or dress doll. Sorts objects. Picks up and puts away toys on request. Domestic mimicry. **ADL** Bowel control almost complete. Often has bladder control during the day. Can eat with a spoon and fork. Usually bottle completely discarded.

2 YEARS

Motor development	Eye-hand co-ordination	Communication	Social development
Walks with a heel-toe gait. Swings arms when in a hurry. Runs well avoiding obstacles. Walks up and down stairs (rail), 2 feet to a step. Can jump off a step, 1 foot leading. Tries to stand on 1 foot. Stands on toes momentarily. Can bring chair, and seat self at table. Throws a ball into a basket 60 cm away. Kicks a ball on request. Propels a ride-on toy using feet on floor. Can carry breakables safely.	Hand preference usually obvious. Makes a train of 3 bricks. Tower of 7+ bricks. Picks up and places accurately pins and thread. Imitates a vertical line. Holds a pencil well down shaft — tripod grasp Turns pages singly. Can open a door (turns knob). Can unscrew a lid. Threads shoelace through large hole. Full adult visual acuity. Finds detail in picture book. Vision can be tested with Stycar matching tests (miniature toys).	Vocabulary of 50+ words. Talks continually to self. Makes short sentences with words of 4+ syllables. Picture vocabulary of 7. Names 10 to 12 objects in a box. Refers to self by name. Uses personal pronouns. Echolalia almost constant. Constantly asking names of objects. Begins to ask questions (What? Where?) Obeys two-part commands. Joins in nursery rhymes. Listens to stories. Points to at least 6 body parts. **Performance adaptation** Shows increasing understanding of own body size in relation to environment and closed spaces, e.g. boxes, cupboards. Makes train using 3 bricks. Tower of 7+ bricks. Can undo a screw toy. Completes 3 shape inset formboard. Understands concept of one.	Usually parallel play. Begins to co-operate in play with other children. Constantly demanding attention. Tantrums when frustrated or thwarted. Demands immediate gratification of needs. Recognizes familiar people in photograph when shown. Meaningful use of miniature objects. Defends own possessions with determination — no idea of sharing toys or attention. **ADL** Actively helps to dress and undress. Usually toilet trained by day. Washes hands.

30 MONTHS

Motor development	Eye-hand co-ordination	Communication	Social development
Rises from kneeling without using hands. Can stand on 1 foot. Can stand on tiptoe. Jumps with both feet off a step. Climbs well on easy apparatus. Pushes and pulls large toys about skilfully. Steers a ride on toy, using feet to push. Confident on stairs, using rail, 1 foot per step upstairs, 2 feet per step downstairs. Can cross both feet and both knees when seated.	Holds pencil in preferred hand with good tripod grasp. Imitates a horizontal stroke as well as a vertical stroke. Copies a circle primitively. Copies a T or V. Tower of 8+ bricks. Threads 6 large beads. Handles scissors and tries to cut paper. Re-assembles screw toy — puts lids on. Recognizes minute detail in picture books. Picks up pin, thread, etc. with one eye covered separately. Can test vision with Stycar single letter cards (1st block VOTHX).	Uses 200+ words. Speech shows numerous infantilisms in articulation and sentence structure. Continually asking questions: What? Who? Stuttering with eagerness common. Knows full name. Enjoys familiar stories read. Talks to self continually at play. Repeats one 6-syllable sentence. Knows 'money'. **Performance adaptation** Recognizes self in photographs. Tower of 8+ cubes. Threads 6 beads. Can re-assemble a screw toy. Four square board completed within 1 minute. Repeats 2 digits. Pellets + bottle — puts pellets in one at a time.	Gives first name on request. Knows own sex. Exceedingly active and resistive of restraint. Little understanding of dangers. Still throws tantrums. Emotionally still very dependent on adult. Recognizes self in photographs. More sustained role play, simple make-believe. Plays meaningfully with miniature toys. Puts away toys if encouraged. Names own drawing. Claps in time to music. **ADL** Eats skilfully with spoon and fork. Takes own pants off to go to toilet. Often dry at night (if lifted out).

3 YEARS

Motor development	Eye-hand co-ordination	Communication	Social development
Runs fast indoors and around obstacles as well. Walks in any direction, hauling large objects around. Can walk on tiptoe (6+ steps). Climbs on apparatus with agility. Stands on 1 foot for approx. 5 seconds. Rides tricycle using pedals. Marches in time to music. Can walk on stairs without rail, 1 foot per step upstairs, 2 feet per step downstairs. Can do a standing broad-jump (a few cms). Can throw a ball overhead and catch between extended arms. Kicks a ball forcibly. Obviously appreciates body size and space in relation to surroundings when playing.	Uses a pencil with good control. Imitates a cross (roughly) (also OVHT). Copies a bridge of 3 blocks. Threads 12+ beads. Cuts papers with scissors. Can undo and do up buttons. Folds a square of paper in half. Stycar single letter vision test at 3 metres.	Speech modulating in loudness and pitch. Large vocabulary intelligible even to strangers. Self talk in play decreasing in favour of talk addressed to others. Constantly asking questions (Who? Why?) May know names of colours. Uses plurals and most prepositions. Relates past events as well as present. Recites some nursery rhymes. **Performance adaptation** Matches primary colours. Counts by rote to 10 or more, but little appreciation of quantity beyond 2 or 3. Knows 'big' and 'little'. Repeats 3 digits. Matches geometric forms. Obviously appreciates body size, space, in relation to surroundings.	Gives full name plus age. General behaviour more amenable. Plays well with other children. Shows affection for younger siblings. Enjoys painting with large brush on easel. Likes to help adult. Makes effort to keep surroundings tidy. Vivid make-believe play. Understands sharing. Some appreciation of need to defer satisfaction to future. Plays interactive games. **ADL** Washes and dries own hands. Goes to the toilet alone. Usually dry at night (very variable). Can dress and undress with little supervision.

4 YEARS

Motor development	Eye-hand co-ordination	Communication	Social development
Can run on toes. Climbs ladders, trees, and high playground equipment. Stands on one foot, 3+ times, 6 to 10 seconds. Can hop on one foot. Walks easily up and down stairs alone, alternating feet. Jumps off 2 steps. Standing broad jump 20 to 25 cms. Touches toes with knees straight. Can run to kick a ball. Rides tricycle quickly and turns sharp corners. Good balance — walks along a chalk line. Increasing skill in ball games — throwing, catching, bouncing, using a bat.	Uses pencil in adult fashion. Can thread small beads with a needle to make a necklace. Builds 3 steps with 6 cubes after demonstration. Copies a ladder, cross, square, circle — well. Draws a recognizable person. Takes a train under bridge of blocks.	Speech fully intelligible. Narrates long stories. Constantly asking meanings of words and questions — How? When? Why? Enjoys verbal jokes Recites many nursery rhymes. Repeats sentences of 10+ syllables. Appreciates past, present, and future. Knows morning and afternoon. Comprehends descriptive adjectives. **Performance adaptation** Counts by rote up to 20. Counts objects up to 4 or 5. Repeats 4 digits. Compares 2 towers for height. Compares 2 weights — which is heavier? Compares 2 lines for length. Points to 8 geometric form insets on board.	Loves playmates of own age. Gives name and address. Sometimes confuses fact and fantasy. Names drawing before production. General behaviour independent and strongly self-willed. Inclined to verbal impertinence and quarrelling. Loves dressing up and dramatic play. Understands taking turns. Shows concern and sympathy for others. **ADL** Brushes teeth. Dresses and undresses independently. Washes self in bath. Uses knife and fork fairly well. Helps to set table.

5 YEARS

Motor development	Eye-hand co-ordination	Communication	Social development
Runs fast out of doors. Jumps a 15 cm high rope, both feet together. Can run upstairs and sometimes down. Skips with alternating feet. Can climb on and off a bus unaided. Hops on one foot (16 times). Stands on one foot arms folded. Can walk heel-to-toe. Running broad jump 70 to 75 cm. Can bounce and catch a ball. Climbs trees skilfully and performs numerous stunts. Plays a variety of ball games including those requiring appropriate placements of scoring.	Copies square and triangle, also VTHOXLACUY. Writes some letters from memory. Can tie a single knot. Threads large needles and sews stitches. Fastens buckles. Draws person with features. Draws house with door, windows, roof, and chimney. Colours pictures neatly. Threads 12 beads to a colour pattern. Stycar vision test — copies letters.	Correct grammatical use established. Fluent speech. Constantly asks meaning of abstract words. Enjoys jokes and riddles. Loves stories and being read to. **Performance adaptation** Counts fingers on each hand. Can coiunt 10 to 15 objects. Knows 10+ letters. Knows 10+ colours. Knows different coins. Knows opposite analogies.	Gives name, address and birthday. General behaviour more sensible and controlled. Comprehends need for order and time restraints. Acts out stories. Plays complicated floor games. Chooses own friends. Co-operative most of the time with friends. Can be bossy. Tender and protective of young children and pets. Comforts playmates in distress. Shows definite sense of humour. Can go on errands alone to nearby shops. Doesn't mind leaving mother. **ADL** Can fasten shoe buckles.

Appendix III: Havighurst's stages of developmental tasks

Life phase	Developmental tasks
Infancy (birth to 2 years)	1. Social attachment 2 Sensorimotor intelligence and primitive causality 3. Object permanence 4. Maturation of motor functions
Toddler (2–4 years)	1. Self-control 2. Language development 3. Fantasy and play 4. Elaboration of locomotion
Early school age (5–7 years)	1. Sex role identification 2. Early moral development 3. Concrete operations 4. Group play
Middle school age (8–12 years)	1. Social co-operation 2. Self-evaluation 3. Skill learning 4. Team play
Early adolescence (13–17 years)	1. Physical maturation 2. Formal operations 3. Membership in the peer group 4. Heterosexual relationships
Later adolescence (18–22 years)	1. Autonomy from parents 2. Sex role identity 3. Internalized morality 4. Career choice
Early adulthood (23–30 years)	1. Marriage 2. Childbearing 3. Work 4. Life style
Middle adulthood (31–50 years)	1. Management of household 2. Child rearing 3. Management of a career
Later adulthood (51 years–)	1. Redirection of energy to new roles 2. Acceptance of one's life 3. Developing a point of view about death 4. Dealing with losses

From Havighurst R J 1982 Developmental tasks and education. David Mckay, New York. Reproduced by permission of Random House, Inc.

Appendix IV: Evolution of play behaviour

0–1 year	1–2 years	2–3 years
Space management		
Gross motor activity: reaches, plays with hands and feet, touches hands to feet, crawls; sits with balance; pulls to stand, moves to continue pleasant sensation	*Gross motor activity:* stands unsupported, sits down; bends and recovers balance, walks and runs — wide stance, climbs low objects; broad movements involving large muscle groups; rides kiddie car	*Gross motor activity:* beginning integration of entire body in activities — concentrates on complex movements (i.e., throwing, jumping, climbing); pedals tricycle
Territory: crib, playpen, house	*Territory:* home, immediate surrounds	*Territory:* outside, short excursions
Exploration: of self and objects within reach	*Exploration:* of all unfamiliar things; oblivious to hazards	*Exploration:* Increased exploration of all unfamiliar objects; very curious
Comments:	*Comments:*	*Comments:*
Material management		
Manipulation: predominant — handles, mouths toys; brings two objects together; picks up; hits, bangs; shakes	*Manipulation:* predominant — throws; inserts; pushes; pulls; carries; pounds	*Manipulation:* remains predominant — feels; pats; dumps; squeezes; fills
Construction: not evident	*Construction:* little attempt to make product; relates two objects appropriately (i.e., lid on pot); stacks; takes apart; puts together	*Construction:* manipulation predominates; scribbles; strings beads, puzzles 4–5 pieces
Interest: people, gazes at faces; follows movements; attends to voices and sounds	*Interest:* movement of self — explores various kinesthetic and proprioceptive sensations; moving objects (i.e. balls trucks, pull toys)	*Interest:* explores new movement patterns (i.e. jumping); toys with moving parts (i.e. dump trucks, jointed dolls); makes messes
Purpose: sensation or function — uses materials to see, touch, hear, smell, mouth (i.e., rattles, teething rings, coloured objects)	*Purposes:* experiments in movement — practices basic movement patterns (i.e., rock, walk, run); process important	*Purpose:* process important — less interest in finished product (i.e., scribbles, squeezes play dough); repetition of gross motor skills
Attention: follows moving objects with eyes	*Attention:* rapid shifts	*Attention:* intense interest; quiet play up to 15 minutes; plays with single object or theme 5–10 minutes
Comments:	*Comments:*	*Comments:*

0–1 year	1–2 years	2–3 years
Imitation		
Imitation: of observed facial expressions and physical movement (i.e., smiling, pat-a-cake); emotions (hugs toys)	*Imitation:* of simple actions; present events and adults — self-related mimicry (i.e., feeds self with spoon)	*Imitation:* of adult routines with toy-related mimicry (i.e. child feeding doll); toys as agents (i.e. doll feeds self)
Imagination: not evident	*Imagination:* imaginary objects (i.e. pretend food on spoon)	*Imagination:* personifies dolls, stuffed animals; starts having imaginary friends (i.e., animals, persons)
Dramatization: not evident	*Dramatization:* not evident	*Dramatization:* portrays single character
Music: attends to sounds	*Music:* sways, listens	*Music:* responds to music with whole body (i.e., marching, twirling)
Books: pats; strokes; picks at pictures	*Books:* handles, points to pictures; begins to name pictures	*Books:* likes familiar stories; fills in words and phrases
Comments:	*Comments:*	*Comments:*
Participation		
Type: solitary play (no effort to interact with other children or choose similar activites)	*Type:* combination of solitary, onlooker play (watches others — speaking but not entering their play)	*Type:* parallel play (plays beside others, play remains independent, but child situates self among others, enjoys their presence)
Cooperation: demands personal attention; simple give and take interaction with immediate family or caretaker (i.e., tickling, peek-a-boo); 7–10 months — initiates games rather than follows	*Cooperation:* more complex games with a variety of adults (i.e., hide and seek, chasing); offers toys but somewhat possessive; persistent	*Cooperation:* possessive (much snatch and grab, hoarding, no sharing, resists toys being taken away); independent (does not ask for help, initiates own play)
Language: attends to sounds and voices, babbles; uses razzing sounds	*Language:* jabbers during play — talks to self, often in sing-song rhythm; uses gestures and words to communicate wants; labels objects	*Language:* talkative — very little jabber, begins to use words to communicate ideas, information
Comments:	*Comments:*	*Comments:*

3–4 years	4–5 years	5–6 years
Space management		
Gross motor activity: more coordinated body movements, smoother walking, jumping, climbing, running (accelerates, decelerates)	*Gross motor activity:* increased activity level; can concentrate on goal instead of movement; ease of gross motor ability allows stunts, tests of strength, exaggerated movements; clambers	*Gross motor activity:* more sedate, good muscle control and balance; hops on one foot, skips; somersaults, skates, lifts self off ground
Territory: home, immediate neighbourhood	*Territory:* neighbourhood	*Territory:* likes to be up off ground
Exploration: interest in new experiences, places, animals, nature	*Exploration:* anticipates trips, likes change of pace	*Exploration:* plans and enjoys excursions and trips
Comments:	*Comments:*	*Comments:*

3–4 years	4–5 years	5–6 years
Material management		
Manipulation: small muscle activity — hammers, sorts, inserts small objects (i.e., peg boards); cuts	*Manipulation:* increasing fine motor control allows quick movements, force, pulling	*Manipulation:* uses tools to make things (i.e., cuts more precisely); copies, traces; combines various types of material
Construction: makes simple products (i.e., blocks, crayons, clay); combines play materials, takes apart, arranges in spatial dimension — design is evident	*Construction:* predominates — makes products, specific designs evident, builds complex structures; puzzles 10 pieces	*Construction:* predominates — makes recognizable products; likes small construction, attends to detail (i.e, eyes, nose, fingers apparent in drawings); uses products in play
Interest: anything new; find motor manipulation of play materials	*Interest:* takes pride in work (i.e., shows and talks about products, compares with friends likes pictures displayed); complex ideas	*Interest:* in reality — manipulation of real life situations (i.e., miniature things); making something useful — props for play; permanence of products; toys that 'really work'
Purpose: beginning to show interest in result or finished product	*Purpose:* product very important — uses to express self; exaggerates	*Purpose:* replicate reality
Attention: longer span — around 30 minutes; plays with single object or theme 5–10 minutes	*Attention:* amuses self up to one hour, plays with single object or theme 10–15 minutes	*Attention:* concentration for long period of time; plays with single object or theme 10–15 minutes
Comments:	*Comments:*	*Comments:*
Imitation		
Imitation: more complex imitation of real world — part of dramatization	*Imitation:* more complex imitation of real world as part of dramatization	*Imitation:* more complex imitation of real world as part of dramatization
Imagination: assumes familiar roles — domestic themes, past experiences	*Imagination:* prominent — able to use familiar knowledge to construct a novel situation (i.e., expanding on the theme of a story or TV show)	*Imagination:* prominent — continues to construct new themes but emphasis on reality — reconstruction of real world
Dramatization: imitates simple action and reaction episodes — mirrors experience, emphasis on domestic and animals; portrays multiple characters with feelings (mostly anger and crying); little interest in costumes	*Dramatization:* role playing for or with others; portrays more complex emotions; sequences stories — themes from domestic to magic; enjoys dress-ups	*Dramatization:* sequences stories — emphasis on copying what occurs in real world; costumes important; props; puppets
Music: sings simple songs — not necessarily on pitch plays instruments	*Music:* sings whole songs on pitch; musical games (i.e., Farmer in the Dell); good rhythm	*Music:* meaning of songs important; enjoys catchy tunes, songs that tell stories; dances reflect interpretation of music
Books: new or information books; pictures important, relates own experiences to story	*Books:* listens better — doesn't need physical contact with book, looks at books independently — repeats familiar stories	*Books:* looks at books independently or with peer; describes picture to tell story; must be credible
Comments:	*Comments:*	*Comments:*

3–4 years	4–5 years	5–6 years
Participation		
Type: associative play (similar activities with groups of 2–3, no organization to reach a common goal, more interest in peers than activity)	*Type:* cooperative (groups of 2–3 organized to achieve a goal, i.e., assigns roles for pretend play)	*Type:* cooperative (groups of 2–5, organization of more complex games and dramatic play)
Cooperation: limited — some turn taking; asks for things rather than grabbing; little attempt to control others	*Cooperation:* takes turns; attempts to control the activities of others (often self-centered, bossy)	*Cooperation:* social give and take evident (i.e., compromises to facilitate group play); rivalry seen in competitive games
Language: uses words to communicate with peers, interest in new words (repeats them, asks their meaning)	*Language:* very talkative — plays with words; fabricates — capable of long narratives; questions persistently; communicates with peers to organize activities	*Language:* very prominent in socio-dramatic play (uses words as part of play as well as to organize play); interest in present, relevant how, what for questions
Comments:	*Comments:*	*Comments:*

Revised by Bledsoe & Shepherd (1982) from Knox (1974), A play scale.

EXPLANATION

Purpose: The purpose of the Play Scale is to give an adequate description of normal play behaviour through the ages 0–6 years.

Method: Play behaviour is described in terms of yearly increments and in terms of four dimensions. These are defined as follows:

1. Space management — This is the way in which the child learns to manage his body and the space around him; through the processes of experimentation and exploration. The bases for the repertoire of activity are the basic postural mechanisms.

2. Material management — The manner in which the child handles materials and the purposes for which he uses materials. It includes the manner in which the child learns control and use of material surroundings.

3. Imitation — This is the way in which the child gains an understanding of the social world around him, and learns how to express and control his feelings through the processes of observation and imitation.

4. Participation — This is the amount and manner of interaction with persons in his environment, and the degree of independence and co-operation demonstrated in play activities.

Use of scale: The scale is constructed with the yearly increments along the horizontal axis and the dimensions along the vertical axis. The child's play is assessed in terms of the descriptions that are most like the observed behaviour. Play is assessed in two separate half-hour sessions, or four 15 minute sessions. Knox (1974) also suggested two outdoor observations and two indoor observations, however Shepherd (1989) believes this is ideal but impossible for clinicians in today's world of occupational therapy. A plus is used to designate those statements which best describe the behaviour; a minus is used when the behaviour is absent. An NA is used if the opportunity to observe a particular behaviour does not arise. Space is provided under each dimension for any comments by the observer, including such things as stereotyped behaviour, absence of any form of play, and any interfering factors.

Scoring: The age manifested by the child's behaviour is computed by taking the mean of each dimension shown and then computing an overall mean which is designated as a play age.

A play quotient can be computed with the following formula:

$$\frac{PA}{CA} \times 100 = PQ$$

Of greater importance are the results derived from theoretical analysis, of the data. The descriptions of each dimension and the observer's comments are helpful in determining trends of behaviour, particular emphases in play, and the relationships amoung the four dimensions and factors.

Limitations of the scale: The scale was administered to a pilot population and has the following limitations:

a. The scale was designed to show general trends of behaviour rather than ability levels.

b. The play descriptions for each age were assumed to be valid because they were compiled form valid studies with established norms. To prove the validity of this scale, the items need to be tested further on groups of normal pre-school children.

REVISION, RELIABILITY and VALIDITY STUDIES

Reference: Bledsoe, Nancy and Shepherd, Jayne. "A Study of Reliability and Validity of a Preschool Play Scale", *AJOT*, Vol 36, # 12, Dec., 1982, pp 783–788.

Methodology: The scale was used on 90 subjects (48 males and 42 females) ranging in age from 4 months to 6 years. Six groups corresponding to the age groupings on the scale were used with 15 children in each group. The subjects were also tested on the Partens Social Play Hierarchy and on the Lunzers Scale of Organization of Play Behaviour.

Shepherd J 1989 Pers comm.

Reliability measures:
1. *Inter-rater — significant at the .0001 level*
2. *Test-retest — significant at the .0001 level*

Validity — concurrent;
1. Scores correlated with chronological age — significant at .0001
2. Scores correlate with scores on Partens Social Play Hierarchy — significant at the .0001 level.
3. Scores correlate with scores on Lunzers Scale of Organization of Play Behaviour — significant at the .0001 level

Appendix V: Guides to selecting play material and equipment

Play materials for development of strength and skill

Infant: 3–12 months	Toddler: 1–3 years	Preschool: 3–5 years
Bright coloured ribbons, bright coloured balloons	Push and pull toys (flat, one piece type)	Push and pull toys and take apart toy interest continues
Bright coloured, large, strongly strung plastic or wooden beads	Take apart, push and pull toys. These come in many forms with detachable disks, squares, triangles and cylinders	Wagon (large enough to sit in), wheelbarrow, sled, tricycle, large rubber ball, wagon and block sets, boxing gloves, slides, trapeze sets, graduated sized boxes
Plastic measuring spoons, bright coloured beaded animals or people	Take apart toys (colour cones, block sets, animated figures, cone trees, and many others)	
Dumbell rain rattles, ordinary sewing spools, brightly coloured blocks (at least 1.5 cm square)	Kiddie car, hobby horse, mallet and peg set, large clothespins, large wooden spoons	
Teeter swing, walker, play pen		

Note emphasis on bright colours. This is indicated because control over eye movements is the earliest motor control. Play materials for development of strength and skill must of necessity be sturdy and well built. The same toys can be used for a long period of time, if so built, only the use of the toy will change, and the toy itself need not be discarded for another new toy or another type of toy.

6–8 years	9–12 years	13–15 years	16–18 years
Tricycle, scooter, wagon, swing, sled, croquet set, soft ball, catcher's mitt, small bat, hammer, nail and wood design set, tenpin game, water toys	Swing and trapeze, bicycle, sled, baseball and bat, catcher's mitt, football, croquet set, roller skates, indoor dart games, bathing suit and swimming equipment, boxing gloves, boy scout axe and knife	Swing and trapeze, bicycle, sled, baseball and bat, catcher's mitt, football equipment, tennis equipment, basketball, archery sets, rollers skates, shuffle board, swimming equipment, trapping equipment	Tennis equipment, sled, croquet set, tennis equipment, volley ball, golf clubs, badminton set, basketball, archery set, boxing gloves, ice skates, shuffle board, swimming equipment

In the normal, healthy child, vitality fairly effervesces in every move. Because of this excess energy, the materials listed here will develop the muscles of the entire body as well as encourage sportsmanship, co-operation, conformity to rules of the game and preparation for sports participated in by adults.

Materials for constructive and creative play.

Toddler 1–3 years	Preschool: 3–5 years	Primary: 6–8 years
Take apart toys, block sets, boxes of graduated sizes, spools, clothespins and boxes	Wooden bead and apron sets, 5 to 10 piece puzzle with large pieces	Clothespins, box and spool interest continues
	Clothespins, spools, boxes, sandbox, sewing cards, hammer, nail and wooden piece design sets, finger painting	Village building blocks, tinker toys, simple embroidery sets, paper construction
		Small carpentry set: hammer, nails, square, saw, screwdriver
		20 to 75 piece jigsaw puzzle, beadwork: large plastic and wooden beads, slottie animals

Constructive and creative play in the small child is simple and without detail. Larger muscles are used rather than small muscles which have not yet fully developed. Much supervision is usually given, and too little opportunity for experimentation is possible because of this excess supervision. Introduce this type of play early in the child's activity, as it takes such a great part in his school curriculum and interest later. This simple, constructive play serves as a basis for more complex constructive play later.

9–12 years	13–15 years	16–18 years
Building logs, tinker toys, village building blocks, 75 to 275 piece jigsaw puzzle, garden tools	Same materials of interest but used in a more complicated way	Same activities but still more detailed
		Hobbies have very definitely begun to develop. Many of these hobbies have proved to be of occupational value and of value in everyday living as well
Modelling sets: boat, airplane, train, house, animal and bird	Crocheting materails, knitting materials, beadwork — $\frac{1}{4}$ diameter plastic beads or Indian seed beads	
Sewing materials, paper construction, embroidery materials, oilcloth designing	Oilcloth constructions, leather crafts, reed and raffia crafts, wood burning (pokerwork) sets, plastic moulding	Wood carving, metal crafts

More precise finger control is now in evidence. Eye and hand co-ordination are well developed, and more precision work is possible. Imaginative play continues, but hobbies play the big role in constructive play beginning at about 12 years. This type of play should be encouraged more and more in the handicapped child, so that real skill will be apparent for job placement and for life work. Well made, hand made articles are in great demand, and prices will be paid willingly for good work.

Materials for dramatic and imitative play

Toddler: 1–3 years	Preschool: 3–5 years	Primary: 6–8 years
Cuddle toys, preferably of slip skin type	Lacing shoe toy, village building blocks, small wooden cars, trucks, boats, soldiers, airplanes and trains	Same toy materials are of interest but the dramatic play is much more complex
Soft dolls: rag, stocking, character of cotton stuffed type		Kitchen utensils: mixing bowl, dishes, spoons and forks
Blocks: commercial square blocks of scrap wood and spools	Paper dolls, soft dolls, doll house, doll house furniture, housekeeping equipment: broom, dustpan, dishes	Toy guns and telephones, medical kits with candy pills, play thermometer and nurse's cap, dress-up clothes, mother's clothes, cowboy outfits, Indian costume, policeman's garb, Hallowe'en costumes
Clothespins and boxes, stiff, heavy backed picture books	Doll bed, doll carriage, picture books, dancing lessons	
		Pets are excellent for teaching responsibility; child will imitate parents in caring for pets: dog, cat, and rabbits
		Dancing lessons, toy musical instruments

The child is a great imitator. The 12-month-old baby quickly imitates expressions of elders as well as treatment of toys, as shown in loving of cuddle toys and putting toy dog in bed with him for nap. By imitating, the child learns how to do things. In the small child there is little real dramatic play until about 5 years. Up until that age it is merely an imitation and not true dramatics.

9–12 years	13–15 years	16–18 years
Make-up kits, character dolls, materials to make dolls, doll's houses and furniture, music lessons, pets of all kinds	Materials to make cuddle toys and character dolls, materials for one act plays, decoration and furnishing for own room, desk and chair	Same materials of interest but use much more complicated and with definite pecuniary benefits in mind
		Hobbies play a major role, cuddle and character dolls

The 9- to 15-year old is striving in every way to be like the adult. The 16- to 18-year old considers himself an adult and acts accordingly as much as possible. Acceptance of more responsibility is important, and duties will be carried out in same manner as has been observed by child watching adults. Operettas and class plays are important in grade and high school. Many activities listed under constructive and creative play can be listed here, such as imitation of elders in all types of activities.

Toys for social development

Toddler 1–3 years	Preschool: 3–5 years	Primary: 6–8 years
Soft dolls and cuddle toys Wagons	Wagons, tricycle, dishes, jingo game, Old Maid or Snap	Marbles, dominoes

Social development progresses slowly. Even those in nursery school show lack of social awareness at times. Solitary play is most enjoyed up until about 4 to 5 years. Interference of another player is not appreciated. It is important, however, that the child learns early the presence of other people in play and work. This is a social world, and little can be accomplished without some help from others. Children should be taught early, by 18 months at least, to share toys with others. Selfishness can be avoided if such training is started early in life.

9–12 years	13–15 years	16–18 years
Card and board games of all kinds Dancing lessons, parties, group games	Card and board games, correspondence clubs, picnics and hikes, clubs	Card and board game interest continues; interest in club groups much more decided Books and magazines, dancing, lunch box socials

Activities of a social nature are generally participated in now in numbers rather than by two people only. However, best friends and pals will chum together, spend much time together and enjoy their many secrets with each other. Hi-Y, Girl Reserves, Boy and Girl Scouts, Campfire Girls, 4-H Clubs and any number of other organizations have done much to make youth conscious of its social responsibilities. Theatre parties, birthday parties, holiday get-togethers, and dancing groups, also, aid the young man and woman to abide by social ethics.

Artistic development — arts and crafts

Toddler: 1–3 years	Preschool: 3–5 years	Primary: 6–8 years
Color cones, large coloured beads, block bus with shaped many coloured removable parts	Large jumbo crayons, coloured blocks of various sizes and shapes, finger painting, peg boards, large coloured beads	Mosaic games, pegboards, bead board, spool board, blocks, smaller crayon, more detailed pictures to colour, clay and wax modelling, finger painting Tracing equipment, water colouring equipment, splatter painting, easel

Art work of temporary measure is most enjoyed at these ages, such as the design made by mosaic games, peg boards and the like. If the design is not just what the child wishes, he can quickly and easily dismantle it and try again. Also wax and clay models and blackboard work can be changed at will. Youngsters who wish their work to be lasting will enjoy finger and splatter painting and crayoning.

9–12 years	13–15 years	16–18 years
Crayons and rather complicated pictures to colour, water colours and brush, pastel painting, charcoal painting, ink painting, enamel painting, tempera paints, wax and clay modelling, splatter painting	Interest continues in all the arts but of more detailed and complete nature Indian bead work, woodburning (pokerwork) equipment, soap carving, reed and raffia, crepe paper artistry, leather tooling Linoleum designing, potato blocking, blueprint designs	Artistic interests have developed into hobbies of practical application for making a livelihood. Interest continues in all arts and crafts mentioned and becomes more detailed and complex

The true beauty of art and colour is now beginning to be really appreciated. Art of lasting qualities will be desired, and striving for perfection will be uppermost in most young minds. Making equipment to carry out art work as well as the constructive and creative work might also be classified as a form of artistic development. Many artistic abilities and interests will be carried on into adulthood and followed either as a profession or hobby.

Toys to stimulate knowledge and aid in school activities

Toddler 1–3 years	Preschool: 3–5 years	Primary: 6–8 years
Pictured and coloured blocks, any coloured wooden toy. Pictured boxes of various sizes and colours	Same toys as in other tables with gradual change in use and more understanding of colour, numbers, pictures, etc.	Design sets such as hammer nail and wood sets
Pictures and picture books	Large jumbo sized colours, blunt scissors, pencils and pencil box, mosaic games, finger painting, take apart toys, mallet and peg sets, push and pull toys, large ball, letter and number forming	Garden tools, sewing cards, building blocks of all types simple embroidery, dolls and dolls' house, toy musical instruments, medical kits, pets, marbles and dominoes, card and board games, chalk and blackboards, tracing equipment, crayons, pencils and inks, books

All toys and activities listed in previous charts may be found under this heading, since all play activity aids in some degree with school activities and stimulates knowledge. School seems to be a combination of all the other five classifications of activities. For the older age groups, materials from the other charts may simple be listed as aids to stimulate knowledge.

Appendix VI: Guides to occupational therapy resources

THERAPISTS' RESOURCE MATERIAL

Play and the hospitalised child. A selected bibliography. Publication of the Association For The Welfare Of Children In Hospital.
AWCH 5 Union St Parramatta 2150 NSW (Australia) or local branch.

Cerebral palsy interaction games for severely handicapped children without speech. Spastic Centre of NSW (Australia) publication.
Available from The Spastic Centre, 6 Queen St Mosman 2088 NSW

Bluma S et al The Portage Guide to early education. Checklist and resource cards.
The Portage Project, CESA 12, Box 564, Portage, Wisconsin 53901 USA.

RESOURCES FOR FAMILIES

Children with spina bifida, at school — one of a range of booklets published by the British Association for Spina Bifida and Hydrocephalus.
Available from 30 Devonshire St London WIN 2EB and from local Spina Bifida Associations.

Baker B L Brighton A J, Heifetz L J, Murphy D M. 1977. Early/intermediate/advanced self help skills (3 manuals)
Research Press, 2612 North Mattis Ave Chapaign I11 61820.
Attwell A, Clabby D A The Retarded Child: Answers To

Questions Parents Ask. A multi-media film strip series.
Western Psychological Services, 12031 Wilshire Boulevard, Los Angeles Calif 90025.

EVALUATION MATERIALS
GENERAL DEVELOPMENTAL ASSESSMENTS

Assessment	Age range	Areas assessed	Reference/Source
Griffith Mental Development Scales (approved users)	0–8 years	Comprehensive, standardised assessment of developmental maturity. Scale 1 covers years 0–2. Subscales examine locomotor personal social, hearing and speech, eye-hand co-ordination and performance skills and yields a general developmental age score. Scale 2 covers years 2–8. Subscales cover the above areas plus 'practical reasoning'. Useful to achieve a profile of early developmental maturity.	Reference: Griffith R 1970 The abilities of Babies, 2nd edn. Young and Son, Somerset Griffiths R 1970 The Abilities of Young Children. Young and Son, Somerset Source: The Test Agency, Cournswood House, North Dean, High Wick, Bucks, UK.
Gessell Scales	0–5 years	Standardized diagnostic developmental maturity assessment, usually combined with parent interview and neurological assessments. Scales assess development in the areas of motor adaptive, language, eye-hand and performance skills, and provide a standarized developmental quotient.	Reference: Gessell A 1950 The First Five Years of Life. Methuen, London

Assessment	Age range	Areas assessed	Reference/Source
Miller Assessment for Preschoolers (MAP)	2.0–5.9 years	Standardized screening tool, designed to detect developmental delays. Areas assessed include sensory and motor abilities, co-ordination, cognitive skills and combined abilities	*Source:* Australian Council of Educational Research (A.C.E.R.), Frederick Street, Hawthorn, Victoria, Australia, or local supplier.
Vineland Social Maturity Scales (Doll, 1965)	0–25 years	Refer to entry under Activities of Daily Living.	
Vulpe Assessment Battery	0–6 years	Developmental assessment/ analysing performance, individualized programming. Assessment of basic senses and functions, gross motor, fine motor, language behaviours, congnitive processes and specific concepts, organizational behaviours, ADL and assessment of environment.	*Reference:* Vulpe S G Vulpe Assessment Battery. National Institute on Mental Retardation of Canadian Association for Mentally Retarded.
Denver Developmental Screening Test	4 weeks–6 years	Screening test which charts general developmental maturity. Indicates need for comprehensive developmental assessment.	*Source:* Ladoca Industries, 833 Grotto Avenue, Providence, Rhode Island 02906, USA.
Hawaii Early Learning Profile	0–36 months	Screening test which assesses cognitive, expressive, language, gross motor, fine motor, social-emotional and self-help development. Accompanied by a guide that provides therapy program ideas.	*Reference:* Setu Furuno, O'Reilly A O, Hosaka C M, Inatsuka T T, Allman T L, Zelsloft B 1979 Hawaii Early Learning Profile. University of Hawaii *Source:* VORT Corporation, P O Box 1175C, Palo Alto, California, 94306.
The Pupil Education Behaviour Readiness Evaluation (PREB)	3–6 years	Standardized screening test that elicits information on a child's development skills required for success in school.	*Source:* Teaching Resources Inc, 100 Boylston Street, Boston, Mass., USA.

MOTOR SKILLS ASSESSMENT TESTS

Assessment	Age range	Areas assessed	Reference/Source
Bruininks-Oseretsky Test of Motor Proficiency	4.5–14 years	Standardized test of gross and fine motor functioning. Provides age equivalent scores for motor development, both unilateral and motor skills. A shortened form is included for screening purposes.	*Source:* ACER (Australia) and J. A. Preston Corporation, 60 Page Road, Clifton, New Jersey, 07012.
Joint Motion — Method of Measuring and Recording	0–adult	A detailed guide to the physical examination of range of movement of all joints of the human body. Comprehensive clearly illustrated manual provided.	*Reference:* American Association of Orthopedic Surgeons 1976 Joint motion, method of measuring and recording. Churchill Livingstone, Edinburgh
Erhardt Developmental Prehension Assessment	0–15 months	Measures development of prehension in relation to chronological age — yields a "prehensile score".	*Reference:* Erhardt R P 1982. Developmental Hand Dysfunction. Laurel, Maryland, Ramsco Pub. Co. *Source:* RAMSCO, P O Box N, Laurel, Maryland, 20707.

Assessment	Age range	Areas assessed	Reference/Source
Reflex Testing Methods for Assessing CNS Function (Fiorentino)	0–adult	The classic guide to assessing reflex development. A well-illustrated manual provides guidelines for examination of reflexes and reactions of children with normal and delayed development.	*Reference:* Fiorentino M R 1972 Reflex Testing Methods for Evaluating CNS Function. Illinois, Thomas Springfield.
Milani-Comparetti Motor Development Screening Test	0–2 years	Guide to reflex development in human infants, comprehensive testing procedures and interpretations of testing.	*Reference:* Milani-Comparetti A, Gidoni E 1965 Pattern Analysis of motor development and its disorder. Developmental Medical Child Neurology 9: 625–630. *Source:* The Meyer Children's Rehabilitation Institute, University of Nebraska Medical Centre, Omaha, Nebraska.
Neurological Dysfunctions of Children (Kuhns)	3–10 years	Screening test that identifies need for further diagnostic assessment e.g. suspected learning disability. Test consists of 16 tasks that the child is asked to perform.	*Reference:* Kuhns J W 1979 Neurological Dysfunctions of Children. McGraw-Hill Inc. *Source:* Publishers Test Service CTB/McGraw-Hill, 2500 Garden Road, Monterey, California, 93940.
Reflex Evaluation (Barnes, Crutchfield and Heriza)	0–28 weeks	A quick screening test that depicts the child's skills on horizontal continuum to assess presence or absence of reflex activity. Assists early detection of neurological problems.	*Reference:* Barnes M R, Crutchfield C A, Heriza C B 1982 The neuro-physiological basis of patient treatment, Vol 2, Reflexes in motor development. 3rd edn Atlanta, Ga, Stokesville Publishing Company
Test of Motor Impairment (Stott, Moyes and Henderson)	5–14 years	Measures minor problems of co-ordination and motor skills. Standardized test items are arranged in yearly levels.	*Reference:* Stott D H, Moyes F A, Henderson S E Text of Motor Impairment. NFER/Nelson, Darville House, 2 Oxford Road East, Windsor, Berks, UK. *Source:* ACER (Australia)

TESTS OF COGNITIVE AND PERCEPTUAL MOTOR INTEGRATION

Assessment	Age range	Areas assessed	Reference/Source
Southern California Sensory Integration Tests (SCISIT) (Certified users only)	4–10.11 years	Aims to detect sensory-integrative dysfunction in learning disabled and clumsy children. Standardized. Assesses the skills of visual perception, tactile ability, motor performance. Should be used in conjunction with Ayres' Clinical Observations and Post-Rotary Nystagmus Test.	*Reference:* Ayres J 1972 Sensory Integration and Learning Disorders. Western Psychological Services, Los Angeles. *Source:* ACER (Australia) and Western Psychological Services
P.S.R Evaluation for Severely Multiply Handicapped Children	0–10 years	Assesses developmental maturity of the multiply handicapped child using auditory-language and visual-motor scales. Test items emphasize conceptual understanding rather than motor performance.	*Reference:* Mullen E M, Danella E A, Myers M A 1977 Meeting Street School. *Source:* Meeting Street School, 667 Watermen Avenue, East Providence RI, 02914, USA

Assessment	Age range	Areas assessed	Reference/Source
Frostig Developmental Test of Visual Perception	4–8 years	Screen young identified learning disabled children for perceptual problems. Produces perceptual quotient. Standardised and measures five operationally defined perceptual skills: eye-hand co-ordination, figure ground, shape constancy, position in space and spatial relationships.	*Reference:* NFER/Neilson, Darville House, 2 Oxford Road East, Windsor, Berks, UK. *Source:* Frostig M & Associates
Visual Discrimination Test (Wepman, Morency and Seidl)	5–8 years	Standardised test of pre-reading abilities, easy to administer. Interprets measure of a child's ability to discriminate between similar visually perceived forms. No verbal responses are required.	*Source:* Stoelting Co, 620 Wheat Lane, Wood Dale, Illinois, 60191.
Developmental Test of Visual-Motor Integration (VMI) (Beery)	2–15 years	Standardized test measures the degree to which visual perception and motor behaviour are integrated. Essentially a pencil and paper test.	*Reference and Source:* Berry K E 1967 Developmental test of Visual-Motor Integration: Administration
Quick Neurological Screening Test	5–adult	Screening test of neurological signs that may indicate the need for further diagnostic assessment. Areas assessed include: motor control, spatial organization, visual and auditory perception, balance and vestibular function.	*Reference:* Mutti M, Sterling H M, Spalding W V 1978 Quick Neurological Screening Test. Academic Therapy Publications Inc., Novato, California. *Source:* Special Child Publications, P O Box 33548, Seattle, Washington, 98133.
Motor-free Visual Perception Test (Colarusso and Hamill)	5–8 years	The MVPT avoids motor involvement so is useful for assessing children with motor difficulties. Areas assessed include spatial relationships, visual discrimination, figure-ground, visual closure and visual memory.	*Reference:* Colarusso R P, Hamill D D 1972 MVPT. Academic Therapy Publications, Navato, Cal. *Source:* Dominie School Centre, 8 Cross Street, Brookvale, 2100, Sydney, (02) 93 0201.
Perceptual Skill Assessment (Brereton and Sattler)	3.5–4 years 4–8 years	A comprehensive guide to assessing perceptual skills of cerebral palsied children. Two scales apply to two age ranges.	*Reference:* Brereton B, Le gay, Sattler J 1967 The Basic Abilities Evaluation. Cerebral palsied basic Abilities. Manual and film. The Spastic Centre, Mosman, NSW, Australia.
The Meeting Street School Screening Test	6–13 years	Standardized screening test to aid early detection of learning disabled children. Assesses the basic perceptual skills required for learning.	*Reference:* Identification of Children with Learning Disabilities: The Meeting Street School Screening Test. Rhode Island: Crippled Children and Adults Society Inc. *Source:* Ladoca Industries, 833 Grotto Avenue, Providence, Rhode Island, 02906, USA.
Auditory Discrimination Test (Wepman, Morency, Seidl)	5–8 years	A quick standardized screening test for young children that gives an indication of auditory discrimination.	*Source:* Stoelting Co, 620 Wheat Lane, Wood Dale, Illinois, 60191, USA.

Assessment	Age range	Areas assessed	Reference/Source
Visual Memory Test (Wepman, Morency, Seidl)	5–8 years	A standardized measure of the child's short-term memory. No verbal responses required. Assesses pre-reading skills.	*Source:* Stoelting Co, 620 Wheat Lane, Wood Dale, Illinois, 60191, USA.

ASSESSMENT OF PSYCHOLOGICAL CHARACTERISTICS, PLAY SKILLS, SELF-CONCEPT AND BODY IMAGE

Assessment	Age range	Areas assessed	Reference/Source
Progress Assessment Chart of Social and Personal Assessment (PAC — Gunzberg)	0–adult	PAC and PEI yield a comprehensive picture of social behaviour functioning by assessing developmentally arranged social skills. For use with intellectually handicapped clients.	*Reference:* Gunzberg H C 1973 Primary Progress Assessment Charts of Social Development. MacMillan Publishing Company, Bristo, Ind.
Symbolic Play Test (Lowe and Costello) (approved users only)	1–3 years	Diagnostic tool for examining early concept formation and symbolization in infant development. Provides an indication of the maturity of a child's nonverbal thought processes through the use of play materials.	*Reference:* Lowe M, Costello A J 1976 Trends in the Development of Representational Play in Infants: An Observational Study. Journal of Child Psychological Psychiatry. 16(1): 33–47.
Self Esteem Inventory (Coopersmith)	8–15 years	Evaluates the child's attitudes towards self in social, academic, family and personal areas. Quickly administered to individuals or groups. Standardized.	*Reference:* Coopersmith S 1981 SEI Consulting Psychologists Press Inc., 577 College Avenue, Palo Alto, California, 94306, USA.
The Play History (Takata)	1.7–19 years	An open-ended questionnaire to be completed by the parent that aims to identify play experiences for the child in his/her environment.	*Reference:* Takata 1969 The Play History, American Journal of Occupational Therapy. 23(4): 314–318. *Source:* C. J. Behnke, M. S. OTR, Occupational Therapy, Bergen Pines Co, Hospital, Patamus, New Jersey, 07652
Play Skills Inventory (Hurff)	8–12 years	An evaluation tool containing play situations from which sensory, motor, perceptual and intellectual behaviours can be assessed.	*Reference:* Reilly M 1974 Play As Exploratory Learning. Sage Publications, Beverly Hills
Knox Preschool Play Scale	0–6 years	Assess play deficits and problems.	*Reference:* Bledsoe N P, Shepherd J T 1981 A study of reliability and validity of a Pre-school Play Scale. AJOT 36: 12, p783–788.
The Play Report (Seagoe)	5–11 years	Questionnaire, assesses play preferences in the categories of "informal and individual", "adult-oriented", "informal-social" and "individual competitive" play. Useful to identify play style and to aid psychological assessment, competitive play.	*Source:* May, V. and Seagoe, 15–410 Brownwood Place, Los Angeles, California 90024, USA.

Assessment	Age range	Areas assessed	Reference/Source
Goodenough-Harris Drawing Test (Draw-a-Man)	3–15 years	The child is asked to draw pictures of self, a man and a woman. Scored by checking the presence or absence of various bodily characteristics of the drawings. May be individually or group administered. Standardised. May indicate problems in body image and self concept, or perceptual difficulties.	*Reference:* Harris O B 1963 Goodenough-Harris Drawing Test. Harcourt Brace & World Inc. *Source:* Harcourt Brace Janovich Inc., New York, New York, USA.
Piers-Harris Self Concept Scale	5–adult	Children answer yes or no to a series of statements about themselves in social, academic and family situations. Standardized.	*Reference:* Harris O B Goodenough-Harris Drawing Test. Harcourt Brace & World Inc. *Source:* Harcourt Brace Janovich Inc., New York.

ACTIVITIES OF DAILY LIVING ASSESSMENTS

Assessment	Age range	Areas assessed	Reference/Source
Pediatric Assessment of Self-Care Activities	0–adolescence	Basic assessment of ADL activities. Contains sample assessment forms.	*Reference & Source:* Coley I A 1978 Pediatric Assessment of Self-Care Activities. Mosby: St Louis.
Primary Progress Assessment Charts of Social Development (PAC) (Gunzberg)	0–adult	Primarily designed for use with intellectually handicapped clients. Contains measures of social and self-care competence. Charts also available specifically for Down's Syndrome clients.	*Reference:* Gunzberg H C 1973 Primary Progress Assessment Charts of Social Development. MacMillan Publishing Company, Bristo, Ind.
Western Cerebral Palsy Questionnaire for Parents	0–12 years	Assessment of ADL activities for cerebral palsied children.	*Reference:* Finnie N 1974 Handling the Young Cerebral Palsied Child at Home. Heinemann, London
Activities of Daily Living Assessment (Copeland, Ford and Solon)	0–adult	ADL assessment designed for use with intellectually handicapped clients.	*Reference:* Copeland M, Ford L, Solon N 1976 Occupational Therapy for the Mentally Retarded Child. University Park Press, Baltimore
Vineland Social Maturity Scale (Doll)	0–25 years	Assessment of: 1 General self-help activities 2 Self-help in eating 3 Self-help in dressing 4 Self direction 5 Occupation 6 Communication 7 Locomotion 8 Socialisation Assesses levels of social competence on 117 items arranged in ascending order of difficulty. A social age and score can be derived from the total score.	*Reference:* Doll E A 1965 The Vineland Social Maturity Scale. Circle Pines, Minn, American Guidance Service
Purdue Perceptual-Motor Survey (Kephart, Newell)	5–adult	A screening instrument to assess perceptual motor abilities such as laterality, directionality and matching. Standardised.	*Reference:* Roach G, Newell, Kephart C Tests for gross-motor functions in children. *Source:* Stoelting Co, 620 Wheat Lane, Wood Dale, Illinois, 60191, USA.

Appendix VII: Guide to practical resource materials

The following guide is not exhaustive, but it will assist therapists who are new to working in the area of early intervention. The guide is classified into materials for a therapist's private use for programme planning; materials suitable to use with families; and materials designed specifically for parents.

PROGRAMME MATERIALS FOR THE THERAPIST

- Bluma S, Shearer M, Trotman T, Williard S 1976
  Portage guide to early education. Portage Project, Wisconsin

The Portage Guide to Early Education is useful for the therapist working with infants and young children. It comprises three parts:
1. A checklist of behaviour based on normal development.
2. A card index presenting each of the checklisted behaviours with suggested teaching techniques.
3. A manual of instructions.

1. The checklist presents a sequential listing of behaviours across colour coded areas of:

DATA GATHERING AND RECORDING

INFANT STIMULATION	}	0–4 months
SOCIALIZATION SKILLS		
LANGUAGE SKILLS	}	0–6 years
SELF-HELP SKILLS		
CONGNITIVE SKILLS		
MOTOR SKILLS		

The items to be checked are behaviourally defined, specifying what the child is required to demonstrate to be credited with a particular item as an entry behaviour. Beside each checklist item is a recording space to indicate mastery of the skill, date achieved and comments.
2. The Card Index comprises 721 cards, colour coded and numbered to correspond with the individual items of the checklist. The checklist item becomes the title of the card and each card lists several activities for teaching the title behaviour.
3. The manual gives directions to using the checklist and card index. For example, directions are given about where to begin testing and when to stop. There are guides to writing objectives, and to facilitating prerequisite skills for the learning of attention, imitation and compliance. The use of correction procedures is explained.

Evaluation of the Portage system

Schemes such as the Portage guide should always be regarded as guides, and not absolute recipes. The colour coding and · compact presentation of the materials makes the Portage Guide to Early Education easy to interpret and administer. The manual provides clear directions on how to utilize the materials. The limiting factor is that there are no directions on how to administer each checklist item. The results, therefore, will not only reflect the level of child functioning, but the skill of the trainer. A list of materials required for use in testing would also expedite the assessment procedure.

The checklist items are finely graded and specified in month age-ranges for young infants. The materials were designed for use with both non-handicapped and delayed preschool children. However, the developmental level of the activities makes the Portage Guide relevant for use with older children and adults who are severely handicapped. Although the materials were developed in conjunction with the home-based Portage project, they are equally suitable for centre based programmes.

- Sheridan M 1977 Spontaneous play in early childhood from birth to six years. NFER Publishing (illustrated)

This book discusses the function of play and outlines the stages of the development of play from infancy through to early school years. Mention is also made of the play of handicapped groups and emphasis is also given to several specific disabilities. Mary Sheridan presents an easy to read, practical guide suitable for students learning about child development.

- Connor F P, Williamson G G and Siepp J M 1978 Program guide for infants and toddlers with neuromotor and other developmental disabilities. Teachers College Press, New York

A textbook and programme guide for professionals and caregivers working with developmentally disabled children and their parents. The book discusses the fundamentals of developmental programmes and the importance of assessment and reassessment. Additionally the developmental sequence of normal and atypical children, and intervention approaches for five areas: movement, prespeech, language, cognition, and social emotion are outlined. Planned programmes and service delivery are also discussed. A very useful book for the beginning therapist because of its practical programmes for intervention as well as its thorough coverage of developmental and theoretical aspects.

- Forrester B J, Brooks G P, Hardge B M, Outlaw D D 1971 Materials for infant development. George Peabody College, Nashville

Focuses on materials that facilitate infant growth and development. The first part discusses early child development and provisions for the infant. Lists materials that can be used, or easily made, to promote development; materials that are readily found in most homes and occupational therapy departments and hence the book has practical application for use by parents at home or therapists doing home visits. Also many ideas could be incorporated into therapy programmes in the hospital setting. A lengthy booklist covers books for infants/toddlers through to older children and would be an asset to an occupational therapy department.

- Baratta-Lorton M 1972 Workjobs. Addison-Wesley, Menlo Park

Useful for therapists and parents. Gives useful ideas suitable for therapy and ideas that could be given to parents. Provides a variety of cognitive activities such as matching, sorting, distinguishing similarities and dissimilarities, relating parts to the whole, as well as suggesting tactile and motor activities.

- Capon J 1975 Basic and 'perceptual' lesson plans for perceptual-motor programmes in preschool and elementary grades 4th edn. Perceptual-Motor Plans Level I
- Mayer C A 1978 Sunshine series: Basic development and developmental disabilities. Easter Seal Society, Anchorage

Excellent as a quick reference especially for students and new graduates. The booklets cover the following areas:

1. Early motor development
2. Intellectual development
3. Emotional development and behaviour
4. Speech and language development
5. Development and learning
6. Motor disabilities
7. Intellectual disabilities
8. Visual disabilities
9. Learning disabilities
10. Hearing disabilities
11. Language disabilities
12. Emotional and behaviour disabilities
13. The handicapped child in the normal preschool class

- Klein M D 1983 Pre-Dressing Skills. Therapy Skill Builders, Tuscon, Arizona. An excellent text which makes use of clear drawings, developmental charts, equipment descriptions and adaptive techniques to teach dressing skills.

MATERIALS FOR USE WITH THE FAMILY

- Carr J 1980 Helping your handicapped child. A step-by-step guide to everyday problems. Penguin, Harmondsworth

A practical book for people who work or live with mentally handicapped children. The teaching style is based on the method of behaviour modification and tasks to be taught are broken down into component parts for ease of teaching.

- Baker B L, Brightman A J, Heifetz L J, Murphy D M 1977 Early self-help skills. Research Press, Champaign
- Baker B L, Brightman A J, Heifetz L J, Murphy D M 1977 Intermediate self-help skills. Research Press, Champaign
- Baker B L, Brightman A J, Heifetz L J, Murphy D M 1977 Advanced self-help skills. Research Press, Champaign

A graded practical skills training series designed for use by parents of children with special needs. It discusses guidelines for choosing skills to teach children and pays attention to making priorities. Activities are broken down into component parts. Also deals with topics such as rewards, modelling, backward chaining and keeping progress charts.

- Forrester B J, Hardge B M, Outlaw D D, Brooks G P, Boismier J D 1971 Home visiting with mothers and infants. George Peabody College, Nashville

Considerations that underlie performing home visits are discussed, particularly in relation to infant growth and development in gross-motor, fine-motor, cognitive, language and personal-social skills. Attention is also paid to planning, implementing and evaluating the home based program.

- Foster M 1974 Promoting infant development: A guide for working with parents. George Peabody College, Nashville

Compiled for home visitors and other people working with parents of infants up to 12 months of age. The sequence of development during the first year is outlined, and activities which promote the development of language acquisition, motor development, personal social skills and cognitive development are discussed. Set out to provide quick reference for students and beginning therapists.

- Foster M, Scanlan J, D'Antonio A H 1974 Training for home intervention. George Peabody College, Nashville

Aimed at developing the home visiting skills needed for teaching parents effective ways for managing and teaching their children. Particularly useful for the paediatric occupational therapist. Topics discussed include: child development information, the home visiting process, educational materials and activities. Useful checklists and parent-child assessments are outlined. References at the end of most chapters, and a recommended reading list for the home visitor.

- Hardge B, Gray S W 1975 Helping families learn: A home-based program. George Peabody College, Nashville

A practical book covering many aspects of home-based programmes. Some topics dealt with include: the role of the home visitor and objectives, conducting home visits, materials for use, father involvement, behaviour management skills, coping styles and developing effective teaching styles. Activities are also suggested for enhancing the development of motor activities (large and small), perceptual-cognitive, personal-social and language skills for the six month to five-year-old. As well as being a practical guide to home visits, the suggested activities and skills could be used as reference ideas for hospital-based programmes.

MATERIAL DESIGNED SPECIFICALLY FOR PARENTS

- Gordon I J 1970 Baby learning through baby play. St Martin's Press, New York (Illustrated)
- Gordon I J, Guinagh B, Jester R E 1972 Child learning through child play. Sidgwick & Jackson, London
- Klein M D 1987 Feeding Position Stickers. Therapy Skill Builders, Tuscon, Arizona. Illustrated stickers depicting frequently recommended feeding positions, such as cup and spoon presentation, jaw control and cheek support. These stickers are 3.5 cm × 3.5 cm and could be used for progress records, and hospital and home programmes. The following stickers are also available from the same publishers:
  - Developmental Position Stickers
  - Neonatal Positional Stickers
  - Baby Position Stickers
- Klein M D (ed) 1990 Parent articles for early intervention. Therapy Skill Builders, Tuscon, Arizona. An illustrated collection of 102 reproducible articles which provides

practical suggestions on therapeutic ways to manage children with special needs. This manual is a valuable and practical reference.

- La Vonne Jaegar D 1987 Home program instruction sheets for infants and young children. Therapy Skill Builders, Tuscon, Arizona. Suggests and illustrates 93 home exercises to reinforce therapy sessions.

- Levy J 1972 Exercises for your baby. Collins, London

An excellent illustrated book suitable for both parents and therapists. The exercises are aimed at strengthening muscle groups. Patterns are given for making wedges and bolsters suitable for use in therapy to provide for example, experience in weight-bearing through elbows. This book is a valuable reference.

Films and audio-visual materials

- Adventure playground for handicapped children credits: The pacemakers (Margery Allen interviewed) London, 12 mins, black and white, video cartridge.

This playground created by Allen is situated in London and is designed for handicapped children of all types to build up their self-confidence by offering them opportunities to take risks and meet challenges without too much adult supervision.

Parallel to this playground is an experimental assessment centre in Gray's Hospital in London where the handicapped children's liabilities and their development is assessed. The purpose is to find out exactly what is wrong (with new techniques) and help them from as early as six months of age.

- First things first: Occupational therapy and the developing child. American Occupational Therapy Association, 16 mm, 15 min, colour; Credits — Sandra Kelly.

The work of the occupational therapist with developmental problems of children from infant to preschool. Their work involves development of motor and perceptual skills in children with growth and developmental problems. Shows what a home visit is and how occupational therapists can work in conjunction with school programmes to help the severely handicapped.

- Making their senses make sense by Center for developmental and learning disorders, University of Alabama, 24 mins, 16 mm colour.

This begins by looking at the various symptoms of a perceptually disabled child, the most obvious being learning disabilities. Also mentions the personality problems which may develop as a result of poor sensory development. Shows children involved in games and activities to improve sensory perception. Methods of improvement and progress are illustrated.

Appendix VIII: Sequential development of prehension

Age (Weeks)	Description	Visual regard	Stimulation
0–12 (Neonate to 3 months)	No approach, ↓ Aimless arm movements ↓ Hand loosely fisted. Arm moves when stimulated	Can't converge or focus ↓ Jerky visual pursuits, gazes at hand on ATNR side of body ↓ ATNR less strong, head rotates with ease, converges at 12.5 cm.	
12 (3 months)	Reflexive, ulnar side strongest. No reaching before eye contract.	Sustained hand regard, head in midline. Converge at 9 cm. Smooth central tracking.	Place objects in hand. Hang toys in crib to stimulate eye contact tracking.
16 (4 months)	Mouthing of fingers; mutual fingering. Retains object placed in hand. No visually directed grasp until both hand and object in field of vision	Close visual monitoring of both hands.	Toys hanging within swiping reach. Toys on floor within visual field and hand reach.
20 (5 months)	Primitive squeeze, raking fingers only, no thumb or palm involved. Immediate approach and grasp on sight.	Rapid co-ordination of visual regard with some success at grasping.	Toys of varied textures, colours, sizes, shapes, and weights.
24 (6 months)	Palmar or squeeze grasp. Still no thumb participation. Eyes and hands combine in joint action.	As above.	Place toys in different positions and distances so that eyes and hands must search.
28 (7 months)	Radial Palmar or whole hand grasp, radial side stronger; thumb begins to adduct; unilateral approach, transfer from one hand to the other.	Long periods of visual regard followed by visual monitoring during reach & grasp. Picks up and visually regards	Toys that can be picked up and transferred — must be washable and suitable for mouthing.

Palmar grasp

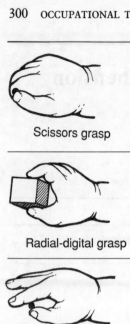

Scissors grasp	32 (8 months)	Inferior scissors or superior palm grasp, known as monkey grasp because thumb is adducted not opposed.	Time spent on visual regard decreases. Visual monitoring occurs while reaching.	Toys with smaller and thinner circumferences to strengthen thumb adductor.
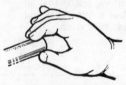 **Radial-digital grasp**	36 (9 months)	Radial — digital or inferior forefinger grasp. Fingers on radial side provide pressure on object. Thumb begins to move toward opposition by pressing toward PIP joint of forefinger. Finer adjustment of digits.	As above	More pliable materials including sand, clay, yarn, tissue paper. Many types of finger food for exploration and self-feeding.
Inferior pincer grasp	40 (10 months)	Inferior pincer grasp. Thumb moves toward DIP joint of forefinger — poking finger. Inhibition of other four digits. Beginning of voluntary release.	As above	Many small objects varied in shape to examine and feel, poke and explore
Pincer grasp	44 (11 months)	Neat pincer or forefinger grasp with slight extension of wrist.	As above	Tiny objects to pick up and drop, e.g. dry cereal.
Pad to pad tripod grasp	52 (1 year onward)	Opposition or superior forefinger grasp. Wrist extended and deviates to ulnar side for efficient prehension. Smooth release of large objects, clumsy release of small objects.	As above	Toys that provide repeated motions of release, e.g. blocks and containers of varying sizes.

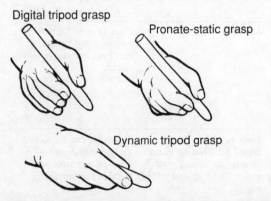

Digital tripod grasp

Pronate-static grasp

Dynamic tripod grasp

• Descriptions based on those of Erhardt, Gesell, Halverson, Perlmutter and Ziviani.

Index